PARENT-INFANT BONDING

PARENT-INFANT BONDING

MARSHALL H. KLAUS, M.D.

Professor of Pediatrics,
Case Western Reserve University School of Medicine,
Rainbow Babies and Children's Hospital,
Cleveland, Ohio

JOHN H. KENNELL, M.D.

Professor of Pediatrics,
Case Western Reserve University School of Medicine,
Rainbow Babies and Children's Hospital,
Cleveland, Ohio

SECOND EDITION

with **57** *illustrations*

The C. V. Mosby Company

ST. LOUIS • TORONTO • LONDON   1982

A TRADITION OF PUBLISHING EXCELLENCE

Editor: Alison Miller
Assistant editor: Susan R. Epstein
Manuscript editor: Diony Young
Design: Diane Beasley
Production: Ginny Douglas

Cover photograph by **Ken Kondo,** *Senior Medical Photographer,* Case Western Reserve University

SECOND EDITION

The C.V. Mosby Company
11830 Westline Industrial Drive, St. Louis, Missouri 63141

Library of Congress Cataloging in Publication Data

Klaus, Marshall H.
    Parent-infant bonding.

    Rev. ed. of: Maternal-infant bonding. 1976.
    Bibliography: p.
    Includes index.
    1. Infants (Newborn)—Family relationships.
2. Parent and child. 3. Infants (Newborn)—
Diseases—Psychological aspects. 4. Abnormalities,
Human—Psychological aspects. 5. Perinatal
mortality—Psychological aspects. I. Kennell,
John H., 1922-   . II. Title. [DNLM: 1. Child
development. 2. Family therapy. 3. Infant,
Newborn, Diseases. 4. Maternal deprivation.
5. Parent-child relations. WS 105.5F2 K63p]
RJ251.K56 1982   618.92'01'019   81-14056
ISBN 0-8016-2686-2 (Hardbound)   AACR2
ISBN 0-8016-2685-4 (Paperbound)

C/D/D 9 8 7 6 5 4 3 2 1   03/C/341 (Hardbound) 03/B/315 (Paperbound)

CONTRIBUTORS

ROBERTA A. BALLARD, M.D.

Department of Pediatrics,
Mount Zion Hospital and Medical Center,
San Francisco, California

BERTRAND CRAMER, M.D.

Chief of Child Guidance Center,
Geneva, Switzerland

CAROLYN B. FERRIS, R.N.

Department of Pediatrics,
Mount Zion Hospital and Medical Center,
San Francisco, California

NANCY A. IRVIN, M.S.S.A.

Department of Pediatrics,
Mount Zion Hospital and Medical Center,
San Francisco, California

CAROL H. LEONARD, Ph.D.

Department of Pediatrics,
Mount Zion Hospital and Medical Center,
San Francisco, California

MARY ANNE TRAUSE, Ph.D.

Division of Neonatology,
Fairfax Hospital,
Department of Pediatrics,
Georgetown University School of Medicine,
Washington, D.C.

Critical commentators

KATHRYN BARNARD, Ph.D.

Professor of Nursing,
University of Washington,
Seattle, Washington

T. BERRY BRAZELTON, M.D.

Associate Professor of Pediatrics,
Harvard University,
Cambridge, Massachusetts

M.A. CURRY, R.N., D.N.Sc.

Associate Professor,
Department of Family Nursing,
Oregon Health Science University,
Portland, Oregon

TIFFANY M. FIELD, Ph.D.

Mailman Center for Child Development,
University of Miami,
Miami, Florida

ERNA FURMAN

Cleveland Center for Research in
Child Development; Assistant Clinical
Professor in Child Therapy,
Department of Psychiatry,
Case Western Reserve University,
Cleveland, Ohio

MORRIS GREEN, M.D.

Professor and Chairman,
Department of Pediatrics,
University of Indiana School of Medicine,
Indianapolis, Indiana

DORA HENSCHEL

Head Midwife, Charing Cross Hospital,
London, England

NATACHA JOSEFOWITZ, M.S.W.

Professor of Management,
College of Business,
San Diego, California

EMANUEL LEWIS, M.B.

Consultant Psychiatrist, Charing Cross
Hospital and Tavistock Clinic,
London, England

BETSY LOZOFF, M.D.

Assistant Professor of Pediatrics
and Anthropology,
Case Western Reserve University,
Cleveland, Ohio

RAMONA MERCER, R.N., Ph.D.

Associate Professor, University of
California School of Nursing,
Department of Family Health
Care Nursing,
San Francisco, California

RUTH MERKATZ, R.N., M.S.N.

Assistant Clinical Professor of Nursing,
Case Western Reserve University,
Cleveland, Ohio

KLAUS MINDE, M.D.

Professor of Child Psychiatry,
Hospital for Sick Children,
Toronto, Ontario, Canada

MICHEL ODENT, M.D.

Director, Obstetrical Unit,
Centre Hospitalier Général de Pithiviers,
Pithiviers, France

ROSS D. PARKE, Ph.D.

Professor of Psychology, University of
Illinois at Urbana-Champaign,
Urbana, Illinois

JAMES ROBERTSON

Robertson Centre,
London, England

JOYCE ROBERTSON

Robertson Centre,
London, England

JAY S. ROSENBLATT, M.D., Ph.D.

Director, Institute of Animal Behavior,
Rutgers University,
Newark, New Jersey

ALBERT J. SOLNIT, M.D.

Professor of Pediatrics and Child Psychiatry,
Yale Child Study Center,
New Haven, Connecticut

To **our patients**
and their parents
and to **Susan, David,**
Alisa, Laura, and **Sarah Klaus**
and **Peggy, David, Susan,**
and **Jack Kennell**

FOREWORD

In this second edition Drs. Klaus and Kennell have responded to my challenge in the first edition to keep their work current as new advances are identified. They have expanded the knowledge base to include a review of new evidence from most recent studies and have added several new chapters covering a variety of relevant topics. Taken together these additions clarify and refine the concepts presented in their first edition. In retitling their book *Parent-Infant Bonding* the authors demonstrate an increased recognition and a greater appreciation for the undoubtedly complex human ecological process central to healthy family development.

The theme of this very timely book deals with the issue of "how to make human beings human," starting in the earliest days of life. Its focus is on the genesis of the earliest relationship that a baby develops with his parents—and the factors that may enhance or inhibit this process. It is timely because, in historical perspective, although we have achieved great progress and can take pride in our accomplishments, we have reached a point at which past practices are being reexamined and new directions charted. At such times of ferment it is good to have guidance from experts who are skillful clinicians and scientists aware of the frontiers in the science and art of care of the family of the normal and sick newborn baby. We can be grateful that, with their professional skill, the authors blend a keen sensitivity to the needs of parents of both well and ill newborns, openness in the reexamination of issues, theoretical orientation that permits them to examine and to think critically about the complicated issue of attachment between parent and newborn, and modesty in placing their scientific studies as well as those of others in perspective.

But why are we in a state of rapid modification of practices surrounding the care of the newborn infant and his family? We need to look at the history of medicine since the turn of the century. At that time advances in the natural sciences made possible the modern era of scientific medicine and particularly clinical investigation. Medical education in its modern form emerged, as did the modern hospital system.

That the results of these developments had a major effect on saving the lives of mothers and infants during the subsequent decades is clear. The growing knowledge of microbiology, immunology, nutrition, and metabolism resulted in improved public health practices, with a lowering of infant mortality (deaths under 1 year of age per 1000 babies born) from approximately 100 in 1915 to 13 in 1978.

Although this progress demonstrates great accomplishment, the efforts to apply the new knowledge resulted in an institutionalization and professionalization of obstetrical and infant care that removed mother and baby from intimate contact with each other and with the family. The increasing knowledge and technology in the care of the premature and sick infant has in recent years resulted in the development of the new subspecialty of neonatology or perinatology and intensive care nurseries that, albeit inadvertently, have contributed further to the isolation of mother from newborn and family from one another.

The increasing isolation of babies from mothers and of babies and mothers from the family at a time of a major family event has resulted in disquiet on the part of both parents and professionals, with a consequent critical reexamination of these practices. A better understanding of epidemiology and infectious disease control has made it feasible to think of modifying long-standing practices. Simultaneously, the growing disciplines of infant observation and child development have focused attention on the importance of studying the interactional and deprivational aspects of this earliest period.

We are fortunate that the authors were among the pioneers in reopening the nurseries—especially for the premature and sick infant—to parents and their families. We are fortunate, too, that they have undertaken to study systematically the effects of this process and that these studies continue. Thus their studies and those of others they review strongly favor a more flexible and liberal policy as being beneficial to babies and families. These studies lead them to present a theoretical framework consonant with their developmental orientation. They assert the importance of a parent-infant bonding and identify a sensitive period in the first minutes and hours of life, during which close contact of mother and father with the neonate have profound effects on their infant's growth and development. They go on to suggest a bidirectional interaction in that the newborn signals back, thus setting in motion an initial interaction that may lead to a profound and long-lasting attachment. In this edition the authors deal more extensively with a critical evaluation of the long-term effects of early attachment, since many investigators have raised many questions in light of the long period of dependency of human beings. Attachment clearly is a long-term process with many subtleties.

We are fortunate, too, that the authors have shared with us their sophisticated, yet practical, review of the scientific literature that only long-term immersion in a problem can make possible. There is no oversimplification of relevance in the presentation of animal studies and cross-cultural experiences for our society. Yet there is much to stimulate thought about the issues that are considered.

Finally, we are fortunate that the authors are clinicians deeply immersed in clinical practices as well as investigation. This comes through on every page; from their insights and from the literature they draw many inferences that they pass along to us. Other clinicians may have some differences—as clinicians generally do—but none can say that the suggestions are not drawn from struggling with the many complex problems of a rich clinical experience.

Thus Drs. Klaus and Kennell have presented a blend of science and art in the care of the newborn and his family and an important theoretical framework for the study of the earliest relationship between the newborn and his parents.

Fortunately, the state of our science and art supports care that seems to be more humane. The authors, through their pioneering clinical and research efforts and through the uniqueness of this volume, have done a great service to families and the child-caring professions. The British epidemiologist Dr. Archie Cochran has stated that modern medicine is moving from a predominant concern with curing to incorporating that of caring as well. This edition will undoubtedly continue to serve as a handbook for family care of the normal and sick newborn baby. We can hope that the authors will again accept the challenge to revise and update this book as we travel along the continuum of expanding knowledge.

Julius B. Richmond, M.D.

PREFACE

In the foreword to the first edition of *Maternal-Infant Bonding* Julius Richmond challenged us to continue to revise and update the book. Although only six years have passed since the previous edition was published, this revision has been a much more difficult task than we imagined. A large number of creative research workers have entered the field from a wide range of disciplines, including animal behavior, anthropology, ethology, ethics, history, nursing, obstetrics, pediatrics, psychology, psychiatry, and sociology. This explosion of knowledge has resulted in extensive revisions of all the chapters. We have added a new chapter on siblings and a section on alternative birth centers. In this revision we have been fortunate to be joined by a large number of outstanding critical commentators from the United States, Great Britain, Canada, and France. We have included their thoughtful and perceptive comments in the text and hope they will enliven, broaden, and clarify issues for the reader. As might be expected, we have benefited immensely from thought-provoking discussions with a number of scholars and researchers concerned with parent-infant interaction, birth, bonding, attachment, and infant development. They include Drs. Pat Bateson, John Davis, Robert Hinde, Martin Richards, John Bowlby, James and Joyce Robertson, Selma Fraiberg, and T. Berry Brazelton. We were distressed when the word *bonding* became too popular too rapidly and was confused with a simple, speedy, adhesive property rather than the beginning of a complex human psychobiological process. For many months we tried to change the terminology to parent-to-infant *attachment*. James and Joyce Robertson used the term *bonding* for parent-to-infant attachment in a paper and then charmingly and convincingly explained to us that the word was so well known that it was here to stay. We have been more at peace with its use ever since. We would like to mention our special help from Barbara Korsch. On many occasions she has had the forthrightness to disagree with us wholeheartedly. We would especially like to thank Dr. Richard Behrman, who gave us the time to carry out our research. Again we are indebted to many thoughtful students, including Robin Geller, Sue Swanson, Michelle Walsh, Kathy Masis, and Nancy Wollam-Huhn. Our ideas have been sharpened by Manoel DeCarvalho, Jose Diaz-Rossello, Deborah Jean Hales, Dennis Drotar, Betsy Lozoff, Norma Ringler, a number of neonatology fellows, and our very close and treasured associates who repeatedly confront us and help us work out many of our ideas. Here we would like to make special mention of Steve Robertson and Mary Anne Trause who have been our close colleagues throughout most of the last eight years. We give special thanks to our research associates, Melissa Masoner and Mary Ann Finlon, our research nurses, Carolyn Rudd and Roberta O'Bell, our editor, Connie McSweeney, our former secretary, Betsy Wilber, and our secretary, Dianne Kodger. A special note should be made about our laboratory in Guatemala at Instituto de Nutrición de Centro America y Panama, which continues to be staffed by three superb, dedicated, and thoughtful research workers, Marta Isabel Garcia, Rubidia Méndez Lopez, and Maricela Ochoa de Zelada, our pediatrician associates in this endeavor, Roberto Sosa and Juan Urrutia, and the personnel at Roosevelt and Social Security Hospitals. Our work during the past six years would not have been possible without the generous support of The William T. Grant Foundation, The Maternal and Child Health Grant No. 642-3326, NIH, The Research Corporation, and The Thrasher Foundation.

When we started our research we had no idea that the exploration of birth, interaction, and attachment could be so fruitful and exciting. We hope the reader can capture and share in our enthusiasm about the discoveries reported in the pages of this book. We have been particularly amazed by the richness of the marvelous natural processes that help the human mother progress through labor, birth, and the early postpartum period. We are impressed that many of the advances in pediatrics and obstetrics that have benefited some high-risk mothers and babies appear to disrupt and negate the normal physiological processes in healthy mothers, fathers, and babies.

Marshall H. Klaus
John H. Kennell

PREFACE to first edition

For each of us, learning is a personal adventure; therefore we have deviated from the traditional style and have used several techniques in this book.

One innovation is the use of the patient interview. Some readers may disagree with the inclusion of this material, but we believe a representative interview with authoritative comments is a thought-provoking device worthy of trial. A reading of the text will not be complete without a reading of the interview. It should be emphasized that the comments we have made about each of the three interviews cannot apply to every patient. Since we did not have long-term, in-depth interviews with the parents, there are sometimes many possible interpretations of the parents' comments. They do, however, tell us something about the feelings, thoughts, concerns, and hopes of parents during these difficult days. They have been chosen because they demonstrate or emphasize certain reactions or issues that other parents have repeatedly discussed. Some readers may choose to read the interview first and attempt to interpret the parent discussions before they note our comments. For those wishing a quick review of the subject, we have added a series of recommendations at the end of each chapter.

To demonstrate the many areas of controversy, we have asked expert consultants to comment on each chapter except the first. Some have made notes scattered throughout a chapter. Others have written a single comment, which we have inserted near the case presentation. We strongly urge the reader to consider these short, pithy, thoughtful contributions, since they extend, expand, or differ from our concepts.

This book has been organized in a special pattern that has evolved, in part, as we have developed our understanding of the subject. To understand maternal and paternal behavior in the human, we have found it valuable to learn from the detailed and precise observations of a wide range of animal species, since the requirements of caring for the young may have led to the evolution of similar behavioral patterns in humans and other animals. Because this is so crucial for our understanding, we have presented this information in a separate chapter (Chapter 2). Many studies have been summarized so that the reader may carefully note differences and similarities of parental behavior in a number of species faced with a common task. Chapter 3 describes the studies that provide the theoretical and empirical framework for discussing the care of the human mother and applies this to clinical situations involving care of the normal human mother. Chapter 4 describes studies related to the families of premature and sick infants and makes specific recommendations for their care. For several years we have been interested in Dr. Bertrand Cramer's interpretation of the reactions of parents to their premature infants, and we have included his discussion at the end of Chapter 4. He listens to these parents with the ears of a psychoanalyst having experience in both the United States and Europe. Chapter 5 takes on the painfully sad and difficult problem of a baby born with a malformation, a frequent occurrence in a high-risk nursery. In most pediatric units the greatest number of deaths occur on the newborn service, particularly in the high-risk nursery. The range of parental reactions to the death of a newborn is described in Chapter 6, accompanied by recommended procedures for the physician who has cared for the infant who has died. The latter three chapters (Chapters 3 to 6) first present basic research data, followed by a case study with our comments. Next there are clinical recommendations and a list of practical hints. We hope that the critical comments interspersed in the text will provoke discussion so that the reader will be aware of the many complex and debatable issues that remain unsettled. We conclude with a glimpse into the future.

As we look back, it was the mothers of premature infants who first kindled our interest by showing us that there were difficult problems of attachment after a separation. Our early curiosity was supported and encouraged by thoughtful nurses (especially Jane Cable) who shared their experiences and were willing to take what seemed at the time a hazardous step of allowing parents to enter the monastic doors of the nursery. We gained a richer and deeper understanding of what was going on in the minds of parents of premature infants through long discussions with colleagues in the behavioral sciences (Cliff Barnett, Mary Bergen, Douglas Bond, Anna Freud, Rose Grobstein, Herb Leiderman, Litzie Rolnick, Benjamin Spock).

We were helped immeasurably with our own investigations by the critical suggestions and provocative questions from other investigators concerned with maternal and paternal behavior. Our special thanks go to T. Berry Brazelton, Harry Gordon, Raven Lang, Julius Richmond, Jay S. Rosenblatt, and the late William Wallace.

We have been especially fortunate to work side by side with a series of bright, inquisitive, refreshing medical students who worked long hours and asked searching questions. Each of the medical students made unique contributions. We thank Gail Bongiovanni, David Chesler, Wendy Freed, David Gordon, Guillermo Gutierrez, Deborah Jean Hales, Rick Jerauld, Chris Kreger, John Lampe, Betsy Parke Macintyre, Willie McAlpine, Nancy Plumb, Howard Slyter, Meredith Steffa, Harriett Holan Wolfe, Steve Zuelke, and the many patient and conscientious research associates who made our studies possible, most recently Billie Navojosky and Diana Voos.

Throughout our studies we have been fortunate to have the benefit of the experience and counsel of Joseph Fagan, Robert Fantz, and Simón Miranda, in the Perceptual Development Laboratory of the Department of Psychology. Special thanks should be given to our department Chairman, Dr. Leroy Matthews, who has been most thoughtful about arranging time to prepare this work.

We would like to acknowledge the expert secretarial assistance and devoted efforts of Janet Negrelli, Jackie Stimpert, and Elizabeth Wilber. Editorial work on the book was started by our former associate Robin White, and then as efforts to complete the book intensified in the final months, skillful help was provided by Alisa Klaus, Laurie Krent, and Susan Schafer.

Our close friend, colleague, and counselor Dr. Avroy Fanaroff has supported and assisted us while we have conducted most of our studies. Since 1973 we have had a highly productive association with our colleague, advisor, and critic Mary Anne Trause. Susan Davis, Dennis Drotar, Nancy A. Irvin, Betsy Lozoff, and Norma Ringler have provided special skills and knowledge for some of our studies. In Guatemala our investigations could never have been carried out were it not for the suggestions and leadership of Drs. Leonardo Mata, Roberto Sosa, and Juan Urrutia, the extremely conscientious and devoted work of research field workers Patricia Baten, Marta Isabel Garcia, Rubidia Méndez, and Olga Maricela Ochoa, and especially the collaboration and expertise of Prof. Gustavo Castaneda and the personnel at Roosevelt and Social Security Hospitals.

Our work would not have been possible without the generous support of the Grant Foundation, the Educational Foundation of America, Maternal and Child Health Grant MC-R-390337, NIH 72-C-202, and the Research Corporation.

Marshall H. Klaus
John H. Kennell

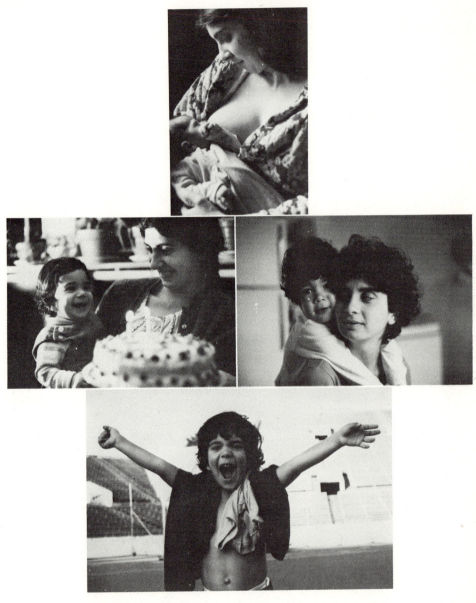

The infant who appeared on the cover of the first edition of this book has grown into a happy, healthy child.

CONTENTS

PARENT-INFANT BONDING

CHAPTER 1

THE FAMILY DURING PREGNANCY

MARSHALL H. KLAUS and JOHN H. KENNELL

I am a man so I can never really know what it is like to see wrapped over there in the cot a bit of my own self, a bit of me living an independent life, yet at the same time dependent and gradually become a person.
Donald Winnicott

In each person's life much of the joy and sorrow revolves around attachments or affectional relationships—making them, breaking them, preparing for them, and adjusting to their loss by death. This book deals with one of these special bonds— the tie a mother or father forms with his or her newborn infant. Individuals may have from 300 to 400 acquaintances in their lifetimes, but at any one time there are only a small number of persons to whom they are closely attached. Much of the richness and beauty of life is derived from these close relationships which each person has with a small number of other individuals—mother, father, brother, sister, husband, wife, son, daughter, and a small cadre of close friends.

Major workers in the field have each described an attachment, bond, or love somewhat differently.

Bonding does not refer to mutual affection between a baby and an adult but to the phenomenon whereby adults become committed by a one-way flow of concern and affection to children for whom they have cared during the first months and years of life. The intensity of bondedness reflects the amount of involvement with the infant that has occurred; it is usually greatest in the mother, somewhat less in the father, and shades off with other family members.*

A mother's love is a pretty crude affair. There's a possessiveness in it, there's appetite in it, there is a "Drat the kid" element in it, there's generosity in it, there's power in it, as well as humility, but sentimentality is outside of it altogether and is repugnant to mothers.†

---

*From Robertson, J.: A baby in the family: loving and being loved, London, in press, Penguin.
†From Winnicott, D.W.: The child, the family and the outside world, London, 1957, Tavistock Publications, Ltd., p. 17.

Whereas Bowlby notes:

> Affectional bonds and subjective states of a strong emotion tend to go together as every novelist and playwright knows. Thus many of the most intensive of all emotions arise during the formation, the maintenance, the disruption and renewal of affectional bonds which for that reason are sometimes called emotional bonds. In terms of subjective experience the formation of a bond is described as falling in love, maintaining a bond as loving someone, and losing a partner as grieving over someone. Similarly the threat of a loss arouses anxiety and actual loss causes sorrow, while both situations are likely to arouse anger. Finally the unchallenged maintenance of a bond is experienced as a source of security and a renewal of a bond as a source of joy.*

The characteristics of the bonding process are not precise or uniform and do not in any way resemble the adhesive properties of the new, rapidly-acting glues. Some misinterpretation of studies in this area may have resulted from a too literal acceptance of the word "bonding" and so has suggested that the speed of this reaction resembles the epoxy bonding of materials. By general consensus a bond is a tie from parent to infant, whereas the word attachment refers to the tie in the opposite direction, from infant to parent. In this book we will use the word "attachment" in two ways—the very specific way just defined, as well as the more generally understood application of the word.

A bond can be defined as a unique relationship between two people that is specific and endures through time. Although it is difficult to define this enduring relationship operationally, we have taken as indicators of this attachment the attachment behaviors such as fondling, kissing, cuddling, and prolonged gazing—behaviors that serve both to maintain contact and to exhibit affection toward a particular individual. Although this definition is useful in experimental observations, it is important to distinguish between attachment and attachment behavior. Strong attachments can persist during long separations of time and distance, even though often there may be no visible signs of their existence. Nonetheless, a call for help even after 40 years will bring a mother to her child and evoke attachment behaviors equal in strength to those in the first year of life.

COMMENT: Some argue that attachment is the qualitative feature of the emotional tie to the partner. The operationalization of the construct (attachment) to determine its presence or absence has to be done by some measure of the interaction between partners. The mother either responds to her infant's cues with affectionate behaviors and evokes the infant's interaction to suggest the infant is a central part of her life, or she does not. The infant either shows preferential response to the mother, responds to her verbal and tactile stimulation or does not. For the infant it is easier to say the tie to the mother is absent. The psychological complexity of adults makes it far more difficult to say a mother has *no* bond to her infant; what seems to emerge is that there are qualitative differences in her ability to express this bond by giving of herself to the child and in perceiving and responding to the infant's cues and needs.
R.T. Mercer

---

*From Bowlby, J.: The making and breaking of affectional bonds, Br. J. Psychiatr. **130**:201-210, 1977.

Attachment is crucial to the survival and development of the infant. The parents' bond to their child may be the strongest of all human ties, and this relationship has two unique characteristics. First, before birth the individual infant gestates within a part of the mother's body and, second, after birth she ensures his survival while he is utterly dependent on her and until he becomes a separate individual. The power of this attachment is so great that it enables the mother and father to make the unusual sacrifices necessary for the care of their infant day after day, night after night: changing diapers, attending to his crying, protecting him from danger, and giving feeds in the middle of the night despite their desperate need to sleep. It is the nature of this bond that we will explore as well as the process by which it develops. This original parent-infant tie is the major source for all the infant's subsequent attachments and is the formative relationship in the course of which the child develops a sense of himself. Throughout his lifetime the strength and character of this attachment will influence the quality of all future ties to other individuals.

> **COMMENT:** Obviously, when the authors speak of attachment between two people, they are not speaking of a "magical" or even a single kind of "bonding"; they are speaking of a kind of working arrangement in which each participant has learned the rules over time, from which each participant derives satisfactions that fuel the ongoing process. In our own work on the attachment process in the first four months, we find that there are four identifiable stages of development in both mother and infant, which evolve and are solidified as they build up the firm bonds of attachment to each other.
> **T.B. Brazelton**

In our professional activity we have the fortunate and unfortunate opportunity to observe daily both sick infants in the intensive care nursery and normal, healthy, full-term infants, and the mothers of healthy, full-term infants as well as those separated from sick infants. Our observations force us to ask the question, "What is the normal process by which a father and mother become attached to a healthy infant?" Recently, we developed an even greater respect for some of the complexities of the process by which this occurs. At the same time we have felt a new excitement as we have appreciated both the opportunities parents have for major psychological growth with the birth of a new infant and the neat orchestration of the many biological systems in both parents and infants that are integrated into the attachment sequence much like a jigsaw puzzle. The crisis of birth in many ways fits the two Chinese characters that represent the word "crisis"—"dangerous opportunity."

> **COMMENT:** The opportunity for parents to resolve their earlier childhood conflicts with the help of health professionals is an example of a "dangerous opportunity." The parents who were abused or mistreated as a child find it difficult to trust that their own needs will be met, or to trust others; if they do not receive professional help, they may reenact their childhood experiences with their own child. With concerned help they can learn to trust and to interact positively with their child.
> **R.T. Mercer**

We agree with the comments that this time period may be specially available for change.

The need for writing this book arose from the background just described and, more personally, from our tenure managing nurseries for normal and sick infants. Our interest in this subject has been stimulated by a number of specific cases. For example, Mrs. D. had been married for nine years and for the past five years had planned to have a baby. The infant, weighing 4 pounds 2 ounces, was born in a medical center after a gestation of 35 weeks. Within a few minutes of birth he was gasping and blue and therefore had to be resuscitated. At this early point the mother wondered if the infant would survive. Three hours later he was transferred to an intensive care unit under the direction of one of us, and within the next 36 hours he was placed on a respirator. Two days later the infant was showing considerable improvement, and the respirator was disconnected. At the end of three days the infant was in an incubator and started to take feedings through an intragastric plastic tube. Two weeks later he was taking feedings well by nipple, and the staff decided that the infant would soon be ready for discharge.

After several days the head nurse came to one of us, explaining that the mother was unable to get even a few drops of milk into the infant, although he could be fed reasonably easily by the nurses. Some suggestions were given to the mother that were unsuccessful. Three days later one of us observed the infant and mother together and noted that she was in a very uncomfortable position and continually jerked the nipple in and out of the baby's mouth. At one point she placed the baby on her knees, picked up his head in her hands, looked at his face, and said, "Are you mine? Are you really mine? Are you alive? Are you really alive?" In retrospect we recognized that this woman believed that her infant would not survive and started to mourn his loss within the first 12 hours after birth. During the first two weeks, while the infant was improving, the mother did not expect him to live. Through similar observations of many other patients, we were repeatedly stimulated to take a closer look at this phenomenon.

It is clear how Mrs. D's interaction with her baby might have easily produced the syndrome of failure to thrive or even child abuse. In fact, she suggested to the hospital personnel that the baby remain in the hospital for a prolonged period, since it took another four weeks for her to develop the necessary caretaking skills. Six months after the infant's birth the mother reflected that those had been the worst six months of her life. One month after the baby finally went home, it was necessary for her to leave him for two or three days so that she could rest.

Another observation raised questions in our minds: A mother who had successfully and skillfully managed two full-term babies was uncertain and anxious as she started to care for a newborn premature infant. She required considerable extra support and instruction to feed the infant and change his diapers and had endless questions during the first three months after he went home.

From our fumbling, early efforts to understand and unravel the mysteries of this process, we have developed our present understanding. We must confess that although our behavioral observations often stimulated certain productive studies, they often misled us in our understanding of a specific phenomenon. For example, when we first permitted mothers to enter the premature nursery to touch their infants in the incubator, we noticed that they would poke at their infants as women poke a cake to test whether it is done, touching the tips of their fingers to their infant's extremities. We wondered about the origins of this behavior. Our thoughts and ideas about it have evolved as we have gone back and forth from the intensive care unit to the normal full-term nursery. As we will see in Chapter 5, poking at premature infants by mothers is possibly an aberration of the normal maternal behavior when the infant appears fragile and an incubator is interposed. When the infant and mother are in a situation more appropriate for their becoming acquainted, this behavior is observed only during the first minutes of contact.

HISTORY OF THE NEWBORN NURSERY

In the early 1900s the high rate of morbidity and mortality of hospitalized children with communicable diseases led to the development of strict isolation techniques for diseased patients and separate wards with protective isolation measures for patients free of infection. Visitors were strongly discouraged because of the belief that they were the source of infection.

The quality of the milk available at the beginning of the century provides an example of one of the prevailing (health) problems of the time. In 1903, at the fifteenth annual meeting of the American Pediatric Society, one of the speakers reported that market milk was still sold over the grocery counter from dippered, unrefrigerated, 5-gallon cans (Faber and McIntosh, 1966). Cultures of this milk showed massive contamination. The victory over summer diarrhea was not achieved until general improvements in milk production and distribution were enforced by law, the most important of which was routine pasteurization of milk, including certification.

In children's hospitals, concern about protecting patients from contagious disorders led to what today appear to be bizarre policies of isolation and separation. In the early 1940s a child was completely separated from his parents during hospitalization. The visiting hours in the major children's hospitals were no longer than 30 to 60 minutes a week. The fear of spread of infection also accounted for the physical barriers observed between individual beds in the older children's hospitals and the physical separation of the obstetrical and pediatric divisions in the large general hospitals. Not only was diarrhea epidemic but respiratory infections were a scourge of children's hospitals and maternity and infant units. As a result of problems of infection, maternity hospitals gathered full-term babies in large nurseries in a fortresslike arrangement. Germs were the enemy; therefore parents and families who might carry them were excluded.

In discussing bonding, it is necessary to note that crucial life events surrounding the development of both attachment and detachment (death) have been removed from the home and brought into the hospital over the past 60 years. The hospital now determines the procedures involved in birth and death. The experiences surrounding these two events in the life of an individual have been stripped of the long-established traditions and support systems built up over centuries to help families through these highly meaningful transitions.

Despite the evidence that epidemics of infection result when recruits are gathered together in a military camp or when young children come together in a summer camp or school, and despite the large number of epidemics of streptococcal, staphylococcal, and *Escherichia coli* infections which occur and persist in central nurseries, it has been difficult to eliminate the central nursery in most maternity hospitals and to establish the practice of keeping individual babies with their mothers to decrease the opportunity for cross-infection. We had a dramatic experience with this in a hospital in Guatemala, where babies who were premature or delivered by cesarean birth were kept together in a central nursery. This resulted in a morbidity of 17 per 1000 infants due to infection. A major earthquake in 1976 forced a change in this policy, and subsequently babies were kept in the same bed with their mothers. Even though the mothers' beds were crowded closely together, the morbidity due to infections dropped dramatically to two or three per 1000 infants (Table 1-1) (Urrutia et al., 1980).

It often seems that practices based on "expert opinion," once established, are almost unchangeable, even though subsequent data and circumstances (such as the availability of antibiotics) make revisions appropriate. On the other hand, a practice such as keeping a mother and baby together, which has been in existence for centuries, makes good common sense, appeals to families, and is now supported by research data, is extremely difficult to introduce and sustain in a medical environment dominated by physicians' concerns about detecting and treating a variety of rare conditions.

If one adopts the standards of what constitutes deprivation and the levels of

Table 1-1. Incidence of infection in full-term infants, Social Security Hospital, Guatemala*

	1975†	1976	1977	1978
Live births	8,456	12,500	14,094	14,302
Infection rate‡	17	3	2	3
	Rooming-in			

*From Urrutia, J.J., Sosa, R., Kennell, J.H., and Klaus, M.H.: Ciba Foundation Symposium 77, Excerpta Medica, 1980, pp. 171-186.
†8 months.
‡Per thousand.

Table 1-2. Deprivation levels over time, related to birth situations*

Birth situation	Deprivation levels, days and weeks postpartum					
	Day 0	Day 1	Day 3	Day 7	Week 8	Week 9
Home, full term	I, no deprivation	I, no deprivation	I, no deprivation	I, no deprivation	I, no deprivation	I, no deprivation
Hospital, full term, rooming-in	III, moderate deprivation	I, no deprivation	I, no deprivation	I, no deprivation	I, no deprivation	I, no deprivation
Hospital, full term, regular care	III, moderate deprivation	II, partial deprivation	II, partial deprivation	I, no deprivation	I, no deprivation	I, no deprivation
Premature, mother allowed into nursery	V, complete deprivation	IV, severe deprivation	III, moderate deprivation	II, partial deprivation	II, partial deprivation (discharge nursery)	I, no deprivation (home)
Premature, regular care (separated)	V, complete deprivation	IV, severe deprivation	IV, severe deprivation	IV, severe deprivation	II, partial deprivation (discharge nursery)	I, no deprivation (home)
Unwed mother, refuses contact	V, complete deprivation	V, complete deprivation	V, complete deprivation	V, complete deprivation	V, complete deprivation	V, complete deprivation

*From Barnett, C.R., Leiderman, P.H., Grobstein, R., and Klaus, M.H.: Pediatrics **45:**197-205, 1970.

deprivation suggested by Barnett and co-workers (1970), it is apparent that many normal births in the United States are associated with several days of deprivation for the mother (Table 1-2). A woman who delivers a premature infant often suffers complete separation from her infant for the first day and even after the first day, moderate to partial deprivation. Using the definitions of Barnett and co-workers (1970), only mothers who deliver their normal full-term infants at home and live with their infants from birth experience no deprivation.

CULTURAL INFLUENCES ON CHILDHOOD

What triggers, fosters, or disturbs a parent's bond to her infant? In an attempt to answer this question, we have gathered information from a wide range of sources including (1) clinical observations during medical care procedures; (2) naturalistic observations of parenting; (3) long-term, in-depth interviews of a small number of mothers, primarily by psychoanalysts; (4) structured interviews or observations; and (5) results from closely controlled studies on the parents of both premature and full-term infants. As we consider the available information, it is important to remember that the necessary controls possible in studies of animal mothers are not always possible in studies of the human mother. Therefore we must delicately tease out information and integrate observations from diverse sources. All studies must be considered within the framework of the social setting. Cultural influences, the values and expectations of both the mother and the observer, as well as hospital structures and policies may all influence the final outcome.

The mother and the observer of the birth enter into the situation with certain biases, with attitudes that have been subtly shaped throughout their lives. Even in the Western world behaviors and practices surrounding birth vary widely.

Beautifully illustrating this variety in birth practices is the town of Termoli, a small community in an agricultural region of Italy. When a woman is about to give birth in the hospital, according to anthropologist Schreiber (1974), the members of the family congregate outside the labor and delivery rooms. Within 5 minutes of birth the parents, grandparents, and, on the average, five other relatives will have kissed the baby. Within the first 20 minutes the mother-in-law, who holds the baby first, returns him to his mother. The news of the birth is quickly dispatched to the parents' home, and a pink or blue rosette, depending on the sex of the baby, is hung on the front door. The birth has been officially announced, and visits by all the near and distant relatives, acquaintances, and neighbors begin. Schreiber found that within six weeks, in a town of 1500 people, 80% of the households had visited the home of a newborn with congratulations and usually a small gift for the mother or baby. In Termoli the birth of a baby brings great pride and tribute to the mother.

COMMENT: Adding to the American woman's feelings of fright and ineffectiveness, is her tremendous loss of expectations for the kind of experience she anticipates for the birth. She grieves for the

loss of her expected childbirth experience when she loses control and an unanticipated cesarean birth is necessary. She feels inferior that she could not perform "up to the standards" of other women. In some cases the hospital staff may have led her to believe she could remain in the labor room with her family for the birth, when in reality there was no possibility for more than one person to be present and giving birth in bed depended on the resident in charge. It is difficult for her to begin mothering when she feels she failed at one of the most important tasks of her life.
R.T. Mercer

However, models or practices that seem to work well in one society are not necessarily optimal solutions for another culture. The success of any one system is not an indication of its universal merit, and what seems to be "natural" is not necessarily "good." It is necessary to emphasize, then, that for cross-cultural data to be meaningful, the system must be examined within the total context of society.

With this caveat in mind, we will begin piecing together components of the affectional bond between a human mother and her infant and determining the factors that may alter or distort its formation. Since the human infant is wholly dependent on his mother or caregiver to meet all his physical and emotional needs, the strength and durability of the attachment may well determine whether or not he will survive and develop optimally.

COMMENT: In most of the Western world there is a pervasive attitude on the part of the medical caretakers of mothers and infants which varies little. This attitude is that the birth of a baby must be treated as an illness or an operation—an attitude that creates an atmosphere of pathology, or of curing pathology at best. The Rosenthal effect of this on mothers' attitudes toward their pregnancy, delivery, and new baby becomes a major issue in understanding how frightened and ineffectual mothers in American culture feel around this event.
T.B. Brazelton

Events that are important to the formation of a mother's bond to her infant are listed as follows:

Prior to pregnancy
    Planning the pregnancy
During pregnancy
    Confirming the pregnancy
    Accepting the pregnancy
    Fetal movement
    Beginning to accept the fetus as an individual
Labor
Birth
After birth
    Seeing the baby
    Touching the baby
    Giving care to the baby
    Accepting infant as a separate individual

By observing and studying the human mother according to these periods, we can begin to fit together the interlocking pieces that lay the foundations of attachment.

COMMENT: I would add another to the list of steps. During pregnancy: Doing the "work" of becoming a mother rather than a "girl" or a married but childless woman. After birth: Accepting her role as a mother; part of her job is to see the needs of the baby as a dependent but also as an individual person who is separate from her and has strengths of his own.
T.B. Brazelton

COMMENT: I also would add to the list of events important to the formation of the mother's attachment. During pregnancy: The acceptance of the coming infant by the mate, and the support of the mate. Current research notes the significant role the mate plays in supporting the woman in the reconciliation of childhood conflicts about her mother. Ballou (1978a, 1978b) observed that the husband played a role in providing the psychological context for the woman to move from the child-mother relationship with her mother to equal partnership—one of the tasks of pregnancy identified by Bibring. During pregnancy the mate functions both as a maternal object who gives and approves and as a paternal object who appreciates the wife's sexuality and protects her while fostering her reconcilication with, and separation from, her mother. Shereshefsky and Yarrow (1973) earlier found that the husband's role of sustaining the woman was highly correlated with her maternal functioning. Westbrook (1978) observed that positive marital relationships affected the woman's attitudes during pregnancy and the first year of motherhood.

Unfortunately, all mates do not have a psychological readiness for this kind of support to the woman during pregnancy. May's research (1980) noted a range of detachment/involvement by mates during pregnancy. Grossman and associates (1980) found the mate's ability for this support and nurturance to be highly predictive, however, of the mother's adaptation during labor and birth, her psychological health, and the quality of her interaction with her infant two months after birth. The infant's mental development was higher at 1 year of age when the father was more satisfied with and enjoyed his marriage more and had experienced less anxiety during pregnancy.

The events of labor and birth also affect the woman's early perceptions of, and interactions with, her infant. We found that women who had unanticipated cesarean births no longer felt the earlier selected names were appropriate for their infants and spoke negatively about their infants during the first 48 hours' postpartum. Peterson and Mehl (1978) also found the woman's birth experience to be the second most significant variable predicting the variance of maternal attachment; length of separation of mother and infant was the first predictor.
R.T. Mercer

BASIC CONSIDERATIONS
Prior to pregnancy

Experimental data suggest that the past experiences of the mother are a major determinant in molding her caregiving role. Children use adults, especially loved and powerful adults, as models for their own behavior. "Playing house," an activity that dominates the waking hours of girls during the preschool years, appears to be a preparatory rehearsal for mothering a real baby two or three decades later. Mothers who watch their preschoolers are continually surprised to find that their daughters imitate their own actions, attitudes, and facial movements in the most minute detail.

Child development literature suggests that children are socialized by the powerful process of imitation or modeling. They may respond to how they themselves were mothered or what they observed. Thus long before a woman herself becomes a mother, she has learned through observation, play, and practice a repertoire of mothering behaviors. She has already learned whether or not infants are picked up when they cry, how much they are carried, and whether they should be chubby or thin. Interestingly, these "facts" that are taken in when children are very young become unquestioned imperatives for them throughout life. Unless adults consciously and painstakingly reexamine these learned behaviors, they will unconsciously repeat them when they become parents.

> **COMMENT:** One of the most tragic aspects of the nuclear family culture in the Western world is that many, if not most, young women are never exposed to caretaking of children before they have their own. Very few new mothers in my practice have even handled an infant or cared for a small child. This leaves them inexperienced and rather helpless when their own baby comes. We need to provide experiences in nurturing smaller children in schools and high schools.
> **T.B. Brazelton**

A young girl in a developing country such as Guatemala has responsibility and experience with the care of young infants until she delivers her own, which allows her to make fine adjustments in her mothering style and gain a wealth of confidence before she herself becomes a mother. Thus the way a woman was raised, which includes the practices of her culture and the individual idiosyncrasies of her own mother's child-rearing practices, greatly influences her behavior toward her own infant. A striking example is the observation that often mothers who batter their children were beaten when they were young. Frommer and O'Shea (1973) have also noted a significant increase in problems of early maternal caretaking when the mother's parents were separated from each other at an early age (less than 11 years).

> A more inclusive assumption is to consider pregnancy as a crisis that affects all expectant mothers, no matter what their state of psychic health. Crises, as we see it, are turning points in the life of the individual, leading to acute disequilibria that under favorable conditions result in specific maturational steps toward new functions. We find them as developmental phenomena at points of no return between one phase and the next when decisive changes deprive former central needs and modes of living of their significance, forcing the acceptance of highly charged new goals and functions. Pregnancy as a major turning point in the life of the woman represents one of these normal crises, especially for the primigravida who faces the impact of this event for the first time. We believe that all women show what looks like remarkable, far-reaching psychological changes while they are pregnant. The outcome of this crisis, then, has profound effects on the early mother-child relationship.*

Hall and associates (1979) also studied women who had come from disrupted families. When one or both of the mother's parents had died, or her parents were divorced or separated, the mother interacted significantly less with their 20-week-old babies than women whose parents were alive and together. Kumar and Robson (1978) noted an association between depression and anxiety early in pregnancy and

---

*From Bibring, G.L.: Some considerations of the psychological processes in pregnancy, Psychoanal. Study Child 14:113-121, 1959.

a previous history of an induced abortion. It should be noted that their observations were limited to women having their first babies and that only in a small proportion of the subjects was there a discernible link between the previous abortion and antenatal depression.

By understanding the genesis of maternal and attachment behavior, perhaps we can better envision interventions that will foster change in those cases where such is desirable for mother and infant.

> COMMENT: It may seem to many that attachment to a small baby will come "naturally" and to make too much of it could be a mistake, since it will make women too self-conscious about a natural step. In general, this is true, but there are many, many women who have a difficult time making this adjustment and for whom an understanding, supportive person will make a critical difference. If we train cadres of people for these supportive roles, we *must* understand the ingredients of attachment in order to help them because each mother-child dyad is unique and has individual needs of its own.
> **T.B. Brazelton**

Pregnancy

During pregnancy a woman concurrently experiences two types of developmental changes: (1) physical and emotional changes within herself and (2) the growth of the fetus in her uterus. The way in which she feels about these changes will vary widely according to whether she planned the pregnancy, is married, is living with the father, or has other children. It will also vary according to the age of other children, her occupation or desire for one, her memories of her childhood, and her feelings about her parents (Bibring and Valenstein, 1976; Boston Women's Health Book Collective, 1976). For most women, pregnancy is a time of strong and changing emotions, ranging from positive to negative, frequently ambivalent. With the realization that she will soon have a baby, particularly if it is her first, the woman must adapt to a dramatic shift in her life-style as she changes from an individual responsible primarily for herself to a parent responsible for the life and well-being of a child. There will also be changes in her relationship with the father, since she will now have to divide her time and attention between two people (Benedek, 1952).

> COMMENT: Birth of a first child is viewed by the woman herself as admission into adulthood. Teenage and older mothers poignantly describe the transformation they feel in having brought a new life into the world and having assumed responsibility for this person's care. Becoming a mother seems to bridge concretely the era from childhood to adulthood.
> **R.T. Mercer**

Acceptance of pregnancy. During the first stage of pregnancy a woman must come to terms with the knowledge that she will be a mother. When she first realizes that she is pregnant, she may have mixed feelings. A large number of considerations, ranging from a change in her familiar patterns to more serious matters such as economic and housing hardships or interpersonal difficulties, all influence her acceptance of the pregnancy. This initial stage, as outlined by Bibring and associates (1961), is the mother's identification of the growing fetus as an "integral part of herself."

Perception of the fetus as a separate individual. The second stage involves a growing awareness of the baby in the uterus as a separate individual, which usually starts with the remarkably powerful event of quickening, the sensation of fetal movement. During this period the woman must begin to change her concept of the fetus from a being that is a part of herself to a living baby who will soon be a separate individual. Bibring and associates (1961) believe that this realization prepares the woman for birth and physical separation from her child. This preparedness in turn lays the foundation for a relationship with the child.

Winnicott (1957) beautifully describes this period when he notes, "Experience shows, however, that a change gradually takes place in the feelings as well as in the body of the girl who has conceived. She'll always say her interest gradually narrows down. Perhaps it is better to say that the direction of her interest turns from outwards to inwards. She slowly but surely comes to believe that the center of the world is in her own body."*

After quickening, a woman will usually begin to have fantasies about what the baby will be like, attributing some human personality characteristics to him and developing feelings of attachment. At this time she may further accept her pregnancy and show significant changes in attitude toward the fetus. Unplanned, unwanted infants may seem more acceptable. Objectively, there will usually be some outward evidence of the mother's preparation. She may purchase clothes or a crib, select a name, and rearrange her home to accommodate a baby.

> **COMMENT:** The developing parental attachment is evidenced during pregnancy as both parents fondly pat and rub the fetus through the thinning abdominal wall, whom they perceive as responding to them by the movement. Immediately following birth the mother's remark, "See, she knows your voice; you've talked to her so much," as the infant turns toward the father's voice, indicates that the parents have spent intimate moments talking to the fetus. During the third trimester the woman seems to embrace her fetus in utero as she sits smiling with her arms around her abdomen.
> **R.T. Mercer**

Recently Lumley (1980) has explored feelings and thoughts of 30 Australian primigravidas during their pregnancies. In the first interview at 8 to 12 weeks' gestation, most women (70%) said they could not believe that the fetus was really there and they never imagined or pictured the fetus. To them the fetus was not a real person. The minority (30%) believed that the fetus was a real person, and they spontaneously imagined the appearance of the fetus. These women were likely to describe the fetus with a feeling of concern in expressive language. They related

---

*From Winnicott, D.W.: The child and the family and the outside world, London, 1957, Tavistock Publications, p. 19.

anxieties about the fetus, such as the fear of miscarriage or abnormality. They predicted severe grief if they were to have a miscarriage.

Fig. 1-1 shows how often the fetus was viewed as a real person and whether they described the fetus as a baby. Interestingly, at 8 to 12 weeks' gestation four times as many women described the fetus as a sort of an animal. Mothers who began to show early feelings of attachment came from larger families and were women whose previous work had been in nursing or teaching. The feelings of bonding were inhibited in the presence of severe symptoms of pregnancy, when the woman's husband was not interested in the fetus, or when the husband did not provide her with emotional support. After the interview mothers were asked to draw an image of the fetus. During the 8- to 12-week gestation period the fetus was shapeless and formless. As the pregnancy progressed, the fetus developed a more human form.

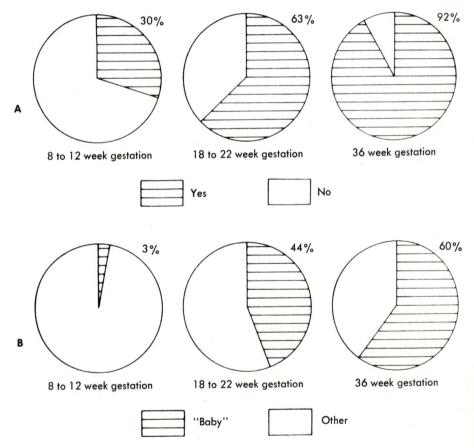

Fig. 1-1. **A,** Is the fetus a real person now? **B,** Those who describe the fetus as a baby. (From Lumley, J.: Birth Fam. J. 7:5-14, 1980.)

Recently the increased use of amniocentesis and ultrasound has appeared to affect parents' perceptions of babies in a rather unexpected fashion. Many parents have discussed with us the disappointment they experienced when they discovered the sex of the baby. Half of the mystery was over. Everything was possible, but once the amniocentesis was done and sex known, the range of the unknown was considerably narrowed. However, the tests have beneficial results by removing some of the anxiety about the possibility of any abnormality. We have noted following the procedure that the baby is sometimes named and parents often carry around a picture of the very small fetus. This phenomenon will require further investigation to understand the significance of these maneuvers to the bonding process.

The production of a normal child is a major goal of most women. Yet most pregnant women have hidden fears that the infant may be abnormal or reveal some of their own secret inner weaknesses.

Brazelton (1973) has clarified the importance of these changes and turmoil that occur during pregnancy for the subsequent development of attachment to the new infant.

> The prenatal interviews with normal primiparas, in a psychoanalytic interview setting, uncovered anxiety which often seemed to be of pathological proportions. The unconscious material was so loaded and distorted, so near the surface, that before delivery one felt an ominous direction for making a prediction about the woman's capacity to adjust to the role of mothering. And yet when we saw her in action as a mother, this very anxiety and the distorted unconscious material could become a force for reorganization, for readjustment to her important new role. I began to feel that much of the prenatal anxiety and distortion of fantasy could be a healthy mechanism for bringing her out of the old homeostasis which she had achieved to a new level of adjustment. The alarm reaction we were tapping in on was serving as a kind of shock treatment for reorganization to her new role. . . . I now see the shakeup in pregnancy as readying the circuits for new attachments, as preparation for the many choices which they must be ready to make in a very short critical period, as a method of freeing her circuits for a kind of sensitivity to the infant and his individual requirements which might not have been easily or otherwise available from her earlier adjustment. Thus, this very emotional turmoil of pregnancy and that in the neonatal period can be seen as a positive force for the mother's adjustment and for the possibility of providing a more individualized environment for the infant.*

> **COMMENT:** This is an excellent example of how physicians would be likely to label a mother as "anxious" or "needing help," when in truth she was undergoing normal anxiety—important to becoming a mother and adjusting rapidly to any kind of infant. We have found that many mothers worry about how anxious they are in pregnancy and with the new baby. Reassuring them that this is normal, healthy, and even a sign of caring becomes a very important step in helping them to see themselves as healthy and ready to mother their baby.
> **T.B. Brazelton**

---

*From Brazelton, T.B.: Effect of maternal expectations on early infant behavior, Early Child Develop. Care **2:**259-273, 1973.

An interesting example of the way in which the adjustment may be handled in another culture occurs in Thailand. For centuries Thai mothers have purchased a clay statue of a mother and infant when they became pregnant. At the time of birth the statue is thrown into the river; thus the image of the mother and infant before birth is literally destroyed.

To understand better the complex events that occur during the perinatal period, we will direct our attention primarily to the mother-infant dyad. It is necessary to repeat again and again that the father, the other siblings, and the extended family are of vital importance to this dyad. Brazelton (1973) suggests that prospective fathers go through an upheaval that is similar to that of the mothers.

Each young man was forced to reevaluate his role as a provider for the family, as an adult male ready to adjust to the responsibility of a dependent, as a model for the new child's learning about masculinity, and as a major support for his wife as she adjusted to her role as a mother. In the process, he was forced back on self-examination and his experience with being fathered. If he was trying to free himself of ties to his own parents, it was hard for him to identify with them as models for his new role. He may have barely adjusted to being a husband, and the new, added expectations became difficult for him to encompass. In our lonely, nuclear family structure in the USA, the young father was often the only available support for his wife. They had moved away from their families, both in physical distance and in psychological expectations, and were unwilling to fall back on them for moral or physical support. There were rarely other supportive figures nearby—such as family physicians, ministers, close friends or neighbors who could help. The father was expected to assume the major supportive role.*

COMMENT: In these days when fathers are eager to play a more active role with wives and their babies, it behooves us to think of the few supports a new father has to help him make his own adjustment. That there is tremendous, valuable energy for attachment to be captured is reflected in a recent statement by Margaret Mead: "No developing society that needs men to leave home and do his 'thing' for the society ever allows young men in to handle or touch their newborns. There's always a taboo against it. For they know somewhere that, if they did, the new fathers would become so 'hooked' that they would never get out and do their 'thing' properly." In our lonely, nuclear families maybe a father's best "thing" is to become more involved with his wife and new baby. I like to have a prenatal visit with both parents and always address at least one major question to the prospective father. Many of these young men tell me that no one has ever asked them anything about the pregnancy or about their role in it before. Isn't this too bad at a time when we are expecting them to play a vital role once the baby arrives?
T.B. Brazelton

Bibring (1959) agrees that what was once a transitional period with carefully worked out traditions for support has become a time of crisis with no societal mechanisms for helping expectant parents cope with the profound changes and developmental conflicts. In the past the structure of the extended family permitted a young girl to observe pregnant women and to be present and help during birth.

---

*From Brazelton, T.B.: Effect of maternal expectations on early infant behavior, Early Child Develop. Care **2**:259-273, 1973.

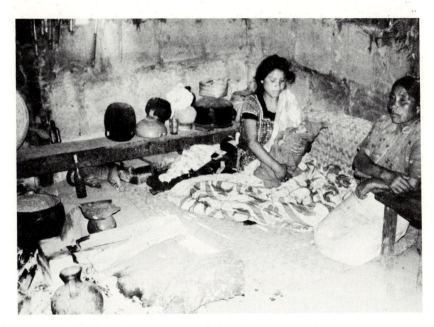

Fig. 1-2. A new mother starting care of her infant under guidance of her mother in the Indian village Santa Maria Cauqué in the Guatemalan highlands.

Thus pregnancy and birth were shared experiences in which every girl participated from an early age. This is still true for the majority of young women growing up in rural and semirural areas of developing countries. Fig. 1-2 shows a new mother in an Indian home in the village of Santa Maria Cauqué in the Guatemalan highlands. In isolated, nuclear families in the United States a young woman and even more, a young man, may have had no experience at all with prospective parents and, although expecting a baby, may not be able to discuss or visit with anyone else involved with pregnancy. With modern hospital deliveries there is the additional fear caused by the strange environment.

> **COMMENT:** The environment of the hospital is particularly strange for parents of other cultures, including poverty-stricken ghetto parents. An example of the strangeness of a university hospital is illustrated by staff nurses who were concerned about an Eastern Indian mother's lack of apparent bonding to her second infant following an emergency cesarean birth. The mother, who would have had her own mother to care for her and her infant for six months, and who had this care with her first infant, perceived the treatment of her ambulating and bathing, changing, and feeding her infant so early as harshly inconsiderate.
> **R.T. Mercer**

Since birth has been moved from the home to the hospital to meet better the physical needs of the mother and infant, there has been a growth of a number of organizations that have partially replaced the extended family. These are groups in which both parents learn with other couples about pregnancy, labor, birth, and infant care. Although their stated purpose is to prepare parents for the actual labor and birth, the result is the sharing of hopes, expectations, and fears. They partly substitute for an extended family. The bonds made through shared participation are strong, and couples will often stay in touch with each other for years afterward.

Cohen (1966) emphasizes that any stress, such as moving to a new geographic area, marital infidelity, death of a close friend or relative, previous abortions, or loss of previous children, which leaves the mother feeling unloved or unsupported or which precipitates concern for the health and survival of either her infant or herself may delay preparation for the infant and retard bond formation. After the first trimester, behaviors that are a reaction to stress and suggest rejection of pregnancy include a preoccupation with physical appearance or negative self-perception, excessive emotional withdrawal or mood swings, excessive physical complaints, absence of any response to quickening, or lack of any preparatory behavior during the last trimester.

As the result of recent advances in perinatal care for high-risk mothers, it is necessary to describe a new area of concern—the result of prolonged antenatal hospitalization. Rather than transporting sick or premature babies from the maternity hospital to a medical center for neonatal intensive care, the new practice favors transporting high-risk mothers prior to delivery for sophisticated perinatal care in the antepartum and intrapartum period. Pregnant women with diabetes, hypertension, premature labor, or a slowly growing fetus are hospitalized for prolonged periods of up to a month or more. Studies by Merkatz (1978) noted that they were primarily concerned about the baby they were carrying and only secondarily about their own health. Merkatz' poignant observations of the concerns and the loneliness of these women point up the importance of designing care for them on an individual basis that takes into account the subtleties of their changing family dynamics. No aspect of hospital practice could be more detrimental to these maternity patients than the traditional hospital restrictions on family visitation. It is in this regard that the opportunity for change is the greatest. It is important that a woman hospitalized on the high-risk maternity unit be visited freely by husbands, boyfriends, children, and parents. In some countries this practice is extended to live-in situations. Merkatz (1978) notes that families need privacy and time together particularly when hospitalization has been extended so that family members can assist each other to cope with fear, anxiety, and uncertainty.

COMMENT: This is also a time when the woman's concerns about whether her enforced hospitalization and her illness will affect her unborn baby. Her concerns may even seem unreasonable in their dimension of anxiety. Again, if obstetricians, nurses, and those around her realize that *of course* her concerns reflect the normal turmoil of pregnancy but also are equated with her energy for future mothering, maybe they can be more tolerant and supportive.
T.B. Brazelton

COMMENT: My continued observations and study of hospitalized high-risk mothers suggest that their response to the situation is highly individual. However, for many there is exaggerated fear that the baby in utero is not normal, for example, when the pregnancy problem is labeled as intrauterine growth retardation, or that a catastrophic event can occur at any time which would be life threatening to the baby. Such fears may pose special problems for the mother in the initial acceptance and comfort with the baby after birth. Some mothers have been so frightened that they avoid normal nesting activities before birth and have to catch up with such activities after birth. Others have been too fearful to have indulged in fantasy about the baby's appearance and characteristics or to have considered names for the infant. In some cases the mother's initial perceptions of the infant may be adversely affected. While observing these mothers after birthing normal full-term infants, I am sometimes reminded of the interactions described for mothers and their premature babies.

Another important consideration is that the antenatal hospitalization generally imposes a change in the mother's usual level of activity. She may have been placed on a regimen of bedrest or even if she was permitted full activity, her range of physical effort is greatly restricted compared with that of the home environment. Thus she needs considerable time to regain physical strength after birth and to assume all of the caretaking responsibilities for the infant. When the mother does not have extended family members or friends to assist her, as is often the case for the mobile American family unit, she may be particularly overwhelmed in her new role.
R. Merkatz

COMMENT: The high-risk woman who is hospitalized either in her local hospital or in a medical center in another city is highly committed to her fetus. She may forfeit a degree of renal functioning or otherwise may take years from her own life in order to have a baby. The cost to herself and to her family is indeed great. Corbin (1981) recently observed that the woman with a high-risk pregnancy exerted great effort toward "protective governance" of the pregnancy as she actively assessed the situation and balanced the benefits and risks of various treatment plans in her attempts to control the situation for a favorable outcome. Some women become so distraught with their treatment plans when hospitalized or so lonely and bored away from family that they sign out of the hospital; others demand a trial with medicine dosages that worked for their conditions before, refusing dosages that would be more harmful to the fetus. Such anxiety and disruption in care can be prevented if health professionals plan the sophisticated perinatal care *with her;* a woman who has lived with a chronic illness for several years knows her body's idiosyncratic response and tolerance to regimens rather well.
R.T. Mercer

PRACTICAL OBSERVATIONS AND RECOMMENDATIONS

1. *High-risk factors*. Early in the pregnancy it is important for the physician and nurse to learn what diseases are in the family of the father and mother, to obtain information about any abortions, stillbirths, neonatal deaths or illnesses, experiences with previous pregnancies and births, and the parenting they experienced in their first years of life, and to hear about their major concerns. There is much evidence that the loss of a parent in the first 11 years of life is a major psychological risk factor for new fathers and mothers, and so information about this can be extremely helpful to the nurse or pediatrician who may note unexplained parental anxiety and unreasonable concerns about a newborn infant.

2. *Family ecology*. Major changes in the ecology of the family such as moving to a new community or the death of a close relative, for example, a father or

mother, brother or husband, can have a devastating effect on the pregnancy, early maternal caretaking, and affectionate interaction with the young infant.

3. *Cesarean childbirth*. Recent findings about the importance of the father's presence at a cesarean birth were disclosed at the National Institutes of Health Consensus Development Conference on Cesarean Childbirth (1980):

> In some hospitals, family centered maternity care has been extended to the cesarean birth family, and in these cases there is no evidence of harm to mother, neonate, or father. The presence of fathers in the operating room and closer contact between mother and neonate appear to improve the post-cesarean behavioral responses of the families. One consistent finding from small scale studies of post-cesarean birth families is the greater involvement of fathers with their infants. . . . Hospitals are encouraged to liberalize their policies concerning the option of having the father or surrogate attend the cesarean birth. The healthy neonate should not be separated routinely from mother and father following delivery.*

4. *Family support*. With the development of high-risk obstetrical care centers for pregnant women who require hospitalization for prolonged periods as a result of conditions such as toxemia, diabetes, hypertension, and intrauterine growth retardation, it is necessary to alter hospital practices greatly to permit and encourage strong family support. This will require changes in visiting policies for young siblings-to-be, extra beds for fathers-to-be to stay overnight in the room with their wives, special dining rooms for the family to eat together, and other alterations to make the hospital more like a home. These changes will not come about easily, since they do not fit with the usual medical model. On a number of occasions women who had prolonged prenatal hospitalization told us how everybody seemed interested in the high-risk pregnancy but not in them as persons or the baby as an individual. With this in mind and with the difficulty of changing hospital practices, questions can be raised about the possibility of developing other systems for the care of the high-risk mother in homelike surroundings adjacent to the hospital.

5. *Home health visitor*. Beautifully executed observations by Larson (1980) reveal that if a home health caretaker such as a visiting nurse made contact with the mother before birth and 48 hours after the baby's birth, rather than starting 6 weeks' postpartum, there was a significant change in the mother's ability to parent. Thus interventions in the perinatal period probably should begin during the pregnancy rather than after the mother has taken her baby home. This gives added impetus for pediatricians to arrange visits to meet and talk with the mother during the pregnancy. It also leads to questions about the distinct separation between physical facilities and caretakers that exist for the entire process of birth, with the pregnancy managed by one physician or midwife and the infant cared for by an-

---

*From National Institutes of Health: Cesarean childbirth, Consensus Development Conference Summary, Bethesda, Md., 1980, vol. 3, no. 6.

other health care worker, often with little exchange of information between those involved. We should keep in mind how recently the change was made from a system in which there was one continuous caretaker, the family doctor and/or midwife, who was available to the mother during her pregnancy, labor, and birth and who provided the care for both the mother and baby during the postpartum period.

6. *Psychiatric disturbances.* Evidence from a small number of individual case observations and studies suggest that close and continuing support for psychiatrically disturbed women that begins in the third trimester of pregnancy and continues through delivery and into the early postnatal period may have a powerful effect on the later parenting and family life of the mothers and fathers.

7. *Prenatal education.* We strongly support the availability of the many prenatal classes in which parents can share with each other, as well as with other couples, their many individual experiences, concerns, needs, and questions and can have time to mull over and appreciate how many of their worries are a normal part of pregnancy. An important component is the opportunity to receive up-to-date information from a childbirth educator. At this time we are unsure about all of the exercises that are taught in these childbirth classes, since there are now a number of innovative procedures that may change the present exercise practices during labor. As an example, Michel Odent (1979) in Pithiviers, France, does not have any special exercises for the pregnant women under his care. These mothers gather three times a month with other members of the family, sing together for an hour, and talk about their pregnancy and the birth process, but there are no exercises. The advantages and disadvantages of exercises during labor will obviously require further investigation to see what will be most appropriate for the largest number of mothers and fathers.

> **COMMENT:** One of the most critical aspects of childbirth education classes is the group experience. Mothers and fathers have an opportunity to share experiences and concerns and to see how universal their own anxiety is. They form lateral attachments within these peer groups that not only serve them through the critical months of pregnancy, but during labor and delivery and, eventually, in the adjustment to the newborn. We will do well to continue these classes for new parents to enable them to share experiences in the early perinatal period.
> **T.B. Brazelton**

CHAPTER 2

LABOR, BIRTH, AND BONDING

MARSHALL H. KLAUS and JOHN H. KENNELL

How long does the fire of love in a woman endure when the eyes and touch are no
longer there to kindle it?
Dante

At the present time sweeping and fundamental changes in maternity practices
relating to labor, birth, and the early postnatal period are under way. No account
of the research in this period would be complete without exploring the current
debate and controversy, or what might be termed the revolution in maternity care
(Arms, 1975; Chard and Richards, 1977; Dunn, 1976; Kitzinger and Davis, 1978;
Oakley, 1980). This revolt against professional medical practices is unprecedented.
The following is a list of some of the practices presently undergoing change and
some outcome measures that deserve evaluation. In the next pages we will indicate
that some of these practices do affect outcomes, but many of the practices require
further evaluation.

Practices undergoing change	*Outcome measures*
Mother's position during labor	Maternal medication
Constant support of a woman during labor	Anesthesia
Parents' control of birth	Length of labor
Birth environment	Perinatal complications
Childbirth education	Infant mortality
Ultrasound	Parent-infant bonding
Electronic fetal monitoring (all mothers)	
Cesarean section	

In a book entitled *The Structure of Scientific Revolutions*, Kuhn (1962) noted
the following:

Normal science, the activity in which most scientists inevitably spend almost all their
time, is predicated on the assumption that the scientific community knows what the
world is like. Much of the success of the enterprise derives from the community's willingness to defend that assumption, if necessary at considerable cost. *Normal science,* for

example, often *suppresses fundamental novelties* because they are necessarily subversive of its basic commitments. Nevertheless, so long as those commitments retain an element of the arbitrary, the very nature of normal research ensures that *novelty shall not be suppressed for very long.**

From the long history of science, if maternity practices are like other scientific fields, Kuhn would predict optimistically that the advances and procedures which are most valuable clinically will win out in the long run. However, Jordan (1980) notes that "any way of doing birth consists of beliefs and practices which are mutually dependent and internally consistent. The work of maintaining this dependency and consistency and thereby the system's efficient operation, is done through a continuous process of justification which draws for its standards on the local definition of birth." She notes "the extraordinary extent to which practitioners buy into their own system's moral and technical superiority," and argues that it will not necessarily be medical or scientific consideration which will determine the correctness of any medical intervention. She notes further that "In the American system medical professionals . . . favor the standard package set of obstetric practices . . ." and that this "does not make them right or wrong in any simple way. Rather it must be understood as their unselfconscious participation in . . . practices which are grounded in the culture's definition of birth as a medical event. We find ourselves here in a fuzzy realm where the science of medicine shades into the culture of doctoring." She adds, importantly, "that birthing systems themselves are a part of a larger cultural system" and "would suggest that any given controversy is decided not on the basis of the kind of evidence that is produced by the biomedical research (though that evidence will be put in the service of the enterprise) but rather its status will depend on how well it fits with the socio-political realities and the ideological belief system of its time and place." Since it is possible that valid scientific evidence for events in this period may be obscured, suppressed, and not fully evaluated if it is not in tune with our society's system of beliefs, we are not as optimistic as Kuhn.

The statue shown in Fig. 2-1, *A*, is one example of how strongly most of us are influenced by a biased view of the world. The photograph illustrates how this statue, made in Mexico about 1500 years ago, has been displayed in Louisiana (a museum outside of Copenhagen, Denmark). Note that if it is placed as shown in Fig. 2-1, *B*, the seeds on the mother's shoulders will not be in a position to fall off and her toes will be curled appropriately. For nearly 20 years this Mexican statue was placed incorrectly so that the woman labored on her back, a position not originally intended by the artist but one that fitted the commonly held view of the "normal science" of modern obstetrics.

---

*From Kuhn, T.S.: The structure of scientific revolutions, Chicago, 1962, University of Chicago Press. Copyright 1962, 1970 by the University of Chicago.

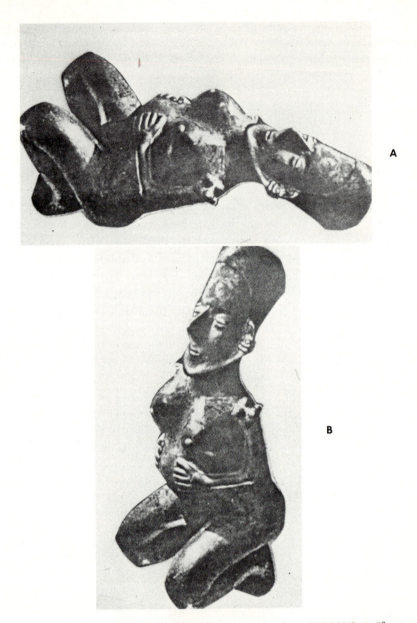

Fig. 2-1. A, Mexican statue exhibited in Denmark 20 years ago (A.D. 200-1200). **B,** If statue is placed in erect position, seeds on the shoulder will not fall off, the mother's breasts are appropriate, and her toes are properly curled.

In the pages ahead we will explore the presently available data and related theories on labor, birth, and the early postnatal period in an effort to discover the role of the many complex variables involved in the bonding process. The practices listed earlier must be evaluated for their biomedical, physiological, and behavioral components and outcomes. To understand how these components may be interrelated and why they cannot be considered in isolation, we will examine the effects on the mother, and subsequently on the child, of the presence of a supportive companion (doula). The studies presented will illustrate how behavioral and medical outcomes can be altered by changing just one, apparently trivial, aspect of the birth process. They also demonstrate that each of the biochemical, physiological, endocrinological, and behavioral systems involved are often linked in a complex arrangement. Finally, based on the evidence from the available material, we will make some practical clinical recommendations concerning the care of parents and infants during labor, birth, and the postnatal period.

SUPPORTIVE COMPANION (DOULA)

In 1974 we went to Guatemala to carry out studies on mother-infant contact, and we spent many days and nights on the obstetrical division in two exceedingly busy maternity hospitals that each delivered 50 to 60 babies every day. The routine on these divisions was established by physicians and nurses from the United States. Hospital policies did not permit any family member or friend to be present in the labor and delivery rooms, apparently as a consequence of the large number of deliveries and the limitation of space.

Prior to the earthquake that destroyed one of the Guatemalan maternity hospitals in 1976, we carried out a pilot study in which we asked an untrained woman to stay with mothers during labor and birth. As a result, we observed dramatic changes in the women during labor. They became quiet and peaceful. Three of the first 10 women gave birth in bed, an unusual event in this hospital where the obstetrical staff had extensive experience with the usual length and course of labor in primiparas and the manifestations of imminent delivery. We noted that several of the women in this pilot study had milk dripping from their nipples when their baby was brought to them following the birth. Up to that time we had not seen this occur in the approximately 100 women who labored and gave birth without a supportive companion.

Of the 150 human cultures studied by anthropologists, in all but one a family member or friend, usually a woman, remained with a mother during labor and birth.* In Santa Maria Cauqué, Guatemala, it is standard for the native midwife, both grandmothers, the husband, and occasionally the father-in-law to be present.

---

*Raphael, D.: Unpublished data.

In 98% of cultures studied there is a tradition of postpartum confinement of the mother and baby together. Before childbirth moved from the home to the hospital, it was also the practice for family members to support the mother actively in labor, often with the assistance of a trained or untrained midwife. Although more fathers, relatives, and friends have been allowed into labor and delivery rooms in the past 10 years in the United States, a considerable number of mothers still give birth in some hospitals without the presence of family members or close friends. There has been little systematic study of this issue since Newton and Newton (1962) reported that mothers who were quiet and relaxed and had better emotional relations with their attendants during labor and birth were more pleased at the first sight of their babies.

> **COMMENT:** Although the presence of another woman during childbirth is close to a human universal, her role is not always a gentle and comforting one. In 73% of 59 cultures for which detailed information was available, the childbirth companion performed potentially uncomfortable manipulations on the laboring women, such as kneading, pressing, bouncing, and manual dilatation of the cervix.
> **B. Lozoff**

Our first study in Guatemala was designed to investigate the effects of a continuous supportive companion (doula) on the length of labor, perinatal complications, and maternal-infant interaction in the first hour after birth in an obstetrical setting in which mothers routinely labor alone (Sosa et al., 1980). In this unit primigravid mothers in labor were admitted to an observation ward when regular uterine contractions were present and the dilatation of the cervix was 1 to 2 cm. Women in early labor with no known medical problems were eligible, and the assignment of women to the control or experimental group was made on a random basis after the woman was admitted to the study. Control mothers followed the hospital routine, which consisted of monitoring the labor by infrequent vaginal examinations and auscultation of the heart and assistance to the mother during delivery. Electronic fetal monitoring was not available in this unit.

The continuous support provided to the experimental group by untrained lay women consisted of physical contact (e.g., rubbing the mother's back and holding her hand), conversation, and supplying the mother with a friendly companion who, although previously unknown to her, would not leave her during the entire labor. A mother was removed from the study if there was prolonged labor or evidence of fetal distress during labor or the delivery required an intervention (e.g., Pitocin, cesarean birth, or forceps), or if the infant was asphyxiated (Apgar less than 8 at 5 minutes), meconium stained, depressed, stillborn, premature, malformed, or had any evidence of illness such as respiratory distress. Mothers were enrolled in the study until there were 20 in the control group and 20 in the experimental group. There were no significant differences between the groups in terms of marital status, the age of the mothers, the babies' birthweights, or sex distribution.

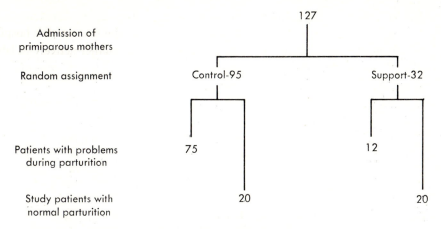

Fig. 2-2. Design of the study.

It was necessary to admit 95 mothers to the control group but only 32 to the experimental group to obtain the final sample of 20 in each group (Fig. 2-2); that is, 75 women were assigned to the control group who were subsequently eliminated from the study for one or more of the reasons described previously. In the experimental group only 12 women were excluded for these reasons. It should be noted that each woman was listed only once (for the first problem identified). Thus, if meconium staining was noted and neonatal asphyxia was observed, only the meconium staining would be noted. Statistical analysis revealed that there was a significantly lower incidence of problems of labor and birth for the group of mother-infant pairs who had the supportive companion (Table 2-1).

> **COMMENT:** Are all companions equal? The kind of relationship between the companion and the delivering mother needs to be examined more closely. A husband, for example, might make an even better support person than a stranger. The history and quality of the husband-wife relationship would be critical and, especially for first-time fathers, preparation for the doula role would be important.
> **R.D. Parke**

Stimulated by the results of this first study on the short-term benefits of a doula, we designed a second study to explore the long-term advantages of having a doula during labor and birth (Klaus et al., 1981). Two hundred and forty-four primiparous, full-term, healthy Guatemalan mothers in early labor were randomly assigned either to the doula group or control group. The mothers who gave birth without perinatal problems were then randomly assigned to early (first hour) or late (2 to 3 hours) suckling. Research workers who did not know the previous experience of the mothers made home visits to the women in both groups at one, three, and six

Table 2-1. Perinatal problems for mother-newborn pairs in first study

	No doula		Doula	
	Percent	Number of mothers	Percent	Number of mothers
Cesarean birth	27.3	26	18.7	6
Meconium staining	25.3	24	9.4	3
Asphyxia	5.3	5	0.0	0
Subtotal	57.9	55	28.1	9
Drugs and forceps	21.0	20	9.3	3
TOTAL	78.9	75	37.4	12

Subtotal row: $p < .01$; Drugs and forceps row: $p < .30$; TOTAL row: $p < .001$

Table 2-2. Perinatal problems for mother-newborn pairs in second study

	No doula		Doula	
	Percent	Number of mothers	Percent	Number of mothers
Cesarean birth	19.2	40	12.0	10
Meconium staining	17.3	36	10.8	9
Asphyxia	2.4	5	1.2	1
Subtotal	38.9	81	24.0	20
Drugs and forceps	21.0	48	7.2	6
TOTAL	59.9	129	31.2	26

Subtotal row: $p < .05$; Drugs and forceps row: $p < .01$; TOTAL row: $p < .001$

months to assess feeding practices, to evaluate the infant's health status, and to make anthropometric measurements of the infant. Table 2-2 demonstrates that significantly more perinatal problems (cesarean birth, meconium staining, fetal distress) occurred in the control group (59.9% vs. 31.2%; $p < .001$). This replicates the findings of our first study. The presence of the doula and/or early suckling did not affect the length of breastfeeding or anthropometric measurements. A number of common pediatric illnesses (e.g., diarrhea, upper respiratory tract infection) did not differ between the control and doula mothers. However, significantly more of the infants born to control mothers were hospitalized in the first 6 months of life with pneumonia or diarrhea (6/67 vs. 0/49; $p < .01$). These observations suggest that present maternity practices which require women to labor and give birth without support may result in iatrogenic disease of the mother and infant.

LENGTH OF LABOR

The mean number of hours from admission to the observation ward until delivery for the mother-infant pairs retained in the study was significantly decreased for the experimental groups as compared to control groups in both studies (Table 2-3).

Following the birth, mothers in the two groups of the first study were observed

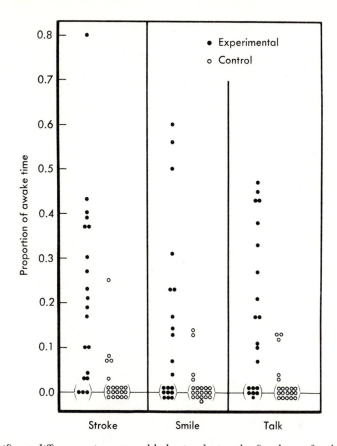

Fig. 2-3. Significant differences in maternal behavior during the first hour after birth between the experimental (doula) and control groups during awake time.

Table 2-3. Mean length of labor in hours

	No doula	Doula	P
First study	19	9	<0.001
Second study	14	8	<0.0001

alone with their infants for 22.5 minutes by observers who did not know their previous experience (Fig. 2-3). The amount of time the mother remained awake during the observation period was greater for the experimental group (p<.02). During the awake time, these mothers did not differ in the amount of simple touching of the infants. However, there was a significant difference in the amount of stroking, smiling, and talking observed, with the experimental mothers being more involved in these activities than the control mothers.

The surprising findings of increased complications and labor length for the control group raise the possibility of an association between acute anxiety and an arrest of labor and fetal distress. The studies of human and primate mothers suggest that one explanation for this is an increased catecholamine level (Fig. 2-4). Epinephrine has a direct effect on uterine muscle, decreasing uterine contractions and thereby increasing the length of labor (Zuspan et al., 1962). Lederman and associates (1978) noted that plasma epinephrine levels and self-reported anxiety at the onset of phase two of labor were significantly correlated in 32 normal primigravid women. Physiological elevations of plasma epinephrine were associated with decreased uterine contractile activity at the onset of labor (3 cm of cervical dilatation) and a longer duration of labor from 3 to 10 cm dilatation. However, fetal asphyxia is probably secondary to the effect of epinephrine on uterine blood flow. Barton and co-workers (1974) noted significant reductions in blood flow (up to 50%) to the sheep uterus with injections of epinephrine or norepinephrine. Catecholamines injected into pregnant rhesus monkey mothers by Adamson and associates (1971) resulted in fetal asphyxia but had no such effect when injected only into the fetus. Myers (1975) noted that psychological stress alone to pregnant monkeys, without pain or physical contact, resulted in severe fetal asphyxia with significant reductions in fetal arterial pH and oxygen tension. Therefore we can hypothesize that the presence of a supportive companion in the experimental group of mothers reduced catecholamine levels. With increased levels in the control group, there was decreased uterine contractile activity and a significant reduction in uterine blood flow.

The findings in these studies suggest the importance of human companionship during labor and birth. Labor was significantly shortened, perinatal problems were reduced, and some aspects of maternal behavior in the first hour of life after birth were enhanced.

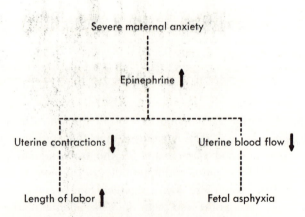

Fig. 2-4. Effect of epinephrine on uterine muscle contractions and blood flow, an explanation for the increased length of labor and fetal asphyxia.

Observations of the effectiveness of a supportive companion on the mother and fetus raise the possibility that human companionship may have influenced the results in electronic fetal monitoring studies. Four control studies of fetal monitoring reported an increased cesarean section rate, presumably due to fetal distress (Chalmers, 1979; Haverkamp et al., 1976; Kelso et al., 1978; Renou et al., 1976). Haverkamp and associates (1976) suggested that the control group of patients in their study had more individualized nursing care and close physical contact for auscultating the fetal heart, and as a result experienced less anxiety. They proposed that the added attention and physical contact might have contributed to the favorable outcome in the group that received individualized nursing care rather than electronic fetal monitoring. In O'Driscoll's technique for the "active management of labor" (1975) he guarantees a personal nurse for every mother throughout labor who never leaves her; he considers this crucial for the management of labor. This technique so shortened the duration of labor that no increase in nursing staff was required to provide this personal attention for 8000 patients each year at the Rotunda in Dublin.

The results of the present investigations suggest that further studies of any labor intervention must ensure that both groups receive the same amount of attention and support from nursing and medical personnel. How often has false labor or the phenomenon of a woman's labor slowing dramatically after entering the hospital been due to her reaction to the many strange, inhibiting, or frightening aspects of the hospital environment? An untrained woman provided the friendly support in our Guatemalan study, but a similar or greater benefit might be expected when a family member or friend remains with the mother throughout the labor and birth. This low-cost intervention may be a simple way to reduce the length of labor and perinatal problems for women and their infants during childbirth, and it vividly illustrates the intimate interactions of maternal behavior, physiology, biochemistry, and medical problems.

COMMENT: To be left alone during labor is not only terrifying, but a severe threat to the woman's self-concept. To be supported is to be valued at a time of intense ego-centrism and fear. The kind of care a woman receives during this vulnerable time is crucial to her subsequent evaluation of the experience, her later maternal behavior, and her self-concept.
M.A. Curry

COMMENT: In contrast to nonindustrial societies in which an experienced female family member is present during labor, the most likely candidate for a supportive person in the United States is the father. Yet only 30% of world cultures allow the father to be present during childbirth. Is there a particular reason for excluding husbands throughout the world? Is the laboring woman especially reassured by the presence of a woman who has borne children herself? Questions such as these remain to be researched, but perhaps continuous comforting companionship is the crucial factor, regardless of the companion's childbearing experience.
B. Lozoff

Analysis of observations recorded in our 1972 study of low-income, inner-city mothers in Cleveland suggested importantly that the effects of a supportive companion on maternal behavior may last beyond the first hour after delivery (Trause et al., 1978). In that study the mothers who were awake in the first 40 minutes of contact with their babies were more affectionate and attentive to their infants at 1 month than mothers who fell asleep in the first minutes of contact. There are, however, some difficulties in using the study results to argue for long-term effects of a supportive person, since in that investigation those mothers who fell asleep were also more heavily medicated. In our Guatemalan doula study, none of the mothers in the final sample received any medication. In addition, contact between mothers and infants in the Cleveland study was limited to every 4-hour feedings for 20 minutes by hospital routine plus 5 hours of continuous contact each day, in contrast with almost continuous contact from birth in our two doula studies.

COMMENT: These studies are not only important in demonstrating that changes in childbirth practices could and do affect outcome in mother-infant interaction in general, but they answer one of the criticisms I often hear—"Do these changes in obstetrical practices help mothers of lower socioeconomic groups, as well as middle-class mothers?" I am under the impression that they will be even *more* meaningful to mothers who are from stressed circumstances, who are used to being shoved around by society, and who often have undervalued themselves as people. These changes are obvious ones to individuate each laboring woman and to encourage her to place more value on herself as a person and as a prospective mother.
T.B. Brazelton

HOME BIRTHS

In sharp contrast to the woman who delivers in the hospital, the woman giving birth at home seems to be in control. Immediately after the birth she appears to be in a remarkable state of ecstasy. We have called this *ekstasis*. The exuberance is contagious, and the observers share the festive mood of unreserved elation after the birth and groom the mother. Particularly striking is the observer's intense interest in the infant, especially in the first 15 to 20 minutes of life.

Preliminary studies of home births have been made from videotape recordings and films, as well as from long discussions with perceptive midwives (Lang, 1976; Mills, 1974). One midwife, Raven Lang, has made observations of 52 home births. The hands-and-knees position was used in 37% of the births. Some midwives prefer a lateral position, which allows the mother to watch the birth of her own infant. The observers are also extremely elated during the birth and offer encouragement and support to the mother; in the first 15 to 20 minutes of life there is intense interest in the infant. Lang also noted that the observers of the labor and birth became more attached to the infant than other friends of the family who did not witness the birth. We believe that this is one of the important principles of bonding. In the past, when maternal mortality was high, this served an essential function by ensuring a substitute mother.

COMMENT: The birth position reported in home births in the United States is unusual in nonindustrial societies. Only 4% of other cultures adopt hands-and-knees as the preferred position. In 90% of cultures the woman's torso is upright, as she sits, kneels, or squats with support. The elation

and orgasmic sensations described in home births have not been reported elsewhere. This lack may reflect inadequacies in the anthropological data or may indicate that our home-birth experiences are invested with the participants' excitement and determination to do something contrary to the expectations of their own society.
B. Lozoff

These home births that were studied in a select population show a somewhat different pattern of interaction, only fragments of which are visible in hospital births. To summarize the findings in a home birth:

1. The mother is an active participant.
2. She immediately picks up the infant after birth.
3. A striking elevation in mood is observed in association with excitement of the others who are present.
4. Everyone present is drawn to look at the infant for prolonged periods.
5. The mother is groomed.
6. Breastfeeding starts within 5 or 6 minutes, beginning with prolonged licking by the infant.

COMMENT: In many cultures the first 30 minutes after birth are devoted to the mother herself. She seems to need and prefer a recovery period of her own before she becomes interested in the infant. This makes a good deal of sense, and I think the ecstasies we see may, in larger part, be related to her relief at having finally made it to the end of labor. This euphoria can certainly be mobilized to attach to the infant, and in American culture, where so many roadblocks have been institutionalized, mothers who are experiencing home births may be demonstrating behaviors that are signs of relief at having their bodies intact. I am not entirely in favor of home births, although I see their value at the present time—as a way for a mother to establish herself as being in control of this important event in her life. But if anything happens to her baby because she has made such an independent decision, in the face of excellent medical care, I can see that she must blame herself forever afterward. That is a big price to pay. I would much prefer that hospitals or hospices make such an attractive, homelike, family situation available that there was no need to push for home births. In other words, if home births are on the rise, the medical system has no one to blame but itself.
T.B. Brazelton

EFFECT OF DRUGS IN LABOR

To understand better the attitude and behavior of mothers and mother-infant interaction in the first hours and days of life, we need more studies on the effects of various delivery procedures and anesthetic interventions. For example, research is now under way on the effects of drugs administered to the mother during labor and birth on the behavior of newborn infants. It seems clear that most anesthetics do depress infant responsivity and thus are likely to influence the first interchanges between mother and child. In our own experience we have been amazed at the differences between large numbers of infants born in other countries with no maternal analgesia or anesthesia and the neonates in the United States delivered under minimal analgesia and conduction anesthesia. The latter infants need to be treated as postsurgical (or postanesthesia) patients for many hours, with head positioned low, repeated suctioning, and close watching (Brazelton, 1961; Richards and

Bernal, 1971). If mothers in developing countries received such drugs, one wonders how many babies might be lost due to problems of airway secretions associated with a lessened sensitivity of the cough, gag, and other reflexes.

> **COMMENT:** Certainly a depressed infant is less likely to be responsive either on initial contact or during feeding situations, and he becomes less stimulating and responsive to a mother who is trying hard to mobilize herself to attach to her new infant. We found breastfeeding and weight gain significantly delayed for mother-infant pairs who had premedication in large doses in a study we did in 1961.
> **T.B. Brazelton**

There is also a need for a comprehensive study of the overall effects of conduction anesthesia and obstetrical practices, such as episiotomies, on mother-to-infant attachment. The relief of pain for a short period of time has to be weighed against the effects of altering this unique experience in the life of a woman, which under unmodified conditions, is reported to be frequently associated with orgasmic sensations and followed by a period of particularly heightened perceptions. In contrast are the sometimes hectic, painful, and awkward maneuvers needed to administer conduction anesthesia as labor progresses rapidly; the relatively common postspinal headaches that keep mothers lying on their backs and limit interaction with their infants for three to five days; and the effects of episiotomy repairs on the comfort, mobility, and ability of the mother to care for her baby. These negative factors must be balanced against the relatively brief period of potential intense pain associated with natural childbirth. The contrast in the postpartum activity and comfort between mothers who have delivered in the United States with medication and anesthesia and those in the Netherlands and Guatemala who have had none has been impressive. Mothers in Guatemala go home from the hospital to take over full care of their babies one or two days after birth.

> **COMMENT:** In a more recent study (1978) we found that epidural and spinal medications did not significantly affect the behavior of neonates unless they were associated with other prenatal or perinatal complications as well.
> **T.B. Brazelton**

· · ·

At this point we need to ask some important questions. Does natural childbirth improve or alter mother-to-infant attachment? Does the presence of the father during birth enhance mother-to-infant and father-to-infant attachment? Does the father's presence during childbirth also affect the closeness of the relationship between mother and father? What are the effects of allowing a mother to choose her position or to control the events in the birth? These questions lead us further into the bonding process and the parents' participation with their newborn infant in the early postnatal period.

COMMENT: Other basic questions need to be asked, such as: Are there differences in families who choose natural childbirth, and if so, how does this alter attachment? How can we best support the woman who is alone during pregnancy and labor? The families who may be the most vulnerable to problems with parenting—the poor, unsupported, and socially isolated—are the ones who are least likely to attend childbirth classes or insist on an alternative birth room. Thus, although the father's presence may affect the mother-father relationship and enhance attachment, what about the families that are too fragmented to even make the decision to be together during this time?
M.A. Curry

EARLY POSTNATAL PERIOD

A major impetus to the study of parent-infant bonding occurred 15 to 20 years ago, when the staffs of intensive care nurseries observed that small prematures who were sent home intact and thriving would sometimes return to the emergency rooms failing to thrive or battered by their parents. Careful studies show an increase in the incidence of child abuse and failure to thrive without organic disease. The latter is a syndrome in which the infant does not grow, gain weight, or show motor or behavioral progress at a normal rate during the first months at home but then shows rapid gains in all aspects of development when given warm, affectionate care during hospitalization.

Table 2-4 presents observations on the incidence of early neonatal separation in infants who were battered or failed to thrive without organic disease. In some instances it was necessary to reanalyze the data from a number of studies (Table 2-4) to highlight the significant association between early separation and the subsequent development of these disastrous conditions. The incidence is threefold to fourfold greater in infants who have been separated from their parents, although many

Table 2-4. The incidence of early neonatal separation in infants who have been battered or exhibit failure to thrive without organic disease

	Authors	Number in study	Percentage separated
Failure to thrive	Ambuel and Harris, 1963	100	27
	Shaheen, Alexander, Truskowsky, and Barbero, 1968	44	36
	Evans, Reinhart, and Succop, 1972	40	22.5
Battering	Elmer and Gregg, 1967	20	30
	Skinner and Castle, 1969	78	13
	Klein and Stern, 1971	51	23.5
	Oliver, Cox, Taylor, and Baldwin, 1974	38	21
	Fomuford, Cinqford, and Louy, 1975	36	41.5
	Lynch,* 1975	25	40

*Separation in 35 sibling controls (6%).

causes other than separation might also contribute to these distressing outcomes. Looking at this question in a prospective study of 255 infants discharged from a regional newborn intensive care unit, Hunter and associates (1978) found an eight-fold increase in the incidence of maltreatment (3.9%) for premature and ill new-borns compared with 0.5% for all infants. These facts and the occurrence of other parenting disorders are a continuing stimulus that compels us to attempt to unravel the mysteries of parental bonding.

Before we consider studies of the individual factors involved, it is necessary to emphasize that there are many influences on parental bonding behavior. A mother's and father's behavior toward their infant is the result of a complex combination of their own genetic endowments, the infant's responses to them, a long history of interpersonal relations with their own families and with each other, past experiences with this or previous pregnancies, the absorption of the practices and values of their cultures, and probably, most important of all, the way in which each was raised by his or her own parents. The mothering or fathering behavior of each woman and man, the ability of each to tolerate stresses, and the needs each has for special attention and support differ greatly and depend on a mixture of these factors.

COMMENT: One of the biggest dangers of overemphasizing the conditions around labor and birth as critical to "bonding" is that parents who may not be able to carry them all out do feel that magically they have lost their chance. They feel even more failure because of too magical an emphasis on the conditions of labor and birth. That would be too bad, since the very reason for the changes recommended and reinforced by these studies is to upgrade labor and birth as an experience for all women. Hence, it is important, it seems to me, to emphasize that the initial bonding experience is only the beginning of the real "work" of attachment between a mother and baby. There is plenty of time and plenty of resources to come in order to really "make it" with a baby.
T.B. Brazelton

Fig. 2-5 is a schematic diagram of the major influences on parental behavior and the resulting disturbances that we hypothesize may arise from them.

Included under *Parental Background* are the following:

1. Parent's care by his or her own mother
2. Endowment or genetics of parents
3. Practices of the culture
4. Relationships within the family
5. Experiences with previous pregnancies
6. Planning, course, and events during pregnancy

Included under *Care Practices* are the following:

1. Behavior of physicians, nurses, and hospital personnel
2. Care and support during labor
3. First days of life, separation of mother and infant
4. Rules of the hospital

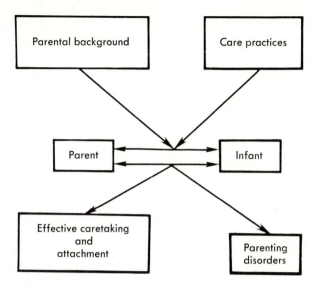

Fig. 2-5. Diagram of the major influences on parent-infant attachment and the resulting outcomes.

Included under *Parenting Disorders* are the following:

1. Vulnerable child syndrome, child abuse, and failure to thrive
2. Disturbed parent/child relationships
3. Some developmental and emotional problems in high-risk infants

Some of these determinants—the parenting the father and mother received when they were infants, the practices of their culture, their endowments, and their relationships with their own families—are already well ingrained in each of the parents at the time the infant is conceived. We originally believed that the effects of these particular determinants were fixed and unchangeable. However, Robert Harmon and Robert Emde from Denver have argued with us that the effects of some of these early life experiences on parental attitudes and behavior may be changed, both *favorably* and *unfavorably*, during the crisis of birth. We agree. Other determinants such as the attitudes, statements, and practices of the nurses and physicians in the hospital; whether the mother is alone for short periods during her labor; whether or not there is separation from the infant in the first days of life; the nature of the infant himself; his temperament; and whether he is healthy, sick, or malformed will obviously all affect parenting behavior and the parent-child relationship.

> **COMMENT:** Psychologically, pregnancy is a "turning point"—a time when the woman is confronted with the enormous developmental tasks of becoming a mother. It is also a time of great emotional lability. Thus the potential for remarkable personal changes exists. Those who have the

opportunity to share in this unique period should be acutely aware of their potential, not only to facilitate favorable changes but unfavorable changes as well.
M.A. Curry

Parenting disorders may range from mild anxiety, such as persistent concerns about a baby after a minor problem that has been completely resolved in the nursery, to the most severe manifestation—the battered child syndrome. It is our hypothesis that some of these problems may result in part from separation and/or other unusual circumstances that occur in the early newborn period as a consequence of present hospital care policies. Experience during labor and hospital practices during the first hours and days of life are the most easily manipulated variables in this scheme. Data on the effects of manipulations in this period will be discussed critically in this chapter.

COMMENT: If hospital personnel are aware that parents will suffer real disappointment when they must give up on their wishes for an ideal labor and birth, they can help make up for it. One marvelous effect of Klaus and Kennell's elegant research has been that most hospitals are sensitized to the fact that they must change to be most effective for new parents. Even when they haven't changed, the personnel are likely to be ready to think about changes and to try to make up for them when they can't be made.
T.B. Brazelton

SENSITIVE PERIOD

Many difficulties arise in attempting to determine systematically whether or not there is a sensitive period in the human. Human maternal behavior is determined by a multitude of factors; for instance, the intelligence and reasoning abilities of a mother may enable her to overcome potential difficulties associated with an early separation from her infant.

Because so little was known about this time period in normal parents, most of the studies designed to determine the effects of early separation have focused on parents of full-term infants. In general, these studies have addressed the question of whether there is a sensitive period for parent-infant contact in the first minutes, hours, and days of life which may alter the parents' later behavior with that infant. In many biological disciplines these moments have been called sensitive periods, vulnerable points, or susceptible periods. In most of the examples of a sensitive period in biology, the observations are made on the young of the species rather than the adult. One striking analogy of the importance of time-related events in the mother-child relationship is the effect of maternal thalidomide ingestion on the induction of limb deformities in the fetus. There are only a few days in early gestation during which thalidomide ingestion in the mother will produce malformations in the fetus. At other times in gestation other substances such as adrenal steroids have been shown to alter lung maturation.

Before describing the evidence for a sensitive period in parents, it is necessary to emphasize some of the concepts noted by Bateson (1979). He comments, "It seems inconceivable that all the phenomena that attract the name 'sensitive period' or one of its synonyms arise in the same way. Nevertheless much of the discussion about sensitive periods rests on the implicit assumption that one explanation would do for the lot." Thus using the term "sensitive period" helps in describing the timing of the function but does not tell anything about what the mechanism is that brings it about or, in Bateson's words, "the job remains of discovering how the results were generated." He notes "the extent to which a sensitive period is replicated may frequently depend on the degree to which conditions in which it was first described are copied. Even small changes can cause the evidence to evaporate. These alterations in conditions, however, are worth investigating because they probe the systems." He notes that "the more powerful are the protective mechanisms, the more stable will be the consequences of the initial experience and the more robust will be the sensitive period phenomenon." He also points out that after a period of rapid reorganization there is a period of withdrawal and isolation from the group. A possible example of this may be the period of 7 to 10 days after birth when the mother and baby are isolated together in 70% of human cultures (Barnett, 1972).

It is interesting to note that early clinical observations suggest the existence of a sensitive period. This period, during which the parents' attachment to their infant blossoms, we have named the maternal sensitive period.

During this enigmatic period, complex interactions between mother and infant help to lock them together. This must be distinguished from another sensitive time later in the first year, during which the infant establishes a stable, affectionate relationship with his mother (Bronfenbrenner, 1968; Yarrow, 1961). In this section we must emphasize that we are focusing on the process of bonding from parent to infant. Data from the several clinical observations and controlled studies performed throughout the world lend support to the principle of a unique period in the human shortly after birth.

COMMENT: Whereas a great deal of effort has been devoted to defining the temporal boundaries and the important events that define a sensitive period, less attention has focused on specifying the variables that define "bonding." Defining a critical set of variables that help tell us whether or not bonding is indicated would be helpful. Probably bonding behaviors are not static, however, and will shift across developmental stages of both mother and baby. Nor should we expect the same set of behaviors always to be present for all parents. Just as there are differences in babies in their temperament and even in their tolerance for different types of stimulation, perhaps parents differ as well. Some mothers may be talkers and others, touchers. Sensitivity to these stylistic differences of parents will have to be part of this search for a better definition of the concept of bonding.
R.D. Parke

Clinical support for a sensitive period

In a remarkable accident in an Israeli hospital, two mothers were inadvertently given and consequently took home and cared for the wrong babies. At the time of the two-week checkup, the error was discovered and efforts were made to return the babies to their own families. Each mother had become so attached to the baby she had cared for during the first 14 days that she was reluctant to give him up. Their husbands, on the other hand, strongly supported correcting the error because of facial and other characteristics unique to the individual families. Their behavior illustrates some of the characteristics of a sensitive period as Bateson noted, in that it "narrows social preferences to that which is familiar and therefore tends to prevent fresh experiences from further modifying those social preferences."

Studies of the effects of rooming-in have also confirmed the importance of contact during the early postnatal period. An increase in breastfeeding and reduction in anxious phone calls was noted when rooming-in was instituted a number of years ago at Duke University (McBryde, 1951). In Sweden, mothers randomly assigned to rooming-in arrangements were more confident, felt more competent in caregiving, and appeared more sensitive to the crying of their own infants than mothers who did not have rooming-in (Greenberg et al., 1973).

All these clinical reports suggest that the events occurring during the first hours after birth have special significance for the mother. Nursery practices in many modern hospitals in the United States do not generally acknowledge this and, instead, separate mother and infant immediately after birth to monitor the mother in an adult recovery area and the infant in a transitional care nursery.

> **COMMENT:** All mothers are ambivalent to some degree in the beginning. A "sensitive period" in the human would certainly be less rigidly determined by timing, by critical events, and by all of the things that describe a critical or sensitive period in animals. We would all prefer to think of the human mother as more flexible, as able to be more plastic to recover from stress, and so on. But maybe we are expecting a great deal of most mothers under the stress of the present medical system in the United States. Can't we change it so we can use a mother's reaction to labor and birth as a way of measuring her ability to mother her baby? If she appears stressed under optimal conditions, it might be more predictive of her inability to mother successfully.
> **T.B. Brazelton**

Winnicott (1964) comments in a different vein.

I think that an important thing about a young mother's experience of early contact with her baby is the reassurance that it gives her that baby is normal (whatever that may mean). You may be too exhausted to start making friends with your baby on the first day, but it is well that you should know that it is entirely natural that a mother should want to get to know her baby right away after birth. This is not only because she longs to know him (or her), it is also—and it is this which makes it an urgent matter—because she has had all sorts of ideas of giving birth to something awful, something certainly not so perfect as a baby. It is as if human beings find it very difficult to believe that they are good enough to create within themselves something that is quite good. I doubt whether any mother really and fully believes in her child at the beginning. Fathers come into this too for he suffers just as much as mother does from the doubt that he may not be able to create a normal healthy child. Getting to know your baby is therefore in the first place an urgent matter because of the relief that the good news brings to both parents.*

---

*From Winnicott, D.W.: The child, the family and the outside world, London, 1957, Tavistock Publications, Ltd., p. 24.

It is assuredly difficult to isolate and demonstrate the effects of the events during a short period of time on maternal attachment. Nonetheless, we believe that the following studies suggest strongly that what occurs in the early postpartum period may greatly help in the development of a parent's bond to the child.

Studies supporting the hypothesis of a sensitive period

In the past 15 years, 17 separate studies have focused on whether additional time for close contact of the mother and full-term infant in the first minutes, hours, and days of life alters the quality of the maternal-infant bond over time. Fig. 2-6 illustrates the timing of the contact in these studies. In three studies (A) the extra time was added not only during the first 2 hours but also during the next 3 days of life. In one study (B) the additional contact was added on days 1 and 2. In 13 studies (C) the additional mother-infant contact occurred only in the first hour of life. Table 2-5 describes these 17 studies in detail. It includes critical comments on the studies. We have gone into this detail because the results of these different investigations have stimulated extensive discussion about the significance of contact during these early hours. Because hospital practices have recently been altered on the basis of these 17 studies, it is essential to explore in depth their design, ecology, and outcome measures and their strengths and weaknesses.

Early and extended contact

GROUP A STUDIES. In the first study, Klaus and associates (1972) observed that a group of poor, primarily single, primiparous, inner-city mothers who had 16 hours of extra contact with their infants in the first 3 days of life fed their infants with more affection prior to discharge and at 1 month were more supportive and affec-

Text continued on p. 46.

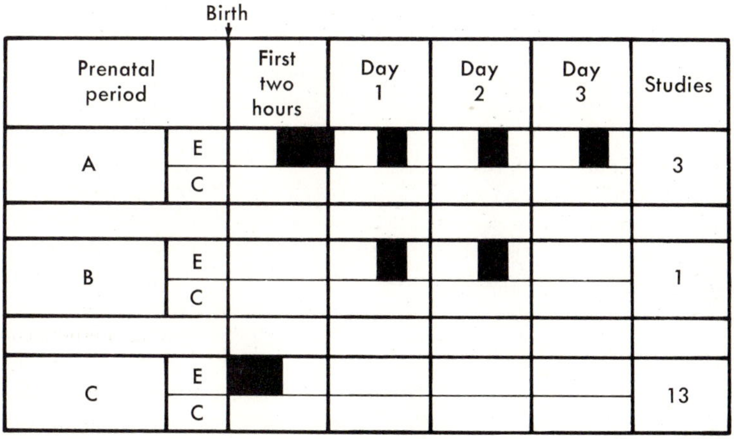

Fig. 2-6. Time patterns and number of three types of controlled studies in which one group of mothers has additional contact (E) with their infants compared to another group with routine contact (C).

Table 2-5. Early and extended contact in 17 studies.

Number of mothers	Study and sample	Extra contact (E.C.)	Hospital routine (H.R.)	Results	Comments
GROUP A STUDIES					
28	Klaus et al., 1972 low-income U.S. mothers and infants, bottle feeding Kennell et al., 1974 Ringler et al., 1975	1 hr with nude newborn within 3 hr of birth and 5 extra hr of contact daily for 3 days (n = 14)	Glimpse of baby at birth, brief contact for identification at 6-12 hr, 20-30 min contact every 4 hr for feeding (n = 14)	1. At 1 mo E.C. mothers demonstrated more soothing, fondling, eye-to-eye contact during feeding 2. At 1 yr E.C. mothers soothed the infant more during physical examination 3. At 2 yr E.C. mothers used fewer impera- tives and more words/proposition	Beginning evidence of early sensitive period for maternal bonding
200	Sousa et al., 1974	Early and continuous contact; infant crib beside mother; enthusiastic nurse encouraging breastfeeding (n = 100)	Glimpse of baby at birth 12-24 hr separation, 30 min contact every 3 hr; infant in nursery (n = 100)	1. At 2 mo 77% E.C. mothers lactating; 27.4% H.R. mothers lactating	Differences in care other than E.C. between H.R. and E.C. mothers might explain results
202	Siegel et al., 1980 low-income U.S. families	97 early and extended contact	105 routine care	1. At 4 and 12 months 2.5%-3.2% of variance explained by E.C.; 10%-22% of variance explained by	

				Results	Comments
				background variables; no difference in child abuse (10 control, 7 E.C.)	
GROUP B STUDIES					
301	O'Connor et al., 1980 low-income U.S. mothers and infants	6 hr of extra contact daily for 2 days (n = 143)	20 min every 4 hr for feeding (n = 158)	During 17 mo follow-up, more H.R. children (10) experienced abuse, neglect, abandonment, nonorganic failure to thrive; 2 E.C. infants admitted for parenting failure	Extra contact affected both later mothering and child health
GROUP C STUDIES					
12	Johnson, 1976 middle-class mothers	Initial breast feeding 1 hr	Initial breast feeding at 15 hr	At 2 mo, 5 out of 6 E.C. mothers breastfeeding; 1 out of 6 H.R. mothers breastfeeding	
60 68 40	Sosa et al., 1976 poor Guatemalan mothers Roosevelt I Roosevelt II Social Security	45 min of skin-to-skin contact (1 hr of life)	Early separation Roosevelt for 12 hr, Social Security for 24 hr	Duration of breastfeeding for E.C. mothers longer at Social Security and Roosevelt II; E.C. babies showed greater weight gain 1 yr at Social Security	Roosevelt I E.C. and H.R. mothers showed significant difference in socioeconomic index determined at home visit
19	Kennell, Trause, and Klaus, 1975	45 min of skin-to-skin contact (1 hr of life) (n = 9)	Glimpse at birth 12 hr separation (n = 10)	At 12 hr E.C. mothers demonstrated more attachment behaviors	Design inadequacy; study observations made when H.R. mothers first held infant

Continued.

Table 2-5. Early and extended contact in 17 studies—cont'd

Number of mothers	Study and sample	Extra contact (E.C.)	Hospital routine (H.R.)	Results	Comments
42	de Chateau and Wiberg, 1977a, 1977b middle-class Swedish mothers and infants, breast feeding	15 min skin-to-skin contact and suckling within 20 min of birth; then treated according to H.R. (n = 22)	Nurses care for baby for 30 min after birth; wrapped infant then placed in crib next to mother for 1 ½ hr; mothers and babies then separated except for every 4 hr feeds for 3 days; on days 4-7 daytime rooming-in (n = 20)	1. At 26 hr E.C. mothers sitting up, holding and cradling their infants more than H.R. mothers 2. In hospital E.C. mothers carried their infants more on the left side and less in their hands away from their bodies 3. At 3 mo E.C. mothers kissed, and looked *en face* more, cleaned babies less, and breast fed more 4. At 3 mo E.C. babies smiled and laughed more and cried less	As little as 15 min early extra skin contact affected both maternal and infant behavior; more synchronous and positive mother-infant interaction apparently established
60	Hales et al., 1977 very low-income Guatemalan mothers and infants, breastfeeding	Early contact 45 min of private skin-to-skin contact within minutes of birth (n = 20); delayed contact 45 min of private skin-to-skin contact at 12 hr (n = 20)	Glimpse of baby at birth, 12 hr separation, then daytime rooming-in for 2 days (n = 20)	At 36 hr early E.C. mothers showed more affectionate behaviors (smiling, kissing, *en face*, talking, fondling) and especially more *en face* than either delayed E.C. or H.R. mothers; no	Maternal behavior at 36 hr altered if mother-infant pair has early skin-to-skin contact

100	Ali and Lowry, 1981 poor Jamaican mothers	45 min early contact (n = 50)	Routine care (n = 50)	difference in keeping babies close or caregiving At 12 wk E.C. mothers showed more gazing, standing near infant, and vocalizing; solely breastfeeding	
62	Carlsson et al., 1979 middle-class Swedish mothers and infants, breastfeeding	1 hr in bed with nude infant immediately after birth with suckling; then treated according to H.R. (n = 22) or allowed demand feeding, extra contact, and nursing support (n = 20)	Infant placed in crib next to mother's bed for 4 hr; then every 4 hr contact for feeding (n = 20)	On days 2 and 4 E.C. mothers, regardless of later ward experience, showed more physical contact and physical affection (rubs, pets, rocks, touches, holds close in arms or lap) during breastfeeding than H.R. mothers; at 6 wk no differences during feeding noted	Early skin contact altered maternal behavior first 4 days
48	Kontos, 1978 middle-class Canadian mothers	1 hr of early contact 30-40 min after birth, skin-to-skin for first 1/2 hr, *en face* for second 1/2 hr (n = 24)	Holding wrapped infant 5-10 min after birth then routine care (n = 24)	Significantly greater attachment behaviors at 1 and 3 mo with extra contact	Observers were not always blinded
100	Campbell and Taylor, 1979 middle-class U.S. mothers	1 hr early contact (n = 50)	Routine care; mother-infant together 5 min (n = 50)	No differences in maternal-infant interaction at 3 days or 1 mo	Mothers in routine group have infant for 5 min in first hr
30	Svejda et al., 1980 middle-class U.S. mothers	1 hr of early contact, 90 min at each feeding (n = 15)	Brief contact at birth, 5 min in first hr, 30 min at every feeding (n = 15)	No significant differences in maternal behavior at 36 hr	Mothers in H.R. group had their infant for 5 min in first hr
30	Thomson et al. 1979 middle-class Canadian mothers	Unwrapped baby on mother's chest, 15-30 min suckling (n = 15)	Brief contact at birth (5 min); feedings every 4 hr (n = 15)	Significantly more mothers successfully breastfeeding at 2 mo	Control male/female ratio 11:4 but experiment 6:9

Table 2-6. Characteristics of mother-to-child speech at two years

Measure	2 years	
	Extended contact (n = 13)	Control (n = 12)
Number of words/proposition	4.45	3.69
Mean utterance length	3.47	2.97†
Percentage of		
Adjectives/all words	3.28	4.48
Content words/all words	52.04	61.63†
Questions/sentences	32.38	25.33
Imperatives/sentences	47.76	58.82*
Statements/sentences	13.58	8.01

*$p < .01.$
†$p < .001.$

tionate when the infant cried during a stressful office visit than the control mothers who received their infants for 20 minutes every 4 hours. Similar differences between the two groups of mothers were noted during an office visit at 1 year. In a six-part study of the mothers and infants done at 2 years by Ringler and associates (1975), the extra-contact group of mothers talked to their infants differently (Table 2-6). In this table the total number of mothers whose speech was analyzed in detail has been increased from 10 to 25. (Three of the original 28 patients were lost to follow-up at the end of the second year.) Follow-up studies at 5 years (Ringler et al., 1978) showed a strikingly close correlation in the experimental group only between the infant's language and cognitive development and the mother's speech at 2 years. There was no such correlation for the control group. A significant relationship was also found in the experimental group between the IQ of the mother and the IQ of the child. In that group only women with the most speech at 2 years had children with the most elaborate and advanced speech development at 5 years.*

In the Sousa study (1974) the outcome measure was the length of breastfeeding. The amount of extra contact for the experimental group was similar to that in the first study (Klaus et al., 1972). However, it should be noted that in the Sousa study there was an enthusiastic nurse present who pushed for breastfeeding only for the experimental group. Therefore this study is confounded by two variables—the additional time and an enthusiastic nurse.

---

*It is important to point out a mistake in a previous report about the abilities of the children at 5 years. We reported a difference in the developmental quotient between the children in the experimental group and those in the control group. When the data were reanalyzed as part of another study in 1979, our research assistant discovered that a mistake had been made when the IQ data were correlated with the experimental and control groups. The developmental quotients of several children had been placed in the incorrect group. When the error was corrected and the data were reanalyzed, there was no longer a significant difference.

Some of the most intriguing and thoughtful observations about the effect of early contact have been made by Siegel and associates (1980), who assessed 202 patients in a beautifully designed investigation. The aim of this study was to explore the effect on maternal attachment of early and extended contact as well as the influence of home visits by well-trained paraprofessionals. Observations were made at four and 12 months. There were no significant effects due to the home visit interventions. However, early- and extended-contact mothers showed differences in attachment variables such as acceptance of the infant and consoling of the crying infant at four months as noted in a home visit. These mothers also had significantly increased positive versus negative infant behaviors in the home at 12 months.

A most important contribution of this study by Siegel and associates was the exploration of the variance contributed by the interventions or, to put it more simply, the power of early and extended contact to influence maternal attachment behavior. The investigators calculated that 2.5% to 3% of the variance could be explained by the early and extended contact, whereas somewhere between 10% and 22% of the variance was explained by background variables such as the mother's economic status, race, housing, education, parity, and age. These were low-income mothers. They were primarily multiparous and lived in a rural area of North Carolina. It should be noted that, importantly, there was no difference between the experimental and control groups in the reports of child abuse and neglect in the first year of life. The Siegel study emphasizes the contribution of background variables that are not easily changed. It also shows that some significant, and advantageous parental and infant behaviors are changed by extra contact. Although early and extended contact contributes less variance than might be expected, it can be arranged for all parents at no additional cost.

> **COMMENT:** Siegel and associates' study adds an important dimension to the analysis of attachment behaviors—the influence of background variables. They emphasize how complex this phenomenon really is! Unfortunately, however, these variables aren't so easily or inexpensively altered as early contact.
> **M.A. Curry**

Extended contact—no early contact

GROUP B STUDIES. It is useful to compare the one study in this group by O'Connor and associates (1980) with the large study by Siegel and associates (1980) (Table 2-7). Siegel did not note any difference in parenting disorders, finding 10 in the control group and seven in the extended contact groups. On the other hand, O'Connor noted significant differences in parenting disorders, child abuse, neglect, abandonment, and nonorganic failure to thrive, finding 10 in the control group and two mothers who were given extended contact. O'Connor also noted that mothers who were given 12 additional hours of contact in the first two days had significantly lower hospital admission rates for their infants and fewer accidents and poisonings. Thus there is a disagreement between the Siegel and O'Connor studies concerning

Table 2-7. Child abuse or neglect in the first year of life

Study	Total	Abuse or neglect
O'Connor et al., 1980		
Extended contact	134	2
Control	143	10*
Siegel et al., 1980		
Extended contact	97	7
Control	105	10

*p < .05.

whether additional early contact prevents or alters parenting failures. In examining both of these studies in more detail, it should be noted that only primiparous mothers were included in the O'Connor study, whereas Siegel's mothers were mainly multiparous. The income level of the parents in both the O'Connor study and the Siegel study was low, but in the O'Connor study the families were from the inner city of Nashville, whereas Siegel's families came from the rural countryside.

Although close and detailed follow-up studies such as these are difficult and time consuming to perform and the incidence of severe parenting disorders is relatively low (0.5% to 2%), further investigations of this high-priority area must be carried out. The desire to prevent or eliminate parenting disorders might be compared with a similar goal for paralytic poliomyelitis. Preventive measures may decrease or eliminate the potential difficulty. However, in both situations, once the problem has developed, there is a devastating effect on the individual and on the family, mammoth expenditures of professional time and effort are required, and even under the best of circumstances the final outcome can never be as satisfactory as initial prevention.

Early contact

GROUP C STUDIES. Thirteen separate studies have looked at the effect of additional mother-infant contact in the first hour of life with contact following this period being similar in both the experimental and control groups. In nine of the studies, differences in either the mother or infant were noted in the experimental group.

Breastfeeding

In six of nine studies it was striking that breastfeeding continued for a significantly longer period for those mothers who had contact which involved suckling their babies in the first hour after birth (Table 2-8). It is difficult to distinguish whether it was simply the early contact or specifically the suckling which altered the length of time that these mothers continued to breastfeed. In a study currently in progress in Guatemala, one group of mothers had their babies in the first hour

Table 2-8. Percentage of mothers breastfeeding at 2 or 3 months postpartum after additional early mother-infant contact

Study	Number	Hospital routine	Early contact
Johnson, 1976 (USA)	12	16	100
Sosa et al., (Roosevelt I, Guatemala)	60	92	74*
Sosa et al., 1976 (Roosevelt II, Guatemala)	68	58	70*
Sosa et al., 1976 (Social Security Hospital, Guatemala)	40	59	85
Sousa, 1974 (Brazil)	200	27	77
de Chateau and Wiberg, 1977 (Sweden)	40	26	58
Ali and Lowry, 1981 (Jamaica)	100	27	57
Salariya, Easton, and Cater, 1978 (England)	108	50	60*
Thomson et al., 1979 (Canada)	30	20	60

*No significant difference.

but did not suckle and another group did suckle. There was then a brief period of separation for both groups, after which mothers and babies were reunited 2 to 4 hours after birth. At this time there appears to be no difference in the length of breastfeeding between these two groups. This issue needs further testing because it is not clear whether contact at 2 to 4 hours after birth is equal in effect to contact in the first hour or whether suckling has an additive effect to the early contact.

It might be argued that the length of breastfeeding is not a valid assessment of the strength of bond between mother and infant, since it is culture bound. It should be noted that in all of the studies with the length of breastfeeding as an end point, both the control and experimental groups of mothers came from the same population except for one study in which there were no significant differences. In that investigation (Roosevelt Hospital I, Table 2-8), the control group (randomly assigned) came by chance from a lower socioeconomic group than the experimental group. Fig. 2-7 illustrates the percent of breastfeeding during the first year in two studies. Thus in all but this one investigation the practices of the population under study could not explain the length of breastfeeding. It is important to note further that these studies occurred in different parts of the world and in both low- and middle-income groups.

COMMENT: Too many variables influence a woman's decision to continue breastfeeding to make it a valid assessment of bonding. A woman who discontinues breastfeeding to return to work four weeks after delivery to support her family can be just as bonded as a breastfeeding Swedish mother who has a nine-month, government-paid maternity leave. Similarly, the initial decision to breastfeed must be cautiously used in the assessment of bonding. A mother's decision to breastfeed may be an indication of her willingness to give of herself to her infant, which is a characteristic of bonding. On the other hand, an Indochinese refugee who decides to bottle feed in order to give her infant the best "American start" is giving of herself in an equally healthy, but different way.
M.A. Curry

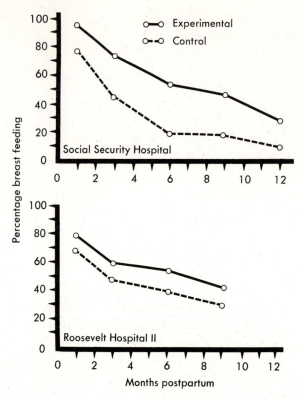

Fig. 2-7. Incidence of breastfeeding in two of the studies during the first year of life.

Differences in study design

Interesting behavioral differences were observed by De Chateau and Wiberg (1977b) in the home at 3 months after birth. They noted that at 3 months early-contact mothers kissed and looked *en face* significantly more and cleaned their babies less during free play. The infants of these early-contact mothers smiled and laughed more and cried less. An interesting confirmation of these findings has been reported by Ali and Lowry (1981) in Jamaica. At 3 months early-contact mothers were more likely to rise and follow when their baby was taken from them, they looked at the baby more frequently during feeding, and they were more likely to talk to their baby. The early-contact children were less likely to cry or be restless during interviews at 6 and 12 weeks. Kontos (1978) found differences between early-contact mothers and control mothers at 3 months, but her study was complicated by lack of a naive observer for some of the observations. On the other hand, Carlsson and associates (1979) noted differences on the second and fourth day after early contact, but not at 6 weeks. In the Campbell and Taylor (1979) study, in which differences were not noted at 3 days or at 1 month following early contact, it should be noted that the mothers in the control group who received routine care had their infants for 5 minutes in the first hour of life. The same was true for the control group of mothers in the study of Svejda and associates (1980). In these two studies it is reasonable to question whether 5 minutes in the first hour was enough contact to result in similar behavior in both the experimental and control groups.

At present there are no appropriate studies to tell us the length of time required in the first hours and days after birth to produce an effect on the behavior of the mother or child in the subsequent days and weeks of life. It is worth reemphasizing Bateson's (1979) admonition about copying the conditions in which a sensitive period was first described: "Even small changes can cause the evidence to evaporate." Could 5 minutes be long enough to affect the mother's later behavior with her infant? To consider this matter further, the patients in both the experimental and control groups in these two studies were well-prepared and motivated middle-class women who delivered in a highly supportive environment. The doula study described earlier (pp. 25-31) indicates that mothers who have had a supportive companion during labor have a greater interest in interacting with their babies in the first hour after birth. In addition, an interested, motivated mother can in 5 minutes see that she has produced a beautiful, healthy baby, and this can trigger feelings of accomplishment and ecstasy and a series of interactions with the baby. In a large number of maternity units a control or routine-care mother who has been totally separated from her child after a glimpse at birth is not sure the baby is healthy or even breathing. She has not experienced the flood of positive feelings that the beauty and responsiveness of her baby could have released, and she may feel lonely, empty, deprived, and worried that the baby has some problem.

Although the timing of the 13 group C studies was similar, it should be noted that the practices in each of the hospitals where they were conducted were often considerably different. In some cases the contact was skin-to-skin. However, Curry (1979) found no difference in maternal attachment behaviors when skin-to-skin contact was compared with contact with a wrapped newborn in the first hour. In some of the studies there was privacy, and in others no privacy was provided during the contact. It is surprising that in all but four of the 13 studies there were statistically significant differences between the control and experimental groups.

Fig. 2-8 shows the position of the mother and baby in just two of the studies. Note in Fig. 2-8, *A*, the mother is dressed and the baby is placed on the bed at the mother's shoulder. In Fig. 2-8, *B*, note that the infant is on the mother's chest. Both mother-infant pairs are alone. These differences during the period of early contact could result in major differences in outcome, but it has been surprising that many of the outcomes, such as increasing the length of breastfeeding, are similar. Many of the differences in outcomes could result from different study designs, which has been suggested by Bateson (1979). In an unpublished report Anisfeld

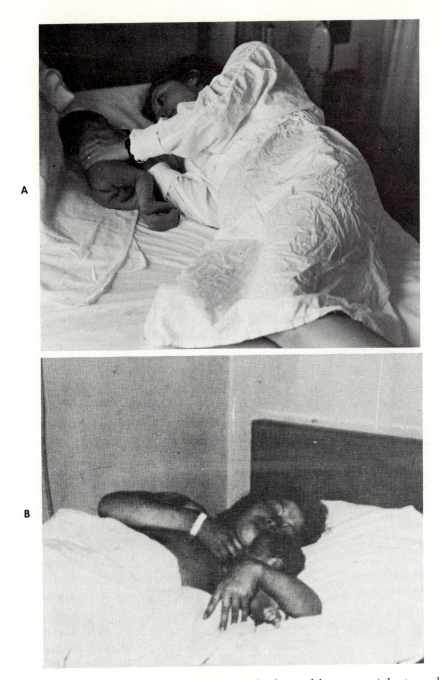

Fig. 2-8. A, A mother and her infant shortly after birth in a labor room. A heat panel (not shown) is above the infant and is maintaining the infant's temperature. **B,** Skin-to-skin contact.

and Lipper (1981) have possibly provided an explanation for some of the variation in the results of the many studies. They noted that early-contact mothers showed significantly higher attachment scores at 48 hours. Further analysis showed the effect was significant only for primiparous mothers of female infants. Additionally, the effect of extra contact was greatest for women who had "low social support." The latter was defined as scoring low if 2, 3, or 4 of the following were present: unmarried, receiving public assistance, no high school diploma, and no support person during labor.

In summary, it is surprising that no matter at what point the early contact was experienced, later differences were observed in the behavior of the experimental group of mothers when compared with the behavior of the control group.

WHEN DOES LOVE BEGIN?

The first feelings of love for the infant are not necessarily instantaneous with the initial contact.

Several years ago a woman who had extensive experience with normal newborn infants told us about the birth of her first baby in a hospital where mothers and their infants stay together throughout the hospital course. She checked her newborn over carefully following the birth and found the baby to be healthy, normal, pink, and breathing easily. She proceeded to feed and care for her baby but did not sense any special reaction to the neonate. Then, 36 hours after the birth, she described a remarkable warm glow that came over her. At that point she suddenly realized that she had the most beautiful, most gorgeous, most responsive baby in the world. And she had strong feelings of love for her infant. Did this come about at the time that her mental image of the ideal expected infant became synchronized with the real baby? (See Fig. 2-14 and pp. 65 and 66.) What are the factors that result in either early or delayed feelings of love for a newborn infant?

The relation between the time when a mother falls in love with her baby and the sensitive period is not clear at present. Several mothers have shared with us their distress and disappointment when they did not experience feelings of love for their baby in the first minutes or hours after birth. It should be reassuring for them and mothers like them to learn about two studies of normal, healthy mothers in England.

MacFarlane and associates (1978) asked 97 Oxford mothers, "When did you first feel love for your baby?" The replies were as follows: during pregnancy, 41%; at birth, 24%; first week, 27%; and after the first week, 8%.

In a study of two groups of primiparous mothers (Robson and Kumar, 1980) (n = 112 and n = 41), 40% recalled that their predominant emotional reaction when holding their babies for the first time was one of indifference. The same response was reported by 25% of 40 multiparous mothers. Forty percent of both groups felt immediate affection. Most of the mothers in both groups had developed affection for their babies within the first week. The onset of this maternal affection after childbirth was more likely to be delayed if the membranes were ruptured artificially, if the labor was painful, or they had been given a generous dose of meperidine (Demerol).

> **COMMENT:** It would be interesting to know the relationship between these reported feelings of love for a baby and behaviors that have been used to index attachment.
>
> One of the serious problems that is only poorly understood concerns the effects of the lag between publicity and practice on maternal behavior and expectations. "Bonding" is now a well-known term to many lay people in our culture, but opportunities for early contact are still not universally available in our hospitals. In addition to encouraging change in hospital practices, perhaps more attention needs to be paid to reassuring parents that a satisfactory and satisfying relationship can develop even without the opportunity for early contact. The parent-infant (father as well as mother) relationship is a continuing process of adaptation to one another's needs, and parents should be aware that "all is not lost" if early contact is not possible.
>
> **R.D. Parke**

Donald Winnicott (1958), who started as a pediatrician and became a distinguished psychoanalyst, has made remarkably perceptive observations that suggest he was describing the sensitive period. From these observations Winnicott proposed that a healthy mother goes through a period of "Primary Maternal Preoccupation."

> It is my thesis that in the earliest phase we are dealing with a very special state of the mother, a psychological condition which deserves a name, such as Primary Maternal Preoccupation. I suggest that sufficient tribute has not yet been paid in our literature, or perhaps anywhere, to a special psychiatric condition of the mother, of which I would say the following things: It gradually develops and becomes a state of heightened sensitivity during, and especially toward the end of, the pregnancy. It lasts for a few weeks after the birth of the child. It is not easily remembered by mothers once they have recovered from it. I would go further and say that the memory mothers have of this state tends to become repressed.
>
> I do not believe that it is possible to understand the functioning of the mother at the very beginning of the infant's life without seeing that she must be able to reach this state of heightened sensitivity, almost an illness, and to recover from it. (I bring in the word "illness" because a woman must be healthy in order both to develop this state and to recover from it as the infant releases her. If the infant should die, the mother's state suddenly shows up as illness. The mother takes this risk.)
>
> The mother who develops this state . . . provides a setting for the infant's constitution to begin to make itself evident, for the developmental tendencies to start to unfold, and for the infant to experience spontaneous movement and become the owner of the sensations that are appropriate to this early phase of life.
>
> Only if a mother is sensitized in the way I am describing can she feel herself into her infant's place, and so meet the infant's needs.*

---

*From COLLECTED PAPERS: THROUGH PAEDIATRICS TO PSYCHO-ANALYSIS by D.W. Winnicott. (c) 1958 by Basic Books, Inc. by permission of Basic Books, Inc., Publishers, New York.

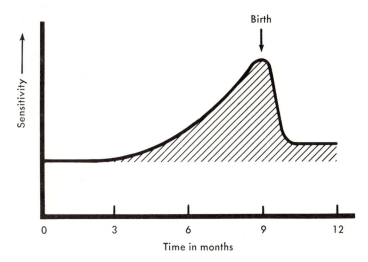

Fig. 2-9. Hypothesized change in maternal sensitivity during pregnancy and in the postnatal period.

Fig. 2-9 illustrates the time of this special state or sensitivity. It rises during pregnancy, is maintained at a heightened level right after delivery, and then decreases in the early months following birth. It is interesting that the timing and course of Primary Maternal Preoccupation are similar to those described for the maternal sensitive period, and both were determined independently using extremely different techniques. We suspect that endocrine changes play a significant role in starting and enhancing both of these processes. Are they initiated by the rise in estradiol and drop in progesterone in the five weeks prior to delivery? Interestingly, the heightened sensitivity of Primary Maternal Preoccupation is sometimes misinterpreted by physicians and nurses as excessive anxiety. Studies of other cultures are important in this regard because in most societies the mother and baby are placed together with support, protection, and isolation for at least seven days after birth. The provision of food, wood, and water and a private time for the mother and infant to get to know each other are common in most cultures.

THE AUTHORS' DILEMMA

We faced a real dilemma in deciding how strongly to emphasize the importance of parent-infant contact in the first hour and extended visiting for the rest of the hospital stay, based on the available evidence. Obviously, in spite of a lack of early contact experienced by parents in hospital births in the past 20 to 30 years, almost all these parents became bonded to their babies. The human is highly adaptable, and there are many fail-safe routes to attachment. Sadly, some parents who missed the bonding experience have felt that all was lost for their future relationship. This was (and is) completely incorrect, but it was so upsetting that we have tried to speak more moderately about our convictions concerning the long-term significance of this early bonding experience. Unfortunately, we find that this had led some skeptics to discontinue the practice of early contact or to make a slapdash, rushed charade of the parent-infant contact, often without attention to the details necessary to the experiences provided for mothers in the studies. There are still large hospitals that have never provided for early and extended contact, and the mothers who miss out are often those at the limits of adaptability and who may benefit the most—the poor, the single, the unsupported, the teenage mothers.

> **COMMENT:** The importance of talking with families who didn't have time with their infant immediately after birth cannot be overemphasized. They need to be reassured that nothing irreversible has occurred. Families can harbor worry and guilt for months and years and may actually believe that the relationship with their child has been permanently damaged. An example is the father who said two years after his daughter was born by emergency cesarean birth, "We're all getting along just fine considering we didn't have the chance to get bonded."
> **M.A. Curry**

We believe that there is strong evidence that at least 30 to 60 minutes of early contact in privacy should be provided for every parent and infant to enhance the bonding experience. Studies have not clarified how much of the effect may be apportioned to the first hours and how much to the first days, but it would appear that additional contact in both periods will probably help mothers become attached to their babies. For some mothers one period may be more important than the other. If the health of the mother or infant makes this impossible, then discussion, support, and reassurance should help the parents appreciate that they can become as completely attached to their infant as if they had the usual bonding experience, although it may require more time and effort. Obviously the infant should only be with the mother and father if the infant is known to be physically normal and appropriate temperature control is utilized. We also strongly urge that the infant remain with the mother as long as she wishes throughout the hospital stay so that she and the baby can get to know each other. We believe that in the near future, placement in the large central nursery will be phased out for most babies. Allowing the infant to be with the mother will permit both mother and father to experience longer periods to learn about their baby and to develop a strong tie in the first week of life.

> **COMMENT:** It should be emphasized that it should be the mother's choice to determine how much time she spends with her infant in the hospital. For some vulnerable mothers, unsupportive care and the constant presence of a demanding newborn can impede, rather than facilitate, bonding.
> **M.A. Curry**

In summary, although there is increasing evidence from many studies of a sensitive period that is significant to the bonding experience, this does not imply that every mother and father develops a close tie to their infant within a few minutes of the first contact. Each parent does not react in a standard or predictable fashion to the multiple environmental influences that occur during this period. This fact is not evidence against a sensitive period but, more likely, represents multiple individual differences of mothers and fathers. When we make it possible for parents to be together with their baby, in privacy, for the first hour and throughout the hospital stay, we establish the most beneficial and supportive environment for the beginning of the bonding process.

COMMENT: The sensitive period appears to be a time shortly after birth during which the events that occur have the potential for affecting the development of attachment. However, it is important to recognize that the development of attachment is influenced by many events, some of which occur even before conception. During pregnancy, feelings of attachment toward the fetus normally develop and are manifested in numerous ways such as acceptance of the pregnancy and interaction with the fetus. Thus some parents may be strongly attached before birth, and the events of the sensitive period will help enhance their bond. For other parents this period may help nurture very early feelings of attachment, and for some it may be a time during which feelings of attachment actually begin. However, the events that foster attachment for some families during this time can have a negative effect on other families. An exhausted mother, for example, may prefer to rest alone and may resent having her infant during this time. It is essential that we don't make judgments about families during this time but evaluate them within the context of their history and their subsequent interactions with their infant.
M.A. Curry

COMMENT: Some hospital authorities have construed the sensitive-period studies to mean that first-hour contact is the only critical time. They have allowed this bonding time and then separated mother and child for the next 24 hours. It cannot be emphasized strongly enough that contact in the first hour and extended contact throughout the early postpartum days are to be encouraged.
B. Lozoff

COMMENT: Perhaps I am oversimplistic in my thinking, but the most obvious result of all of these studies for the clinician is that if we offer choices which can be individuated to the particular mother's and father's needs, we can make them feel an importance and a responsibility at a time when their energies are high to begin the nurturant or bonding role with their new baby. By increasing their self-image at such a time, we may indirectly affect their ability to mother and father their offspring. These are simple and obvious changes to make. If the yield is toward an improvement in the quality of life for families—why can't we make them?
T.B. Brazelton

FATHERS

Parke (1974) has described hospital practices that exclude the father from the early interaction with his infant as reflecting and reinforcing a cultural stereotype. Both American culture and theories have focused on the maternal role in early infancy, largely ignoring the father. However, recent modifications in hospital practices and the renewed interest in home births indicate a changing view of the father's role.

Yogman (1980) made the following observations:

While there are few studies of men becoming fathers, the limited data suggest that the period prior to the birth of the baby is, at least superficially, similar for fathers and mothers. For both, it is a time requiring psychological readjustment as they integrate the roles of child and spouse with that of expectant parent . . . . However, the expectant father does not feel the physical presence of the fetus growing within him and this may stimulate a father to search for alternative evidence of his productivity and creativity, i.e., through increased attention to his work and the provision of financial security for his family . . . . The struggle for the expectant male during the prenatal period is to remain emotionally available to his wife at the same time that he meets his own needs for feeling responsible and productive.*

In this regard, Shereshefsky and Yarrow (1973) found an association between the husband's responsiveness to his wife's pregnancy and her successful adaptation to it.

Greenberg and Morris (1974) have used the term "engrossment" (absorption, preoccupation, and interest) to describe the powerful impact of a newborn on the father. They have identified several specific aspects of the father's developing bond to his newborn, ranging from his attraction to the infant, his perception of the newborn as "perfect," to extreme elation and an increased sense of self-esteem.

Rödholm and Larsson (1979) observed father-infant interaction at the first contact after delivery. They filmed 15 fathers of full-term infants delivered by cesarean birth. The naked infant was presented to the father 15 minutes after birth, and pictures were taken every second. They noted an orderly progression of behavior. The father began touching the extremities and then proceeded to touch the infant with his fingertips, then to use his palms, and finally the dorsal side of his fingers. An increase in eye-to-eye contact was also observed. The percentages of the different behaviors were surprisingly similar to those previously described for mothers. McDonald (1978) noted similar findings.

Parke has observed parents in three different situations: the mother or father alone with the infant at 2 to 4 days of age and the father, mother, and infant together in the mother's hospital room (i.e., triadic interaction). The most striking finding is that these studies have revealed few significant behavioral differences between fathers alone with their infants and mothers alone with their infants.

In a series of studies, Parke (1979) noted that fathers are just as responsive as mothers to infant cues such as vocalizations. Both fathers and mothers increase their rate of vocalizations following an infant vocal sound. However, fathers and mothers differ in the behaviors they show in response to an infant's vocalization. Fathers are more likely than mothers to talk rapidly. However, mothers are more likely to respond with touching when the baby vocalizes. Parke notes that "these data indicate that fathers and mothers both react to the newborn infant's cues in a contingent and functional manner even though they differ in their specific response patterns." He noted that fathers and mothers are not only similar in their sensitivity

*From Yogman, M.W.: Development of the father-child relationship. In Fitzgerald, H., Lester, G., and Yogman, M.W., editors: Theory and research in behavioral pediatrics, New York, Plenum Publishing Corp., vol. I (in press).

to the infant but are surprisingly equally successful in bottle feeding the infant based on the amount of milk consumed.

In the triadic situation the father tends to hold the infant nearly twice as much as the mother, vocalizes more, touches the infant slightly more, and smiles at the infant significantly less than the mother. The father clearly plays the more active role when both parents are present in contrast to the cultural stereotype of the father as a passive participant. In fact, in this triadic interaction the mother's overall interaction declines. It should be noted that all but one of the fathers whom Parke studied had attended labor and birth, and this could be expected to produce an unusual degree of father-to-infant attachment. However, he conducted another study using a similar design but in which the fathers rarely participated in labor and birth. Despite these social and institutional differences, the fathers again played the more active and dominant role with increased holding, vocalizing, and touching.

Parke believes that the father must have an extensive early exposure to the infant in the hospital where the parent-infant bond is initially formed. "There is a lot of learning that goes on between the mother and infant in the hospital—from which the father is excluded and in which he must be included so he'll not only have the interest and a feeling of owning the baby, but also the kinds of skills that the mother develops." Parke reviewed his findings as indicating that the father is much more interested in, and responsive toward, his infant than United States culture has acknowledged.

COMMENT: Our findings should not be interpreted to mean that fathers do not need support. Fathers, as well as mothers, can benefit from information about infant development and infant care techniques. In agreement with Lind, my colleagues and I (Parke et al., 1980) recently found that the postpartum period may be one good time for teaching about fathering. We showed fathers a 15-minute videotape that illustrated infant competencies, encouraged fathers to become involved with their babies, and demonstrated caregiving and play techniques. In contrast with control fathers who saw no videotape, these men were more knowledgeable about infant capacities and were more involved in routine caregiving in the home three months later. However, other researchers have found that father learning is not limited to this early period, and father involvement can be increased by supportive interventions at a variety of later points in the infant's development.

Paternity leaves, which are available to all men in Sweden, would be an excellent way to allow fathers to participate in this early postbirth acquaintance process.
R.D. Parke

In agreement with these observations are the findings of Lind (1973), who noted that paternal caregiving in the first 3 months of life was greatly increased when the father was asked to undress his infant twice and to establish eye-to-eye contact with him for an hour during the first 3 days of life.

Rödholm (1981) has taken advantage of different hospital policies following cesarean birth in two maternity hospitals in Goteborg, Sweden, to study the effect of allowing fathers to handle their newborn infant immediately after birth. These fathers were compared with another group whose infants were kept in an incubator

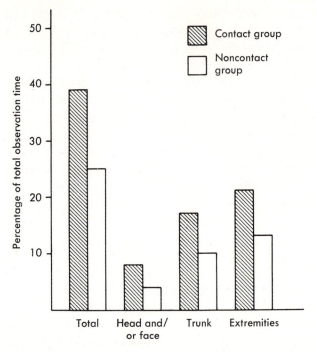

Fig. 2-10. Caressing behavior in 29 early-contact fathers compared with 16 noncontact fathers observed during a home visit at 3 months.

and the fathers were only permitted to look at them. In a play situation three months later the early-contact fathers showed significantly more touching behavior toward their infants (Fig. 2-10) and held them less often with the baby's face directed away from the father than the noncontact group. The presence of the incubator may have had a contributory effect, but these differences suggest that early contact might have altered paternal behavior.

In another controlled study of early contact for fathers in cesarean births Keller (1981) noted that fathers given extended contact displayed more *en face* behavior during feedings at 6 weeks. Their responses on questionnaires were more positive about their infants, and they were more involved in the care of their babies than the control fathers (this was also confirmed by the mothers' reports).

COMMENT: Boyd (1980) found that fathers who were demonstrated the Brazelton Neonatal Assessment Scale had more positive attitudes toward parental involvement in parenting activities.
M.A. Curry

In this period, with many more women at work and more fathers parenting than in times past, there is an obvious shift in the roles of fathers and mothers. Changes in our society and the expectations of young parents have suggested that the role of the father and mother is the same. However, we tend to agree with the thoughts of Winnicott (1964) that each parent has a separate and distinct role. He beautifully describes the role of the father in the following words.

> This is the way the father can help. He can provide a space in which the woman has elbow room. Properly protected by her man the mother is saved from having to turn outwards to deal with her surroundings at the time when she is wanting so much to turn inwards, when she is longing to be concerned with the inside of the circle which she can make with her arms in the centre of which is the baby. This period of time in which the mother is naturally preoccupied with the one infant does not last long. The mother's bond with the baby is very powerful at the beginning and we must do all we can to enable her to be preoccupied with her baby at this time—the natural time.*

Interestingly, Pedersen (1975) noted in his studies that if the father was more supportive of the mother, she evaluated her maternal skills more positively. She was more effective in feeding the baby. However, he wondered that maybe competent mothers might elicit more positive evaluations from their husbands.

> **COMMENT:** Several studies have found a relationship between the mother's perception of her husband's support and her maternal behavior (Curry, 1979; Westbrook, 1978).
> **M.A. Curry**

Furman (1980) further delineates the important and separate roles of fathers and mothers in the development of young children when she notes, "The father's special investment of the mother-child unit is essential to the mother who builds her relationship of devotion to the child with the help of his devotion to them."

> **COMMENT:** This work reminds us that many times mothers and fathers affect their infants not only directly but often indirectly through the mediation of another family member. For example, Pedersen (1975) has found that husband-wife conflict was associated with high levels of negative affect directed toward the infant. Or a parent who is insensitive and impatient in his or her handling of the infant may make it more difficult for the spouse to pacify the infant. We need to treat the family as a social system and pay attention to relationships among all family members.
> **R.D. Parke**

It is important in this period of change that we do not fit the data to our prejudices. It is important to stand back and take a fresh view of the role of the mother and the father with their infant at the same time that the role of the man and woman in professional activities and the working world is changing.

> **COMMENTS:** The fathers I have worked with have told me that their own excitement in being included in labor and birth not only attaches them to the baby differently from the first baby, but it gives them a very different feeling of closeness to their wives—having shared such an intimate, important event.
> **T.B. Brazelton**

---

*From Winnicott, D.W.: The child, the family and the outside world, London, 1957, Tavistock Publications, Ltd., p. 25.

COMMENT: I agree that mothers and fathers often play different roles. Most researchers report that fathers generally contribute less time to caregiving than mothers, whereas fathers, in turn, spend more of their time with their infants in play. And fathers and mothers play differently—fathers are more physical, arousing, and unpredictable, whereas mothers are less physical and more talkative and use toys more in their play. Even male and female adult monkeys show some of the same differences in their interactions with their young. However, these roles are not fixed or unmodifiable, and recent trends have shown that men and women are capable of a wide range of roles in infancy.
R.D. Parke

WHAT PULLS THE PARENT AND INFANT TOGETHER?

We must now attempt to answer the question of why this period is so important. What happens between a parent and a newborn infant that pulls them together and assures the mother's long-term commitment to the relationship? Again we must consider observations from a number of sources to find our answer.

An important step in understanding this period was made when Wolff (1959) described for the first time six separate states of consciousness in the infant, ranging from deep sleep to screaming. The state with which we are most concerned is state 4, the quiet, alert state. In this state the infant's eyes are wide open, and he is able to respond to his environment. Unfortunately, he may be in this state for periods as short as a few seconds. This made original detection of the state difficult and explains why it was not identified until 1959. Fig. 2-11 shows a 6-minute-old infant

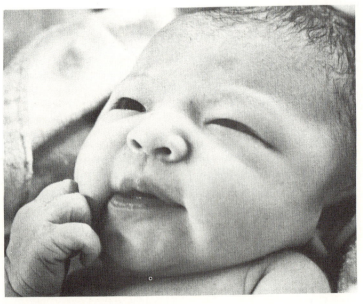

Fig. 2-11. A 6-minute-old infant in the quiet alert state. (Copyright Suzanne Arms, 1981. All rights reserved.)

in the quiet alert state (state 4). However, Emde and Robinson (1981) observed that the infant is in state 4 for a period of 45 to 60 minutes during the first hour after birth. After these discoveries it was possible to demonstrate that an infant can see, that he has visual preferences, and that he will turn his head to the spoken word, all in the first hour of life. After this hour, however, he goes into a deep sleep for 3 to 4 hours (Fig. 2-12). Thus for 1 hour after birth he is ideally equipped for the important first meeting with his parents. Since the quiet alert state also occurs about 10% of the time in the first weeks of life, there are other opportunities for interaction.

Detailed studies of the amazing behavioral capacities of the normal neonate have shown that the infant sees, hears, and moves in rhythm to his mother's voice in the first minutes and hours of life, resulting in a beautiful linking of the reactions of the two and a synchronized "dance" between the mother and infant (Condon and Sander, 1974). The infant's appearance, coupled with his broad array of sensory and motor abilities, evokes response from the mother and father and provides several channels of communication that are most helpful in the process of attachment and the initiation of a series of reciprocal interactions.

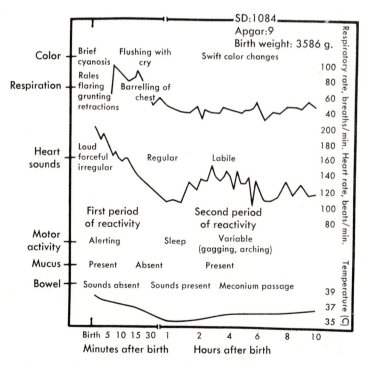

Fig. 2-12. Physiological changes in the normal infant after birth.

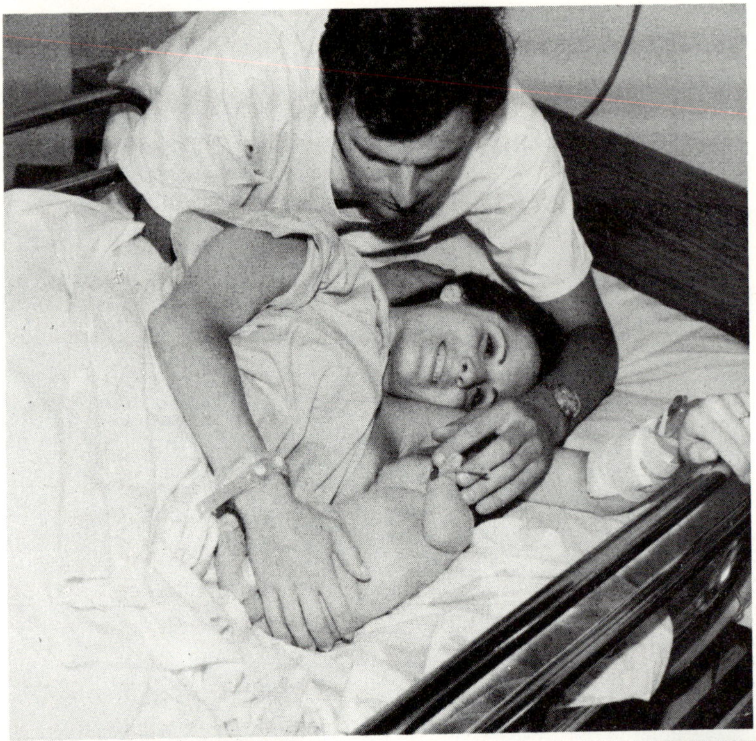

Fig. 2-13. A, A mother nursing her infant a few minutes after birth as the father looks on. **B,** What the mother sometimes sees.

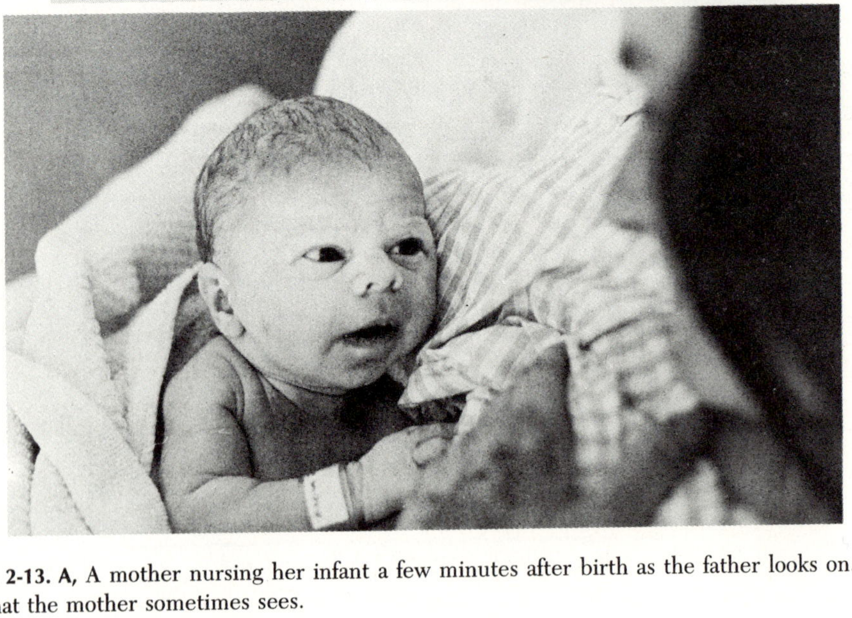

As an example of the infant's role in attachment behavior, Fig. 2-13, *A*, shows a mother nursing her infant a few minutes after birth. The infant often licks the area around the nipple (Lang, 1976). MacFarlane (1975) has shown that six days later this infant will have the ability to distinguish reliably by scent his own mother's breastpad from the breastpads of other women. On the mother's side, she is intensely interested in looking at her newborn baby's open eyes (Fig. 2-13, *B*). The infant is awake and alert and visually follows his mother over an arc of 180 degrees during this special period immediately after birth (Brazelton et al., 1966). The infant's licking of the mother's nipple induces significant prolactin secretion and oxytocin release, which cause the uterus to contract thereby reducing postpartum bleeding. Recent discoveries in endocrinology, ethology, infant development, immunology, and bacteriology have greatly increased knowledge of the reciprocal linkages at many levels between the parent and infant.

Possible explanations or mechanisms for a sensitive period

At present, it is not known why alterations in attachment behaviors have been noted when mother-infant contact is increased for such a short time in the first hours and days of life. The infant's state in the first hour after birth may be a major factor.

To students of behavior, these findings do not fit with previous knowledge or experience. They suggest possibly a new process or principle. How can changes made during just a few hours around birth profoundly alter the later behavior of a woman who has already lived 160,000 to 180,000 hours? What processes can explain the results?

A critical period? Is it a critical period? A critical period has been defined as a relatively brief time in which major changes in organization occur, and following which further change is impossible. The concept is now most often used in connection with anatomical or biochemical changes. Critical periods are thought to occur only early in development and are believed to be irreversible. However, for the past 30 years in many hospitals in the West, mothers and infants have had minimal contact, yet most parents have provided adequate care. We stress *most* and *adequate*, but these terms do not apply to 10 mothers of the 158 control subjects in O'Connor's (1980) study. The term "critical period" does not fit.

> **COMMENT:** There are thousands of mothers who would not only say they were adequate, but superb!! In the past 30 years the stresses on the American family may be more influential in the cause of child abuse than the lack of early contact.
> **M.A. Curry**

Changing the mental image. Before suggesting another possible explanation, it is necessary to note that the process of attachment of mother to infant often begins before fetal movement. However, the onset of fetal movement will often make women accept previously unwanted infants. Other internal processes occur during

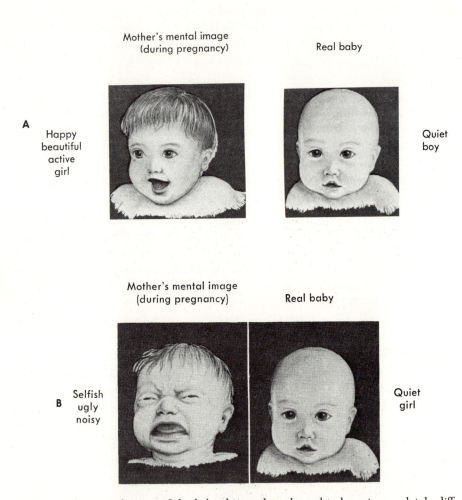

Fig. 2-14. A, The mental image of the baby this mother planned to have is completely different from the baby she has. **B,** The mental image for some women with mothering disorders and the real infant.

pregnancies. Mothers in the West dream of the expected infant. The mental portrait in the mother's mind before birth often includes specific hair color, sex, and so forth, but the real baby is never like the infant the mother has pictured, and during the first days after birth the mother must adjust the mental portrait to match the actual baby.

We believe that every parent has a task to perform during the postpartum period. The mother in particular must look and "take in" her real live baby and then reconcile the fantasy of the infant she imagined with the one she actually delivered (Fig. 2-14, *A*). Many cultures recognize this need by providing the mother with a doula, or "aunt," who relieves her of other responsibilities so that she can devote herself completely to this task.

There is suggestive evidence that many of these early interactions also take place between the father and his newborn child. Parke (1979) in particular has demonstrated that when fathers are given the opportunity to be alone with their newborns, they spend almost exactly the same amount of time as mothers in holding, touching, and looking at them.

The striking reduction in mothering disorders noted by O'Connor (1980) may be the result of changing the mother's mental portrait from that of an angry, ugly, mean infant—often noted in mothers who batter their infant—to that of the actual baby (Fig. 2-14, *B*). Interestingly, Ferholt and Provence (1976) noted that in women with mothering disorders, a distorted mental portrait of the infant is often the most difficult factor to normalize in therapy. Is it possible that the increased contact somehow sets into motion in the mother a sequence of innate behaviors not previously described?

Innate or genetic behavioral patterns? Our human ancestors as we know them were probably carried and nursed frequently for over 99% of our species' existence (Fig. 2-15). For more than a million years they lived as hunters and gatherers (Lee and DeVore, 1976). They had the same skull, the same bone structure, and perhaps some of the same behavior patterns as humans today. The small square in the lower right-hand corner of Fig. 2-15 indicates the approximately 10,000-year period since the agricultural mode began, and the 200-year span of our present industrialized society is represented by an almost invisible dot, a period too short for evolutionary adjustments to occur.

Women carried and breastfed each infant until he was 2 to 4 years of age. To explore this explanation fully, it is necessary to take what appears to be a detour.

Fig. 2-16 presents recent historical data showing how advice to parents about feeding schedules and the length of lactation changed from the year 1550 to the present (Ryerson, 1961). Until the 19th century feeding schedules were rarely mentioned in English-speaking guidebooks for parents. The Industrial Revolution, women leaving the home to work, as well as the studies and guidelines of Emmett Holt in New York may all have contributed to changing the recommendations on

Duration of human subsistence patterns

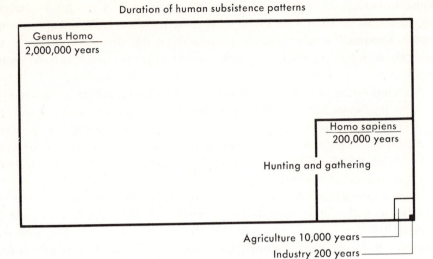

Fig. 2-15. Schematic diagram illustrating the relative time humans have spent as industrial and agricultural societies compared with their long duration as hunters and gatherers. (Modified from Lozoff, B., Brittenham, G.M., Trause, M.A., et al.: J. Pediatr. **91**:1, 1977.)

Parental advice on timing

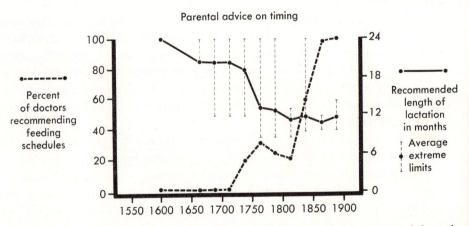

Fig. 2-16. Historical data on feeding schedules and the length of lactation in English guidebooks for parents. (Modified from Ryerson, A.J.: Medical advice on child rearing, 1550-1900, Harvard Ed. Rev. **31**:302, 1961.)

feeding schedules. In 1899 Holt excised the stomachs of 91 babies at autopsy, clamped the stomachs at both ends, filled them with water, and measured their capacity. Dividing this volume into the total 24-hour milk intake, he calculated a 2- to 3-hour schedule, which he then strongly recommended. Interestingly, Holt noted that the stomach of the infant actually empties in 1 to $1^1/_2$ hours. The change to a 2- to 3-hour feeding schedule, which occurred early in this century at the same time that the automobile was becoming popular, might be termed the "gas tank" theory of infant feeding. (If we know the volume of the gas tank and the amount of gas consumed in a period of time, we can then calculate how often it has to be filled.) Physicians likened the gastrointestinal tract to a production line and thus took a simplistic (by our present knowledge) view of gastrointestinal absorption and the multiple complex systems involved with breastfeeding.

Data that should make us reconsider 3- and 4-hour feeding schedules come from the provocative work of Ben Shaul (1962), who has measured the protein, fat, carbohydrate, and water constituents of many different animal milks and related them to maternal care and feeding schedules. Fig. 2-17 indicates that animals fed every 5 to 15 hours, such as the rabbit or deer, have rich, concentrated milk with a low water content. Animals that feed almost continuously, such as primates or herd animals, have a very low concentration of protein and fat in their milk. Animals that provide milk of a medium concentration feed their infants every 2 to 4 hours.

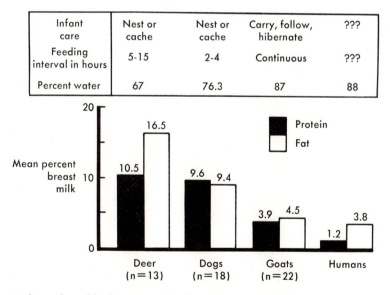

Infant care	Nest or cache	Nest or cache	Carry, follow, hibernate	???
Feeding interval in hours	5-15	2-4	Continuous	???
Percent water	67	76.3	87	88

Fig. 2-17. Relationship of feeding interval to fat and protein concentrations and percentage of water. The differences in fat and protein concentrations between the groups are significant. n = Number of species studied. (Modified from Lozoff, B., Brittenham, G.M., Trause, M.A., et al., J. Pediatr. **91**:1, 1977.)

The differences in protein, fat, and water content between the groups are substantial. Note the considerable change in water content. On this scale the human is far to the right, fitting best as a very frequent feeder. In agreement with these findings are the recent observations of spontaneous maternal milk ejection that show bursts occurring in the intervals between 4-hour breastfeedings. This suggests that the reflex and hormonal mechanisms of the mother may also be set for more frequent feedings. Rigid 3- to 4-hour schedules, which have only recently become part of our tradition, have probably contributed to many failures in lactation.

In our industrialized society the infant is usually physically separated from the mother much of the time, but in pre-industrialized cultures today and for most such cultures in the past, the body of the mother has been kept close to that of the infant. This not only permitted the mother to be available to feed the infant frequently, but to sense the other needs of her infant from his bodily movements.

Thus the sensitive period effects in humans may result from tripping innate or genetic behavioral systems built into the mother's repertoire that can be modified by the baby's behaviors such as suckling the nipple, looking, bodily movements, and so on. It is difficult to believe that these behavioral, immunological, sensory, and hormonal systems, which interact so beautifully, rewarding both mother and infant, are just present by chance. We must consider that other mother-infant interactional components have not yet been discovered.

The effects of increased mother-infant contact in the 17 studies described earlier may be due in part to a recapitulation of what was previously normal human maternal behavior and something that has been present in our genetic makeup for centuries. The remarkable effects of increasing mother-infant contact may in part also make up for the marked deprivation that is a part of present-day routines in modern hospitals.

Multiple factors. Although it was hoped that a single process might explain the findings in these studies, it now appears that many processes are activated to pull the mother to her baby during the first days of life. A possible analogy is the first breath of an infant. For years respiratory physiologists have attempted to unravel why the infant takes its first breath. At present, the data suggest that multiple factors, including low blood oxygen, high carbon dioxide, cooling, cutaneous stimulation, and proprioceptive stimulation, are in part responsible. For the survival of the human infant, mother-infant attachment is essential. Thus it seems unlikely that such a life-sustaining relationship would be dependent on a single process. Keeping the mother and baby together soon after birth is likely to initiate and enhance the operation of known sensory, hormonal, physiological, immunological, and behavioral mechanisms that probably attach the parent to the infant. Fig. 2-18 shows a few of the multiple reciprocal factors that are in play during the first three days a mother is with her infant.

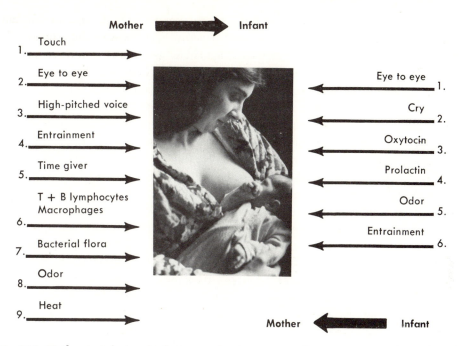

Fig. 2-18. Mother-to-infant and infant-to-mother interactions that can occur simultaneously in the first days of life.

We hypothesize that a cascade of interactions between the mother and baby occurs during this period, locking them together and ensuring the further development of attachment. We suggest that exploration of this important period after birth will unravel many new and significantly interlocking behavioral, immunological, endocrinological, and physiological systems that we are currently only beginning to understand.

Reciprocal interaction

The fascinating question of *why* the development of maternal attachment progresses so rapidly during the early postpartum period can only be answered by minutely examining what happens between the mother and infant during this crucial time. What pulls them together, ensuring their proximity through the many months during which the infant is unable to satisfy his own needs? What are the rewards for the mother's commitment and efforts? In the center of Fig. 2-18 is a picture of a common situation—a mother feeding her infant in the first hour of life. The diagram surrounding the picture, however, belies the simplicity of the scene in a schematic presentation of the multiple interactions simultaneously occurring between mother and child. Each is intimately involved with the other on a number of sensory levels. Their behaviors complement each other and serve to lock the pair together. The infant elicits behaviors from the mother that in turn are satisfying to him, and vice versa, the mother elicits behaviors in the infant that in turn are rewarding to her. For example, the infant's hard crying is likely to bring the mother near and trigger her to pick him up. When she picks him up, he is likely to quiet, open his eyes, and follow. Looking at the process in the opposite direction, when the mother touches the infant's cheek, he is likely to turn his head, bringing him into contact with her nipple, on which he will suck. His sucking in turn is pleasurable to both of them. Actually, this is a necessarily oversimplified description of these interactions. These behaviors do not occur in a chainlike sequence, but rather each behavior triggers several others. Thus the effects of an interaction are more like that of the stone dropped into a pool, causing a multitude of ever-increasing rings to appear, rather than like a chain where each link leads to only one other. In a sense we see a fail-safe system that is overdetermined to ensure the proximity of mother and child.

Because of the limitations of language, the interactions must be described sequentially rather than simultaneously, dispelling momentarily the richness of the actual process for the sake of understanding it. We therefore will have to present each system singly, although it is important to remember that they interlock (Fig. 2-18).

We will first describe the interactions originating in the mother that affect the infant.

1. *Touch.* A most important behavioral system that serves to bind mother and infant together is the mother's interest in touching her baby. Although no studies have yet defined which neonatal characteristics elicit maternal touching, three independent observers have described a characteristic touching pattern that mothers use in the first contact with their newborns. Rubin (1963) noted that human mothers show an orderly progression of behavior after birth while becoming acquainted with their babies. Klaus and associates (1970) observed that when 13 nude infants were placed next to their mothers a few minutes or hours after birth, most mothers touched them in a pattern of behavior that began with fingertip touching of the infant's extremities and proceeded in 4 to 8 minutes to massaging, stroking, and encompassing palm contact of the trunk (Fig. 2-19). In the first 3 minutes mothers maintained fingertip contact 52% of the time and palm contact 28% of the time. In the last 3 minutes of observation, however, this was reversed. Fingertip contact had greatly decreased, and palm contact increased to 62% of the total scored time. Rubin (1963) observed a similar pattern but at a much slower rate. In her study mothers usually took about three days to complete the sequence, but the infants were dressed, which may account for the difference. Rödholm and Larsson (1979) have noted a similar sequence in fathers. Mothers of normal premature infants who were permitted early contact followed a similar sequence of touching their infants

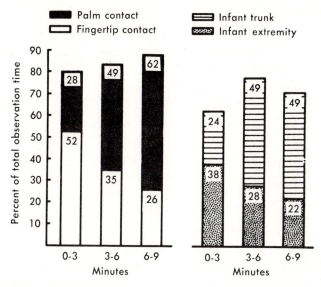

Fig. 2-19. Palm and fingertip contact on the trunk and extremities at the first postnatal contact in mothers of full-term infants. (From Klaus, M.H., Kennell, J.H., Plumb, N., and Zuehlke, S.: Pediatrics **46:**187-192, 1970.)

in the incubator but at an even slower rate; even at the third visit mothers of premature infants were not using their palms. Much more progress in tactile contact occurred in mothers of full-term infants in just 10 minutes.

In a study of home births, Lang (1972) observed that almost always the mother rubs the baby's skin, starting with the face. Rubbing is done with the fingertips and is usually a gentle stroking motion. This occurs before the initial breastfeeding and before delivery of the placenta. The baby is usually offered the breast but often does not suck at first. The most common action for the baby when given the mother's nipple is to continually lick it.

Thus we have fragmentary evidence for what we believe is a significant principle—that human mothers engage in a species-specific sequence of behaviors when first meeting their infants, even though the speed of this sequence is modified by environmental and cultural conditions.

The observation by Rödholm and Larsson (1980) is of special interest in understanding the meaning of the sequence of touching behaviors. They observed that unrelated adults (medical students) have a touching sequence that is similar to fathers. Is this sequence the process by which humans approach an infant? Is it genetically built into our biology? Or how adults approach small objects?

2. *Eye-to-eye contact.* Another interaction that proceeds from mother to child originates in the eyes. The mothers studied by Klaus and associates (1970) ex-

Table 2-9. Percent of total observation time in *en face* position

Initial contact (minutes)	En face (percent)
0 to 3	10
3 to 6	17
6 to 9	23

pressed strong interest in eye-to-eye contact. Seventy-three percent of the mothers verbalized an intense interest in waking the infant to see his eyes open. Some even voiced a relationship between the condition of the baby and his eyes, for example, "Open your eyes. Oh, come on, open your eyes. If you open your eyes, I'll know you're alive." Several mentioned that once the infant looked at them, they felt much closer to him.

The mothers of full-term infants studied by Klaus and associates (1970) showed a remarkable increase in the time spent in the *en face* position from the first to the fifth minute. Table 2-9 shows the percentage of *en face* in mothers of full-term infants. Rödholm and Larsson (1979) noted a similar increase in *en face* in fathers.

Lang (1976) observed in most home births that immediately after the birth of the baby, but before the delivery of the placenta, the mother picked up the baby and held him in the *en face* position while speaking to him in a high-pitched voice.

> COMMENT: Eye-to-eye contact serves the purpose of giving a real identity or personification to the baby, as well as getting a rewarding feedback for the mother.
> **T.B. Brazelton**

In Fig. 2-20 a father of a full-term infant is shown in this position.

There seem to be other mechanisms that foster the rewarding eye-to-eye contact. As Robson (1967) so aptly describes, "The appeal of the mother's eyes to the child (and of his eyes to her) is facilitated by their stimulus richness. In comparison with other areas of the body surface, the eye has a remarkable array of interesting qualities such as the shininess of the globe, the fact that it is mobile while at the same time fixed in space, the contrasts between the pupil-iris-cornea configuration, the capacity of the pupil to vary in diameter, and the differing effects of variations in the width of the palpebral fissure."*

Fantz (1961) reported that the infant can see at birth. An infant born of an unmedicated mother will easily follow a moving hand at an 8- to 12-inch distance. One would expect the seeing infant to focus on the most interesting visual stimulus, which, as described by Robson, may be the human eye.

In the course of performing the Brazelton Neonatal Behavior Assessment on large numbers of infants, we have been repeatedly struck by the greater appeal of the examiner's face than any inanimate object.

---

*From Robson, K.: The role of eye-to-eye contact in maternal-infant attachment, J. Child Psychol. Psychiatry 8:13-25, 1967.

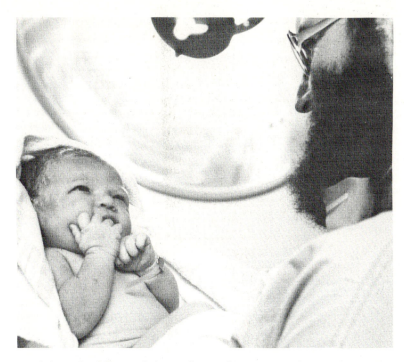

Fig. 2-20. A father of a full-term baby in the *en face* position. (Copyright Suzanne Arms, 1981. All rights reserved.)

> **COMMENT:** The neonatal data on vision (Haith et al., 1969; Stechler and Lantz, 1966) point to the infant's preference for both moving, moderately complex stimuli and those which are ovoid and have the ungarbled contents of the human face. Goren (1975) shows that the neonate at birth will follow an ungarbled representation of a face for 180 degrees, but significantly less (60 degrees) and for less time if it is garbled. He is programmed for the human face at birth.
> **T.B. Brazelton**

3. *Mother's voice*. Illustrating the unique talents of the infant, DeCasper and Fifer (1980) have discovered that within the first three days of life, newborns discriminate between speakers and demonstrate a preference for the mother's voice but not the father's after only limited maternal exposure. Lang's (1976) observation that mothers giving birth at home usually speak to their infants in high-pitched voices prompted us to watch for this phenomenon. Interestingly, after hearing about this, we also have observed mothers speaking to their newborn infants in a much higher pitched voice than that used in everyday conversation. They may turn and speak to the doctor or nurse in their regular voice and then abruptly return to the higher frequency speech as they address their neonates. As Brazelton reported, a neonate alerts and attends to a female voice in preference to a male voice because

of its higher pitch. The mother's use of a high-pitched voice, then, fits with the infant's sensitive auditory perception and his attraction to speech in the high-frequency range. Detailed studies of neonatal auditory function may be found in the work of Eisenberg (1976).

> **COMMENT:** Recently David Phillips and I have found that fathers, as well as mothers, adjust their speech patterns when they talk to their babies. In contrast with the way they talk to other adults, both parents slow their rate of talking, use shorter phrases, and repeat themselves more. This "baby talk" probably helps to attract and maintain the baby's attention more effectively than talking in a normal adult fashion. If this is true, it may be one of the ways that helps babies learn to recognize their parents' faces and voices.
> **R.D. Parke**

4. *Entrainment*. The microanalysis of sound films shows that human communication is not sound alone but also includes movement. When a person speaks, several parts of his body move in ways that are sometimes obvious and sometimes almost imperceptible; the same is true of the listener, whose movements are coordinated to the elements of the speech. When two people are filmed, the microanalysis reveals that both the listener and the speaker are moving in tune to the words of the speaker, thus creating a type of dance. The rhythm or tune of the dance is the pattern of the speech (Condon and Sander, 1974).

Exciting observations by Condon and Sander (1974) reveal that newborns also move in time with the structure of adult speech. "When the infant is already in movement, points of change in the configuration of his moving body parts become coordinated with points of change in sound patterns characterizing speech." In other words, as the speaker pauses for breath or accents a syllable, the infant almost imperceptibly raises an eyebrow or lowers a foot. The investigators demonstrated that live speech in particular is effective in entraining infant movement. Neither tapping noises nor disconnected vowel sounds showed the degree of correspondence with neonate movement as did natural, rhythmical speech. Interestingly, synchronous movements were found with both of the two natural languages tested, English and Chinese. As noted by the authors:

> This study reveals a complex interaction system in which the organization of the neonate's motor behavior is entrained by and synchronized with the organized speech behavior of adults in his environment. If the infant, from the beginning, moves in precise, shared rhythm with the organization of the speech structure of his culture, then he participates developmentally through complex, socio-biological entrainment processes in millions of repetitions of linguistic forms long before he later uses them in speaking and communicating.*

---

*From Condon, W.S., and Sander, L.W.: Neonate movement is synchronized with adult speech, Science **183**:99-101, 1974.

Although the infant moves in rhythm to his mother's voice and thus may be said to be affected by her, on the other hand the infant's movements may reward the mother and stimulate her to continue. The point is that these areas of contact are interactive.

> **COMMENT:** By this subtle entrainment of his movements to the rhythm of her speech, the newborn gives the mother feedback that she can hardly resist. We have found that this synchrony becomes the important ambience for their affective communications thereafter. Their communications become a sort of "mating dance" (cf. swans) when they are analyzed on film by frame-by-frame analysis.
> **T.B. Brazelton**

5. *Time giver.* Synchronous movements are part of a much more comprehensive phenomenon of entrainment between a mother and her baby, which has been identified by the intensive and meticulous studies by Sander and associates (1970). We can speculate that while the baby is in utero many of his actions and rhythms are attuned to those of the mother. This is due to a variety of rhythmical influences—her own sleep-wake cycle, the diurnal rhythms of her hormones, the orderly patterns of the mother's day, the regular beat of her heart, and the rhythmic contractions of the uterus preceding the onset of labor and continuing up to the time that the baby emerges from the birth canal. By carefully monitoring the states and activities of normal infants rooming-in with their mothers during the first 2 weeks of life, Sander has confirmed the existence of those behavioral phenomena in the first hours of life that have been emphasized by others, such as an unusually prolonged, alert state following birth. In addition, he has shown that on the second day there is a breakup of the rapid-eye-movement (REM) and non-REM sleep pattern present on the first day. In succeeding days the length of each period of sleep, the total amount of REM sleep, and the total amount of deep sleep decrease progressively. Concurrently there is an increase in crying, which reaches a peak on the third day. Thus the disruption of birth seems to upset the baby's prior rhythms and throw his systems into a state of disequilibrium. He must reorganize and retrain the biorhythmicity of his states and behavior to fit his extrauterine environment.

By following a steady routine in the early days, the mother helps her infant to reestablish biorhythmicity. As evidence of this, Sander has identified a progressive increase in the co-occurrence of the infant's being in an alert state and his mother's holding him. This increases from less than 25% on the second day to 57% co-occurrence on the eighth day. Cassel and Sander (1975) describe the mother as the time giver *(Zeitgeber)* for the baby for the entrainment of rhythmic neonatal functions. They compare the mother's effect on the infant to the effect of a magnet in organizing and lining up iron filings.

Sander has emphasized that the alert state in a young infant is extremely stable. He has shown that if the baby is in any state other than the alert state and the mother intervenes, it is likely that he will become alert. However, if the baby is already in the alert state and the mother intervenes, there is only a slight chance of a change in state. The high occurrence of the alert state results from the interaction of a sensitive mother with her infant. When he is alert, he is ready to respond to the mother to dance in rhythm to her speech or movements.

6. *T- and B-lymphocytes, secretory A macrophages.* New information about breast milk will emphasize the intricate contributions of the mother to the baby shortly after birth. It has been known for some time that breast milk is a rich source of antibodies, particularly in the colostrum. Breast milk and colostrum contain high concentrations of secretory immunoglobulin A and T- and B-lymphocytes. Secretory immunoglobulin A coats the lining of the infant's intestine with a multitude of antibodies to infectious agents to which the mother has been exposed over her lifetime. Secretory immunoglobulin A is not destroyed by intestinal enzymes and thus provides protection against many pathogens. As an example, if a mother has had a recent enteric infection with salmonella C infection before delivery, cells in the mother's intestinal epithelium will begin to produce antibodies against this organism. Some of these cells will migrate specifically to her mammary gland, where some will be discharged into the colostrum and others will remain in the gland and produce antibodies against salmonella C, which the baby is likely to encounter during his journey through the birth canal and in the early months of life. Similar protection is provided against many other potentially dangerous organisms in the environment. Thus the lymphocytes and antibodies in the colostrum and breast milk specifically protect the baby against this salmonella infection (Pittard, 1979). This explains in part how a newborn infant who is 100% breastfed is protected in precarious environments from infectious agents such as *Shigella*, typhoid, many viral infections, and pathogenic *Escherichia coli*.

7. *Bacterial nasal flora.* During a period of more than eight years in which the bacteriological status of all the infants in a Guatemalan Indian village was carefully monitored, there was no known baby delivered at home under poor hygienic conditions who developed a staphylococcal skin infection in the first two months of life (Mata, 1974). During this same period in Guatemala City, a few miles away, many newborns discharged from the hospital nurseries returned with skin infections due to pathogenic strains of *Staphylococcus aureus* (as occurs in hospital nurseries all over the world). The babies in these nurseries were separated from their mothers for the first 12 hours of life. It is our hypothesis that if mother and baby are kept together in the first minutes of life, the mother gives her baby her own mixture of strains of respiratory organisms, such as the *Staphylococcus*. Then these maternally provided strains grow and populate the infant's respiratory and gastrointestinal tracts. Just as a lawn planted with grass will resist the introduction of weeds after the grass has had a good start, these organisms may prevent the baby from acquiring the hospital strains of staphylococci. This principle of bacterial interference has

been applied clinically by Shinefield and co-workers (1963), who demonstrated that epidemics of pathogenic staphylococcal infection in newborn nurseries could be stopped by placing a benign strain of *Staphylococcus* into the nares of newborns. A similar protection may be accomplished naturally by the mother.

8. *Odor*. The odor of the mother can also affect the infant. MacFarlane (1975) found that by the fifth day of life breastfeeding infants can discriminate their mother's own breastpad from the breastpads of other mothers with significant reliability. Schaal and associates (1980) have confirmed this observation. In the future the olfactory system may be found to play an essential part in attachment to the mother.

9. *Heat*. For completeness, temperature control should be mentioned. In the past the body of the human mother was a reliable source of heat for the infant, although this is a diminishing function. This has been clearly confirmed by the study of Phillips (1974), who found a minimal drop in the infant's temperature when the baby was placed on the mother's chest wrapped and without a heat lamp. Emphasizing the multiple interactions is the observation of Schoetzer (1979), who noted that mothers closely regulate the distance from their face to the infant's during an interaction to a median of 22.5 cm. She notes that this falls within the range defined by Hall (1966) as the intimate distance—where body contact, sensation of radiant heat, and olfaction play a large role in perception of the partner.

• • •

Other studies have emphasized other aspects of the mother-to-infant interaction. Cassel and Sander (1975) pointed out that the infant has an advanced sensory system when he enters the world but is greatly retarded in his motor abilities. Motor dependency results in an obvious need for continuous caretaking from a mothering figure. Most importantly, this dependency serves a second function by involving the infant in interaction, through which he can regulate his circadian rhythms. Although his functions and those of his caretaker are temporarily desynchronized and disorganized in the first days after birth, the baby becomes reorganized by repeated mother-event situations.

Cassel has demonstrated evidence of the newborn's perception of the interaction through experiments in which he has the mother wear a mask and be silent during one feeding on the seventh day of life. The infant takes significantly less milk, scans the room when placed in the crib, and has significant disruption in rapid-eye-movement and nonrapid-eye-movement sleep following the masked feeding compared with the usual feeding.

Meltzoff and Moore (1975) have demonstrated the remarkable finding of neonatal imitation of visually perceived stimuli through facial and manual gestures at two weeks after birth. These findings were obtained by presenting four gestures (tongue protrusion, lip protrusion, mouth open, sequential finger movements) to six infants on four occasions and recording the subsequent performance of the infants. Each behavior occurred significantly more frequently in the 20 seconds after it had been demonstrated to the infant than did other behaviors. Thus the neonate might respond to his mother as early as the first hour with a form of mimicry that begins a fascinating interchange. Surprisingly, her face will imitate the baby's during many interactions in the first year, and thus she will be a "mirror" for the infant. (This is described in greater detail in Chapter 1.)

Using our simplified system, the following interactions originate with the infant.

1. *Eye-to-eye contact*. The visual system provides one of the most powerful networks for the mediation of maternal attachment. This fact is emphasized by the work of Fraiberg (1974) who has described in detail the difficulties that mothers of blind infants have in feeling close to them. Without the affirmation of mutual gazing, mothers feel lost and like strangers to their babies until both learn to substitute other means of communication.

Interestingly, the distance between the eyes of the mother and infant when the mother is breastfeeding or holding him in her arms is about 9 to 10 inches, which is the distance at which infants can best focus on an object. These positions provide repeated opportunities for eye-to-tye contact during a mother's care of her neonate.

Robson (1967) has suggested that eye-to-eye contact is one of the innate releasers of maternal caretaking responses. Some of our experiences have shown how powerful it is. For example, three researchers who were participating in a study with us were required to assist with Brazelton Neonatal Behavior Assessments on infants each day. We were distressed to hear all three say that they did not particularly like babies, found newborns especially unappealing, and planned never to have a baby. They grumbled about learning the behavioral assessments. As they carried out the assessment, each of the women had her first experience with a baby in the alert state who would follow her eyes with his own, and an amazing change occurred. Suddenly each became enthusiastic about "her" baby, wanted to hold him, and came back later in the day and the next day to visit. At night she would tell her friends about this marvelous baby she had tested. In a few weeks all three decided they would like to have and even breastfeed a baby. This anecdote about the three women demonstrates the compelling attraction of a newborn infant moving his eyes to follow an adult's eyes, and the layer upon layer of emotional meaning that the viewer may place on this.

2. *Cry*. The voice of the infant also affects the mother. Lind and colleagues (1973), using thermal photography, reported on yet another biological level where reciprocal behaviors pull mothers and infants together. After being exposed to the hunger cries of healthy newborns, 54 of 63 mothers demonstrated a significant increase in the amount of blood flow to their breasts. The infant's cry causes a physiological change in the mother that is likely to induce her to nurse. To increase the complexity of the system, Morsbach and Bunting (1979) in a neatly designed study

have demonstrated that mothers can significantly identify their own infant's cry soon after birth.

3. *Oxytocin*. The infant can also initiate the secretion of maternal hormones. Breastfeeding the infant or having him lick her nipple leads to the release of oxytocin in the mother, which hastens uterine contraction and reduces bleeding. Each suckling, by as yet an unknown mechanism, calms the mother and also increases the tie the mother has to her infant. Thus after birth the mother and infant are closely intertwined through complex behavioral and physical interactions.

4. *Prolactin*. Hwang and associates (1971) have shown that serum prolactin concentrations increase during pregnancy and decrease rapidly in the postpartum period. Furthermore, whenever the nipple of the mother is touched, either by the infant's lips or by a finger, there is a fourfold to sixfold increase in her prolactin level and then a decrease after breastfeeding begins. Licking, sucking, or perhaps even tactile contact alters maternal prolactin levels.

It is intriguing to consider whether these changes in prolactin levels, which are known to induce the alveoli of the breasts to secrete milk, have other effects on the mother. In birds, prolactin is a love hormone; it appears to activate the close attachment between mother and young. Does the great increase in prolactin also enhance the mother's attachment to her infant? If so, its production through the agency of the child is an efficient biological mechanism serving to promote the survival of neonates.

Evidence that gives partial support to this hypothesis comes from observations in Denver, Colorado, where Avery (1973) has developed a method for inducing milk production in women who have never given birth. Women who have been able to breastfeed their adopted babies have reported the rapid development of strong feelings of closeness and attachment while breastfeeding. In these situations skin-to-skin contact, touch, smell, body warmth, and auditory and visual stimuli all operate together to promote attachment.

Up to this point we have attempted to separate the components of this complex system into effects of the mother on the child or the child on the mother. However, we are now able to approach the fact of interaction operationally. For example, one can hypothesize that the mother is rewarded for her touching by the resulting closeness with her infant, through which she can pleasurably experience his warmth and soft skin. In addition, she can look at him closely and observe his responses to her touch.

5. *Odor*. Interestingly, odor is probably also important. Schaal and associates (1980) noted that on the third and fourth days after birth most mothers recognize their own infant's odor.

6. *Entrainment*. From numerous clinical experiences we believe that an essential principle of attachment is that parents must receive some response or signal, such as body or eye movements, from their infant to form a close bond. We hy-

pothesize that for most parents this takes place in the first days of life, when the infant is in the quiet alert state and moves in rhythm to his parents' speech. We have abbreviated this principle to: "You cannot fall in love with a dishrag."

Maternal and infant behaviors complement each other in several sensory and motor systems, thus increasing the probability of interaction occurring. These behaviors seem to be specific and innately programmed to start the process of locking mother and infant together in a sustained reciprocal rhythm. For example, as we have seen, the mother's use of a high-pitched voice appears to fit perfectly with the infant's especially sensitive auditory perception and attraction to speech in the high-frequency range. Thus, if the observation that humans characteristically speak to newborn infants in a high-pitched voice is correct, nature has provided a means by which stimulation from humans is especially attractive to the young of the species and will easily evoke a response. Similarly, a mother's interest in her new baby's eyes corresponds to his ability to see, to attend, and to follow. Nature appears to have preferentially developed in the occipital cortex the visual pathways so that these sensory and motor functions are ready for the newborn infant to receive stimulation from his mother and to interact with her.

Kaila (1935), Spitz and Wolff (1946), and Ahrens (1964) have established that one of the earliest and most effective stimuli for eliciting a social smile in an infant is a visual configuration consisting of two eyes and a mouth shown *en face*. Goren and associates (1975) demonstrated that this is the innate form preference of newborns, minutes after birth, even before there has been any opportunity for the infant to see human faces. Thus mothers tend to look at their babies in a way that increases the chance that their babies will attend and follow and then, a bit later, smile back. Since smiling is an extremely powerful reinforcer, the visual interaction helps to cement the proximity of mother and child.

It should be noted that Condon and Sander's (1974) studies on entrainment to the human voice were done with infants a few hours old and that all of the babies were bottle fed and were in United States hospitals. Would the entrainment progress more rapidly, would the co-occurrence of the mother's holding and the infant's alerting take place more frequently, and would the breakup in the baby's sleep and awake states be less marked and less prolonged if mother and baby were together continuously from birth and if the baby were breastfed?

Hearing and vision distal systems for communication assume greatly enhanced importance in Western industrialized nations, where mother and baby are separated for many hours of the day. In some developing nations, where the baby remains on the mother's body from birth on, these state changes might well be different. A woman in Africa who carries her baby on her back or side is identified as a poor mother if her baby wets or soils on her after the seventh day—that is, if she cannot anticipate these elimination behaviors and hold the baby away before they occur. This finely tuned awareness of the movements (a proximal system of communication) of the baby is almost inconceivable to those in nations where mother and baby are kept apart much of the day and sleep separately at night.

These observations are especially provocative because they extend the perceptive observations of Bowlby (1958), Ainsworth and Bell (1970), and Ainsworth and associates (1974), who distinguished between executive and signal behaviors. Executive behaviors consist of responses such as rooting, grasping, and postural adjustment, which tend to maintain physical contact between infant and caretaker, once established. Signal behaviors, on the other hand, comprise responses such as crying and smiling, which increase proximity or establish physical contact between infant and mother. We suggest that the signal and executive behaviors act in conjunction with the reciprocal interactions just presented. One of the major advantages of the early interaction is that it helps the parents to become more quickly attuned to the individuality of their own infant and therefore to adapt their behavior to his needs and tempo (Brazelton et al., 1974).

Although individual infants differ in their capacity to receive and shut out stimuli, as well as in their ability to exhibit behaviors to which the environment can respond, we wonder whether some of the individual differences described in later infancy might occur partly as a result of whether the mother is permitted early or late contact. Brazelton and co-workers (1974) and Stern (1974) have started to decode the normal intricate mother-infant interaction at 3 and 4 months of age. We suggest that the amazing synchronization of normal mothers and infants found at that time begins in these crucial first minutes of life.

COMMENT: The complexity of available systems for the mother to use in making the initial attachment to the baby are obviously a kind of fail-safe system for assuring the newborn of a caring environment. We should be aware of the richness of these and utilize as many as we can as we try to lock a new mother into her baby's uniqueness. For, then, if one system is deviant or disappointing, the others can make up to her for it. The complexity of a baby's responses seems to be matched in maternal responses to adapt to and enfold her new individual. As in animal studies, there seem to be especially potent, inborn responses in both baby and mother that set the tone for the initial job of making a firm attachment. Klaus and Kennell have shown us how critical they are and how they can be utilized in the perinatal period to help new parents get going with their new baby.
T.B. Brazelton

In the next section we will consider other major rules or principles for which experimental data and solid evidence are scanty but which we believe play a significant role in this attachment.

1. *Monotropy*. Observations of our nurses working in the premature nursery, discussions with the head nurse at the Matera (a large adoption home in Athens, Greece), and clinical follow-up of twin deliveries suggest another basic principle of attachment—that the phenomenon of mother-to-infant attachment is developed and structured so that a close attachment can optimally be formed to only one person at a time. In the premature nursery we have learned that each nurse has a

favorite, usually liking the other infants but never having more than one special infant at any one time. When the favorite infant leaves the nursery with the mother, the nurse usually is sad, often for two to five days. At the Matera, where the nurses live on the division for four to five months with the children (nine nurses for 12 infants), a nurse has never become attached to more than one infant at a time, although 3000 infants have been raised in the past 15 years. After the discharge of the infant at four to five months, the nurses at the Matera usually go through a prolonged period (four to six months) of grief and mourning responses similar to those which follow the death of a close relative.

In addition to this phenomenon are clinical observations of a number of sets of twins, where the larger twin was discharged and the smaller twin was left in the nursery to grow, which suggests that there is a much higher incidence of mothering disorders in the second twin. In a short observation period in Lausanne, Switzerland, three sets of twins were discharged, the larger first, and the smaller later. Three months later the smaller twins of two of the sets returned. One infant had been battered, and the other failed to thrive. The second mother mentioned that the larger twin was hers but not the second baby. We have seen similar problems in our own unit. This is apparently an important principle that may explain why mothers of twins prefer to dress them alike. Optimally, they may only be able to take in one image or bond to one infant at the end of each pregnancy. This has obvious clinical significance, and we are now attempting to design further observations to test this. It is interesting that in a paper written by Bowlby in 1958 discussing a child's tie to his mother, he stated, "The tendency for instinctual responses to be directed toward a particular individual or group of individuals and not promiscuously towards many is one which I believe so important and so neglected, it deserves a special term. I propose to call it monotropy." This observation about the tie in the opposite direction, mother to infant, has the obvious clinical implication that twins should be kept together and should be discharged at the same time so that simultaneous attachments may be possible.

2. *Infant-mother interaction*. During the early process of the mother's attachment to her infant, it is necessary that the infant respond to the mother by some signal, such as body or eye movements.

> **COMMENT:** Mothers need some reward from their infants—some indication that this is a mutual endeavor. Problems can develop when the infant's signals are disorganized or unclear, or the mother misinterprets them or gives them unrealistic meaning. For example, a mother at the limits of her adaptability, may perceive her infant's tongue thrusting as a deliberate display of rejection. One of our most important jobs is helping parents to recognize, understand, and respond appropriately to their infant's cues and signals.
> **M.A. Curry**

3. *Observing birth*. People who witness the birth process often become strongly attached to the infant.

4. *Attachment-detachment*. Another significant principle which has evolved from many clinical experiences and the work of Evans and associates (1972) is that the processes of attachment and detachment cannot easily occur simultaneously. We have noted in many parents who have lost one of a twin pair that they have often found it difficult to mourn completely the baby who died and at the same time to feel attached to the survivor. The same problem is found when a mother quickly becomes pregnant after losing a neonate. Supporting evidence is the observation of Evans and associates (1972), who discovered that one third of parents who have a failure-to-thrive infant without organic disease have recently suffered from the loss of a close family relative. While mourning the loss of a parent they are unable to care for their newborn adequately. Thus, whenever feasible, it should be recommended that a new infant not be conceived until the grief is finished (six to 12 months).

5. *Early events*. Early events have long-lasting effects. Anxieties in the first day about the well-being of a baby with a temporary disorder may result in long-lasting concerns that may adversely shape the development of the child.

CLINICAL CONSIDERATIONS

Until a century ago, events surrounding childbirth had changed little; elaborate customs served to help parents through the period. In the last century, however, increasing emphasis has been placed on the medical and scientific aspects of birth, but less attention has been paid to the equally valid psychological and social considerations. Has the enormous improvement in medical management, which has dramatically lessened the physical dangers to the mother, contributed to a waning concern about the many other problems a mother faces during pregnancy?

When evaluating clinical data, one must appreciate that evaluation depends on the entire environment, including the social values of the system and the regulations of the hospital. In Russia, for example, a high value is placed on the birth of the human infant, and a woman is honored for having more than three children. But the hospital does not permit the father to be present at the birth or even to visit his wife and baby in the hospital. He does not see the infant until discharge. In Denmark, visiting regulations for fathers are exactly the opposite. Therefore it is not possible to compare the effects of mother-infant contact in the first hours on later maternal attachment in these two systems.

It is also necessary to separate one- and two-phase obstetrical delivery systems. For example, Denmark has a two-phase system. A normal, healthy pregnant woman is usually examined and followed through the prenatal period by a midwife, with a few examinations by a physician, and then often gives birth in a maternity clinic. A maternity clinic does not contain all the facilities usually found in a hospital but is designed somewhat like a home. It has no blood bank and only minimal emergency equipment to care for sick infants. Five to six hours after the birth the mother assumes full daytime care for her infant, coming into the nursery to take her infant. It should be noted that a mother can learn not only from the nurse but also from other mothers as she actually begins to provide for her baby's needs. She gains skill and confidence before she takes him home. The nurse does not usually care for the babies or formally teach. She is available for questions and support.

In this system pregnancy is treated as a normal process and not as a disease. Mothers who have diabetes, toxemia, premature labor, or other complications of pregnancy detected from the first prenatal visits up to the time of birth are monitored by obstetricians and give birth in a hospital.

In the one-phase system, in the United States, Germany, and Switzerland, all mothers with or without complications give birth in the same unit; pregnancy is treated as a disease requiring hospitalization. Therefore, when inspecting data on maternal behavior, it is important to note in which type of setting the studies were done—a one- or a two-phase system.

To minimize the number of unknowns for a mother while she is in the hospital, she and her partner should visit the maternity unit to see where labor and birth will take place. She should also learn about the drawbacks as well as the benefits of the anesthetic (if she is to receive one), the delivery routines, and all the procedures and medication she is likely to receive before, during, and after birth. Advance preparation increases the parents' confidence by reducing the possibility of surprise. For an adult, just as for a child entering the hospital for surgery, the more meticulously every step is detailed in advance, the less will be the subsequent anxiety. The less anxiety the mother experiences while giving birth and becoming attached to her baby, the fewer perinatal complications and the better will be her immediate relationship with him.

Preparing for the birth

The mother needs continuing support and reassurance during her labor and birth, whether from her husband, mother, a friend, a midwife, or a nurse. She also must be satisfied with the arrangements that have been made to maintain her home during her hospitalization. In Holland, when a mother gives birth at home, a mother-helper comes into the home at the time of birth and takes over the care of the family and helps the midwife deliver the baby. This gives the mother the freedom to concentrate on the needs of her baby and enjoy her family in the process, and it relieves the pressure on the father, allowing him to reserve his energies for the family.

COMMENT: Is this not where our system is failing the most? We don't provide families with the support necessary to help them concentrate on and enjoy their infant.
M.A. Curry

Labor and birth

To reduce the amount of tension for the mother, she should labor and deliver in the same room, eliminating the necessity of rushing to a delivery room in the last minutes of labor. It is crucial, as noted earlier, that she be never left alone during labor (pp. 25-30). Once the birth is completed and the mother has had a quick glance at the infant, she usually needs a few seconds to regain her composure and, in a sense, catch her breath before she proceeds to the next task—"taking on" the infant. In standard hospital births this breath catching usually occurs while the placenta is being delivered and while the mother is being cleansed and is having any necessary suturing. It has been our experience that it is best not to give a mother her baby until she indicates that she is ready to take him on. It should be her decision. However, some mothers indicate their desire to hold and nurse their babies within a few seconds. If the delivery table is sufficiently wide and the baby can be kept warm, many mothers will welcome an opportunity for this early contact and nursing.

In many hospitals it is customary to put the baby on the mother's chest for 1 or 2 minutes shortly after birth. Although this is helpful, the lack of privacy, the narrow table, and the short time period do not allow sufficient opportunity for the mother to touch and explore her baby. This first visit ideally should not coincide with a painful experience of suturing the episiotomy.

After birth it is extremely valuable for the father, mother, and infant to be together for about 30 to 60 minutes, either in the delivery room or in an adjacent room. Obviously this is only possible if the infant is healthy and the mother is well. The mother should have the infant with her on the bed so that she can hold him rather than in a bassinet where she can only see his face. She should be given the infant nude and allowed to examine him completely. We encourage the mother to move over in her regular hospital bed or on a wide delivery table, leaving the other half for her partially dressed or nude infant. A heat panel easily maintains or, if need be, increases the body temperature of the infant. Several mothers have told us of the unforgettable experience of holding their nude babies against their own bare chests, so we recommend skin-to-skin contact. If the mother plans to breast-feed, the first nursing can take place at this time. The father sits or stands at the side of the bed by the infant. This allows the parents and infant to become acquainted. Because of the importance of the eyes in the formation of the attachment, we withhold the application of silver nitrate to the eyes until after this rendezvous.

COMMENT: Since some mothers may not be ready for the intimacy of skin-to-skin contact immediately after birth, all possibilities of early contact should be offered with the same enthusiasm, such as holding in a blanket. We must be careful to not transmit either verbal or nonverbal negative messages when parents choose these other options.
M.A. Curry

We leave the mother, the father, and their baby together for about 60 minutes. In Guatemalan hospitals, where drugs and anesthesia are used more sparingly than in the United States, most mothers are awake after 45 minutes of privacy with their babies. The mother and father never forget this significant and stimulating shared experience. It helps to bond firmly the infant to both parents. We must emphasize that this should be a private session with a minimum of interruptions.

> **COMMENT:** Again, maternity personnel must be aware of the *messages* they are transmitting to parents with such institutionalized procedures. They are saying "*You* are the important ones to that baby's survival, not we!" "This is an important thing to do, to get attached." People are subtly influenced by medical priorities. For example, we found that many mothers of premature infants hold their babies out in their laps in a seated position to feed them. On a Brody Closeness Scale the mothers score poorly, until one realizes that they have learned about their babies in premature nurseries where the nurses commonly feed them in this position.
> **T.B. Brazelton**

Affectional bonds are further consolidated in the succeeding four or five days through continued close association and interaction of baby and mother, particularly when she cares for him. Close contact with her husband and other children is also important.

Michel Odent of Pithiviers, France, has developed a model maternity unit that brings together what appears to be the best of both the delivery practices of the past and modern obstetrics as well as a strong dose of humanism that includes utter confidence and respect for the entire family. For many years he has been interested in the position the mother finds most comfortable and efficient during labor and birth. He notices that most mothers walk around during labor until the end of the first stage. They then commonly choose a hands-and-knees position and usually squat supported by the husband and midwife at the time of birth. Mothers are never left alone during the labor. The midwife and/or the husband remain with the mother constantly. The same midwife is present for the entire labor, even though it takes many hours. Odent keeps the room quiet and without bright lights during the labor. It is his impression that it is not beneficial for the mother to follow a set of rules and breathing exercises but that it is important for her to allow "her mid-brain to lead her rather than her cortex." He does not endorse Lamaze or breathing exercises, but the mothers come three times a month with their husbands and parents for an hour of singing sessions and to talk about birth.

Odent has noticed that at the end of the first stage, most mothers will get into a hands-and-knees position, as shown in Fig. 2-21. In this position infants in the posterior presentation usually rotate without forceps. Medications are used only occasionally; for example, oxytocin is prescribed about once a month. The mother sits down after the birth and holds her baby for 45 to 60 minutes, which gives her time to suckle the infant. Then she gets up and walks to her room, carrying the

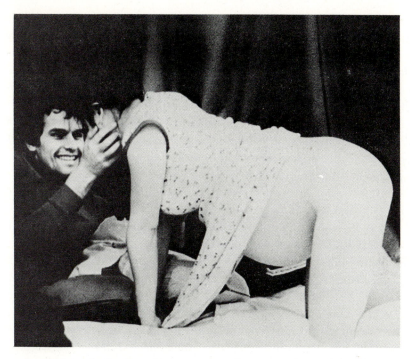

Fig. 2-21. A mother in the hands-and-knees position (a position observed for about 10 minutes when the cervix is fully dilated).

infant in her arms. A quick survey of the charts of 25 primiparous mothers by one of the authors showed a mean labor length of 5.5 hours. Gillett (1979) visited the maternity unit in Pithiviers and reported on a cesarean birth rate of 8.3% for the years 1977 and 1978 and a low perinatal mortality of 9 per 1000 births.

First days of life

The arrangements for the mother and her newborn infant vary greatly depending on the culture. In many parts of the world the mother and infant are together in a small hut for the first seven days. In Holland it is common for the mother to have the infant at home in her own room. In Denmark the infant usually stays in the hospital room with the mother for most of the day. One of the authors (M.H.K.) visited a maternity clinic in Horsholm, Denmark, where mothers go when a normal birth is anticipated. We have chosen to describe this clinic because we believe that several of its practices tend to optimize maternal attachment.

A mother visits one midwife several times during her pregnancy. All of the women give birth in the rooms where they have labored. The clinic has a homelike living room, dining room, and various kitchens on one floor, and the nursery and mothers' rooms are on another. Sometimes women labor in the living room. At the time of the visit to the unit there were 20 mothers in two- or four-bed rooms. Six hours after birth a mother takes over the care of her infant, and the infant is left next to her bed. Many women describe the value of having their babies at their sides, available for viewing with just a turn of the head. Women mention that they look at their infants over and over again whenever they awaken, continually taking them in. In other Danish hospitals that were visited, the babies are at the foot of the beds, where it is difficult for the mothers to observe them continually. In the Horsholm clinic there is unlimited visiting during the whole day, and at lunch hours or teatime mothers come downstairs into the dining room and leave the babies upstairs alone. At night between 8:30 and 10:30 P.M. they take the babies back into the large nursery where they are cared for by nurses overnight, except when they wake and are returned to their mothers for breastfeeding. In the previous year 2100 infants had been delivered in this maternity clinic. Twenty-five were premature infants but none died. The year before there were 1700 births and again no neonatal or maternal deaths. Thus the selection process is effective in picking out high-risk mothers.

One of the most impressive features of this unit can be observed in the morning, when the mothers come to the nurseries to pick up their babies and take over their care. There is much sharing of information about such routine procedures as bathing and diapering between more and less experienced mothers. In this clinic the mother becomes well acquainted with her baby before discharge.

Several features of the birth should be mentioned. There is little anesthesia. The parents are together during labor, there are no stirrups, and the mother's hands are not bound. She has an opportunity to see and hold the baby briefly after birth, and every attempt is made to make it a natural process. Just before birth a general practitioner comes to assist. There is no question that the midwife is in charge, and practitioners usually ask how they can help. The entire birth experience is strikingly different from a hospital delivery in the United States.

At University Hospitals of Cleveland, Ohio, there are a number of different options for housing the mother and infant. The mother can live with the infant continuously, she can have him for a few hours, or he may be kept in the nursery at night and in a bassinet with his mother during the day, from 8:00 A.M. until 11:00 P.M., as in many European and United States rooming-in units. We strongly recommend that the mother have her infant for a long period during the day, for example, at least from 1:00 P.M. until early evening. We also believe that she should see her husband while their infant is in the room and that she be allowed to see her other children. This allows the family to form a new unit around the newborn and decreases the mother's concerns about her other children. This lessens the separation concerns of the siblings, which not only has extremely important preventive benefits for them but also makes for an easier transition when the mother returns home (Chapter 3). Winnicott (1965) again nicely describes what goes on during this period.

> I cannot find words to express what big forces are at work at this critical point, but I can try to explain something of what is going on. There is a most curious thing happening: the mother who is perhaps physically exhausted, and perhaps incontinent, and who is dependent on the nurse and the doctor for skilled attention in many and various ways, is at the same time the one person who can properly introduce the world to the baby in a way that makes sense to the baby. She knows how to do this, not through any training and not through being clever, but just because she is the natural mother. But her natural instincts cannot evolve if she is scared, or if she does not see her baby when it is born, or if the baby is brought to her only at stated times thought by the authorities to be suitable for feeding purposes. It just does not work that way. The mother's milk does not flow like an excretion; it is a response to a stimulus, and the stimulus is the sight and smell and feel of her baby, and the sound of the baby's cry that indicates need. It is all one thing, the mother's care of her baby and the periodic feeding that develops as if it were a means of communication between the two—a song without words.*

In the United States a new mother, particularly a primipara, frequently states that she is unable to take over the strain of caring for her baby for a 3- or 4-hour period until after the fourth or fifth day. In Denmark, where mothers provide total care for their infants in a homelike setting in the hospital, mothers feel able to take over these duties 6 hours after giving birth. How can we account for these differences? Are Danish women healthier? Is this due to fewer episiotomies being performed? Are they given different drugs? Are the opportunities to care for the baby different? Do the mothers come to the hospital with different expectations?

> **COMMENT:** Much of the difference probably results from the fact that in Denmark, and other countries, the prenatal care and five- to 10-day hospital stay is entirely paid for by the state. This not only frees the family from this financial worry but allows the mother to be nurtured in the immediate postpartum period. This allows her to concentrate her energies on her newborn. Furthermore, unrestricted visiting by the family, including siblings, minimizes family disruption and allows the family to adapt to the new member in a supportive environment. Our American system can be a dismal contrast, since new parents are forced to leave the hospital in hours or days because of soaring costs, and not infrequently to a home devoid of supportive family members. Thus it may be for self-preservation that some new mothers in the United States choose to not room-in, believing that a brief time of rest without responsibility may be the best preparation for the task of assuming total responsibility at home alone.
> **M.A. Curry**

Almost every physician or nurse who works in a maternity unit comments on the extreme sensitivity of mothers during the early postpartum period. They may become greatly upset over a minor change in their infant and require assurance

---

*From Winnicott, D.W.: The family and individual development, London, 1965, Tavistock Publications, Ltd., p. 111.

that he is healthy and that their mothering is adequate. After they have left the hospital, mothers may comment about their unusual and unexpected feelings of hypersensitivity. It is this special sensitivity that makes a mother receptive to learning about her infant.

COMMENT: . . . and about her own importance and adequacy as a mother for this fragile, rather unknown infant. By this time she has been stripped of her autonomy and importance as a person, and also as the important figure to the infant.
T.B. Brazelton

The model for the childbirth unit of the future should be more than just a facility where continual contact is provided. The policy of the unit should be to give healthy parents complete responsibility for the care of their infant, with nurses or midwives available as consultants when the mother wishes and asks for help. Homelike birth units have been started in a number of hospitals in the United States.

We have noted that male physicians often find it difficult to answer the many small but important questions raised by new mothers. They frequently consider their pressing duties with sick infants more important and give this other responsibility to nurses. Nurses easily manage this task when they are aware of the importance of questions that may be raised.

Cesarean birth

Cesarean births have greatly increased in frequency in the United States, and many questions have been asked about parents' adaptation following elective or emergency cesarean birth. Should this area be discussed in detail in childbirth classes when in some hospitals the percentage of cesarean births has reached 25% to 30%? What preparation should be made in the hospital for parents with a planned cesarean birth? In our unit in Cleveland, Ohio, we are fortunate to have local anesthesia used for the surgery, and fathers may be present in the delivery room. The father sits behind the mother with the anesthesiologist, receives the infant, holds the infant, and shows the infant to the mother.

Twenty minutes following the birth the mother, infant, and father go to the small labor room where they have privacy and the infant can be placed next to the mother with a heat panel. Here the mother can have the normal 45 to 60 minutes together with her husband and newborn infant. The only procedures interrupting this period are pulse rate and blood pressure measurements, which are made every 10 to 15 minutes. It is usually fortunate that during this period the mother's anesthesia continues so that she is free to explore and enjoy her new infant with her husband. This simplifies an extremely difficult procedure for the families. It occurs before the common depression associated with the surgery, pain, and the failure to have had a vaginal delivery set in. We are pleased to see a number of studies now beginning to explore this especially difficult area.

Postpartum blues

Many physicians and nurses who have had extensive experience with postpartum patients in the average United States hospital report that well over 80% of mothers have postpartum blues, with crying some time during hospitalization. A number of physiological, psychological, and biochemical explanations have been proposed, but none has been conclusive.

Let us look at three scenes:

1. If you suddenly come into a postpartum division in Russia, you might be impressed with the sad expressions on the faces of the women, their spiritless motions and conversation. Note that husbands are not allowed to visit, that mothers see their babies every 4 hours for feedings, and that they do not participate in other infant care.

2. On a surprise visit to one mother's room on a postpartum division in the United States between feedings, you might find the mother cheerily talking on the phone to her mother, but in the next room the mother is quiet with postpartum blues. Note that fathers often visit once a day, that babies are brought often only every 4 hours for feedings, and that siblings are sometimes not allowed to visit.

3. If you come unexpectedly into the maternity clinic in Horsholm, Denmark, you find a quiet, happy, pleasant atmosphere and mutual support as a group of mothers care for their babies and get to know them. Note that babies are with their mothers for the whole day, that the mothers provide all the care, and that fathers and siblings visit freely.

COMMENT: Also the cultural expectations for not showing one's feelings may dominate a mother's behavior in Russia.
T.B. Brazelton

We do not know the etiology of postpartum blues, but our observations lead us to speculate that mother-infant separation, the assignment of most of the caretaking responsibilities to "experts," the concerns about ability to care for the newborn at home, and the limiting of visitors are major factors. For further reading in this area we suggest the work of Brown and Harris (1978).

COMMENT: It is also a cry of helplessness for help in becoming the "ideal" mother that women in the United States have in their fantasies. Certainly in this culture, mothers may need more backup both for their own self-image as competent people and for ongoing support in decision making about goals for their babies. The economy of achieving a start toward both of these by the simple, rather inexpensive changes suggested by this book makes it obvious that lying-in hospitals in the United States should reexamine their birthing practices. One of the most important reasons for such reexamination would be that of giving new parents a more positive relationship with the medical profession. If we do want to reach people early to be more effective with our preventive, outreach programs, we should see these innovations as opportunities for showing that our profession is supportive and interested in them as individuals.
T.B. Brazelton

RECOMMENDATIONS FOR CARE

1. *Special needs*. The special needs of a mother should be assessed through examining the history of her previous pregnancies, her desires and plans for the birth experience and infant, and the type of mothering she received.

2. *Parent preparation*. Group sessions with provision of information about emotional and physical aspects of labor and birth together with special exercises are of value to the parents-to-be. They help to relieve anxiety and allow the parents to share with others the many problems that arise during a normal pregnancy. This enables the mother to turn a passive experience into an active one, to become a participant rather than a "victim."

3. *Need for companion*. It is necessary for a mother to have one person (her husband, mother, a friend, a midwife, a nurse, or an obsetetrician) with her throughout labor and birth for guidance and reassurance. Because the supportive companion does not fit the medical model of care, because it has been a universal feature of childbirth in humans up until this century, because it has positive clinical outcomes (shorter labor, decreased perinatal problems, and increased affectionate maternal-infant interaction in the first hour), and because it makes good sense, there is a real hazard that it will be looked on as unscientific and less important than medical interventions and therefore will not be provided for all mothers in all hospitals. For this reason it is particularly crucial that we insist that *no woman should ever labor or give birth alone*—without a supportive companion.

4. *Enhancing attachment*. To enhance the mother's attachment to her baby the following arrangements should be provided during the birth and postpartum period:
   a. Privacy
   b. Extended periods of father-mother-infant contact
   c. Complete responsibility given to the mother for the care of her baby, with a nurse or midwife available as consultant

COMMENT: The choice of complete responsibility or of forced responsibility are two different things. The latter may be just as detrimental as not having a choice. What is more important than nurturing the mother so she can give to her infant? Helping parents proceed at their own pace, nurturing them, requires more, not less of our time. On the other hand, what could be more rewarding?
M.A. Curry

5. *Eye medications*. We recommend delaying eye medications such as silver nitrate for the infant until after the parents have had an extended period with their infant in the first hour after birth.

6. *First hour*. We strongly suggest that the mother, father, and infant have a period of at least 15 to 20 minutes alone together in privacy after the placenta is delivered and the episiotomy sutured (5 to 15 minutes after birth). We place a heat lamp or radiant panel over the nude infant, and the mother is instructed not to

cover the infant. She may be encouraged to hold him against her bare chest. The period should be long enough so that the mother, infant, and father are able to participate fully in the exciting transformation of three separate individuals into a new family unit. If a heat panel is not available, the dried infant can be placed on the mother's chest and a warmed blanket placed over both of them.

7. *Rooming-in.* The mother and infant should be kept together continuously or have long periods together in the days after the birth (Jackson et al., 1948). We suggest that the infant be in a small bassinet at his mother's side for a minimum of 5 hours a day so that she can learn about the infant's needs and activity. During this period it is necessary that she have control over the care of the infant while the nurse acts as consultant. Reversing the usual pattern of "experts" who correct a mother when she deviates from the usual routine is a step in the direction of increased confidence and competence for the mother. The postpartum period should be a time when the mother interacts with her infant so that she may become acquainted with him, learn about his needs, and be thoroughly satisfied with her own ability to meet these needs before she decides on the time of discharge (obviously only if her physical condition warrants this). The average mother in the United States has had so little previous experience with infants that she is unaware that certain characteristics of breathing, color, and bowel movements are normal. She may worry unnecessarily that many normal features and behaviors are a sign of disease or abnormality. By keeping her baby with her and having the opportunity to talk with other mothers, she will realize that her own infant is normal. Mother-infant contact is particularly important when there has been a separation or an illness in either member of the dyad, for example, after a cesarean birth.

COMMENT: Groups of mothers in hospital can gather, compare their concerns, their inadequacies, as well as their ecstasies. This gives them a great deal of personal support, and a concept of peer support for the future days ahead.
T.B. Brazelton

8. *Early discharge.* Recently hospitals have begun to permit early discharge of mother and baby if the mother is doing well and the infant is completely normal. The studies of Yanover and associates (1976) have shown that this is perfectly safe as long as there is a home visit by a nurse on the first and third day after discharge to answer any questions and check a bilirubin level if necessary. It is especially helpful if there is a supportive woman or husband who is able to take over the household tasks while the mother spends her time caring for the infant.

9. *Parental choice.* We believe it is essential that parents have a choice in the many decisions associated with labor and birth if at all possible, for example, the birth environment, procedures such as shaving the perineum, use and choice of drugs, use of electronic fetal monitor, ambulation and food and drink during labor, the position for labor and birth, who should be present, and so on.

10. *Care by the mother.* We suggest that, when possible, infants requiring additional heat in an incubator remain with the mother, for example, babies who are slightly small for gestational age. We also recommend that bilirubin light treatments take place in the mother's room.

11. *Frequency of breastfeeding.* Mothers who are breastfeeding should be encouraged to feed their infants as frequently as the infant desires. This often is between 8 and 18 feedings per 24 hours. Recent studies by DeCarvalho (1981) of 47 breastfeeding mothers reveal that women feeding more frequently (8 times per 24 hours) in the first 14 days have a larger milk output at 30 days, minimal nipple soreness, and their infants have significantly lower bilirubin levels than women nursing less than 8 times in 24 hours during the first 2 weeks.

12. *Family visits.* The mother needs close contact with her husband or chosen companion and her other children during this period for emotional support. Sadness about separation from her husband and other children often compels a woman to leave before she is physically ready. The separation may have severe immediate and long-term effects on the siblings, especially those under 3 years of age (Chapter 3).

13. *Caretakers.* In the postpartum period even a perfectly normal woman is extremely sensitive to opinions and statements by the nurse and physician concerning the infant's health and her ability to care for the infant. We strongly recommend that nurses, physicians, and other maternity staff be optimistic and avoid criticism of mothers. Much more will be gained by praising a mother for what she does well. The average mother may look at her infant objectively during the first 24 to 48 hours and then suddenly feel that she has the greatest and most handsome baby ever born. This normal process can be enhanced if nurses and physicians can give every mother the feeling that they, too, think her baby is uniquely grand.

> **COMMENT:** What about an opportunity just to let off steam—to cry, to show disappointment, to be a baby, etc. This may be more therapeutic for a mother than back slapping. But I doubt that many physicians can tolerate a mother's negative feelings. Most obstetricians, pediatricians, midwives, and nurses are in this racket because of the generally optimistic outcome.
> **T.B. Brazelton**

After discharge the physician and nurse can be alert to evidence of the quality of mother-infant attachment. Levy (1951) has provided original and extremely helpful suggestions. For example, he wrote about maternal feelings as follows:

> While questioning a mother and writing on a health record, the pediatrician paused and remarked, "That's a very pretty baby." The mother, who had the baby in her lap, looked at him, said "Thank you," and smiled, but she did not look down at her baby. Accumulation of data in this study appears to corroborate the conclusion that the mother's typical response, after praise of the baby, is to look at it, and that absence of the glance indicates less than the usual maternal feeling.
>
> Response to the compliment may be as tangible evidence as response of a knee jerk to a tap on the patella. Both must be done in the appropriate manner; although the

stimuli will never be exactly the same, the response is forthcoming regardless of the difference in personalities that elicit them.*

COMMENT: As physicians, nurses, and other maternity staff caring for new dyads or triads, why do we not encourage all of this automatically? Why have we allowed such rationalizations as "infection," "sterility," and "optimal medical care" to push out these important aspects of childbirth and caring for the newborn and his parents? Surely, we are not all this insensitive to the vital importance of these issues. I believe that we have allowed it to become institutional practice to separate adults from their infants for three very good *unconscious* reasons:

1. As physicians and nurses, we basically like to help people depend on us. If we allow them too much choice or autonomy, our rewards are minimized.

2. To do this most effectively, we must push a pathological model—one in which childbirth and neonatal care are based on treating pathology rather than reinforcing for the strengths that are present in most people and for the odds that are enormously in favor of a good outcome.

3. All adults who care about babies are competitive with all other adults, and each would like to be the primary caretaker of the attractive helpless infant. *Unconsciously* we devaluate the role of parents to fulfill our own role as *the* important caretaker of this new infant. No one would ever admit to this drive, but it is universal. Perhaps we could use this same energy to care for the dyad or triad (mother, father, new infant) if we take Klaus and Kennell's advice and change the training of nurses and pediatricians to orient them toward roles of caretaking for cementing rather than splitting families!

T.B. Brazelton

SUMMARY

An assessment of the needs of the family makes it apparent that the physical facilities available in the United States are often inadequate to meet their requirements fully. Postpartum arrangements in the United States, which bring the infant to the mother for only 20 to 30 minutes out of every 4-hour period, are probably insufficient for some women to develop a close attachment with their infant. After observing other maternity care systems in the Western world, such as those in Denmark, Holland, and Britain, we have come to believe that there are several other essentials that have been forgotten in the United States. The infant should be near his mother so that she can learn how he reacts and may begin to meet his needs as they arise. This permits the mother, during her short hospitalization (three to six days in the United States but seven to 10 days in most European countries), to be prepared to care for the infant completely at the time of discharge (knowing how to feed, clean, soothe, and relax the infant, and how to react to all the little changes such as hiccups, skin changes, burps, and funny noises that appear normally in every infant).

The small amount of time that the American mother has with her infant in the hospital does not give her adequate exposure to him, with the result that she is not fully acquainted with him at the time of discharge. The first days after discharge are described by many mothers as "hellish," or as the most difficult days of their

---

*From Levy, D.: Observations of attitudes and behavior in the child health center, Chicago, 1951, Year Book Medical Publishers, Inc.

lives. Often the mother's idea of what a good mother should be able to accomplish with her baby has been built up to such an unrealistic level by magazine articles and college courses that she may exhaust herself and then have little tolerance for the many minor problems that arise in the course of the early care of her infant. Almost all maternity units in the United States can arrange to keep the baby in a small bassinet at the mother's side during most of the day. We believe that the existing facilities and routines in the United States can easily be adapted (if outmoded state regulations are brought up to date) so that the conditions are optimal for the development of parent-infant attachment in the first days of life.

> **COMMENT:** One of the most useful techniques I have found for relieving new mothers of their anxiety about their own adequacy in the face of the new infant is to show her the strengths of the infant as a potent individual. When she sees that he has a personality of his own, she no longer feels entirely responsible for this "lump of clay," and it becomes an interaction between them rather than her "action" on him. We have used the Brazelton Neonatal Behavior Assessment most successfully for this.
> **T.B. Brazelton**

An alternative birth center in a hospital setting

ROBERTA A. BALLARD, CAROL H. LEONARD, NANCY A. IRVIN, and CAROLYN B. FERRIS

During the past 15 years numerous forces have influenced the way maternity care is provided in the United States. There have been incredible advances in technology and in understanding the physiology of the pregnant woman, fetus, and birth process, as well as the care of the newborn infant. These advances have increased the capacity of health professionals to provide care in the perinatal period and have reduced morbidity and mortality for both mothers and infants. However, learning the requisite physiology and understanding the complex technology take a great deal of the energy of all of the health care personnel involved, and a large proportion of training time is being devoted to the development of technological skills in relation to that devoted to learning skills and services addressing the humanistic concerns.

This trend has pervaded all areas of health care, and it therefore comes as no surprise that consumers of health care have begun to challenge it. The first areas of care to be questioned are those concerned with issues of birth and death. This has occurred concomitantly with a growing consciousness among women of themselves and their rights, their bodies and their experiences, and has led to an increasing interest and support by large groups of concerned individuals for humanizing maternity services. To many consumers the obstacles they encountered in dealing with institutions and traditional practices seemed insurmountable, and they began to choose home-birth experiences to gain the qualities they sought. This choice, while providing many psychological benefits and frequently resulting in a unique and positive beginning with a new child, also denies the use of the true advances in technology and understanding of physiology to those infants who require immediate skilled care around the time of birth.

At the same time, a new understanding of the sensitivity of a mother to her newborn infant around the period immediately following birth has provided a basis for questioning many of the routine procedures used in hospitals that may detract from the experience, especially those related to separation of parents and infant and to the use of anesthesia or analgesia. Thus greater numbers of concerned professionals are seeking to respond to the demands of parents and to develop ways of enhancing both the medical and emotional aspects of maternity care in hospitals. One of the attitudes that has contributed to accomplishing this is the assumption of a "lifeguard" stance by professional personnel. Such a position permits more freedom and control for the parents while the professionals remain in the background

99

to ensure that the newborn infant makes the transition into extrauterine life without damage and that the mother's well-being is protected.

> **COMMENT:** Rather than the approach that "permits more freedom and control for the parents," one would like ideally for professionals and parents to meet on an equal basis and on a basis of trust—not the fear that "if something goes wrong, all further care will be imposed on me," but that "everyone supports me in what I am doing and will help me should I need this."
>
> In fact, the authors have expressed this very clearly under the heading Relevance of the alternative birth center to other kinds of maternity care (later on in this section), and this, I think, is the most important aspect of the chapter.
> **D. Henschel**

An alternative birth center within a hospital is one response to the concerns of both parents and health care professionals.

DEVELOPMENT AND IMPLEMENTATION

In developing an alternative birth center (ABC) program, it is important to seek out as many viewpoints as possible of the needs to be addressed. Therefore, in any community considering changes in maternity services, it is important to recruit an advisory committee comprising consumers, prenatal educators, midwives, nurses from obstetrical and nursery services, obstetricians and pediatricians, and administrative staff. Such a group needs to define the goals for their program and to develop policies and procedures to be used for training staff, for organizing the center, and for providing services. Agreement of the obstetrical and pediatric departments of the hospital staff is needed, and the concurrence of the maternal and child health authorities of the state government or other pertinent regulatory agencies must be obtained. Hospital administrative support and legal counsel's review and recommendations are also necessary. This involves justification of the importance of such a program to the institution's responsible governing body and of the mechanisms by which it will serve the interests of patient care. Consultation with third-party carriers of insurance benefits is also desirable.

> **COMMENT:** I like the clear description of all aspects of development, implementation, and policies. The importance of an advisory committee with members from all interested parties cannot be overemphasized. I would like to suggest adding a sentence about the preparation of all personnel involved, both administrative and medical.
>
> In the United Kingdom the system of maternity care is, of course, very different from that in the United States. Angles other than those described would have to be considered, but here, too, it is high time for making changes in the traditional care given, particularly in attitudes to prospective mothers and parents.
> **D. Henschel**

The background efforts just outlined led to the development of an alternative birth center program at Mount Zion Hospital and Medical Center (MZH) in San Francisco in May, 1976. This program was opened within the regular obstetrical department rather than as a separate service.

ALTERNATIVE TO TRADITIONAL SERVICES AT MZH

The alternative birth center provides a homelike atmosphere within the hospital. The mother moves about as she feels comfortable. There are no routine "preps," enemas, intravenous fluids, or other regimented orders. A standard double bed is provided in the room, as well as comfortable chairs, stereo, plants, and other homelike furnishings. Family and friends are included as desired by the mother. Sterile trays and emergency equipment are housed in attractive wooden cabinets out of sight until needed. A Kreiselman unit is present in the room for resuscitation of the newborn, should it be needed. The room is located immediately adjacent to a high-risk obstetrical suite and close to a tertiary level intensive care nursery. A buzzer above the bed in the birth center sets off an alarm, which is answered by both obstetrical and pediatric staff should there be an unexpected emergency.

CRITERIA FOR USE OF THE CENTER

The criteria for use of the birth center follow:

1. Prenatal supervision by an obstetrician or by a member of the family practice or nurse-midwifery staff with an obstetrician's backup.
2. No findings suggestive of increased risk of complications during labor, birth, or the immediate postpartum period.
3. Childbirth preparation classes.
4. Participation in the orientation program provided by the nursing staff of the birth center.
5. All women must understand that if their labor status changes to one of high risk, transfer to the regular labor and delivery area will be necessary.
6. All women who wish to use the birth center must be accompanied by a support person.
7. An informed-consent form accepting the risks involved in giving birth in the birth center must be signed.
8. A specific plan for family participation, if desired, must be agreed on in advance of admission.
9. The infant's pediatrician must be in agreement with the criteria for care of the newborn in the birth center.

COMMENT: Our view is radically opposite. Semidarkness, silence, assistance by an experienced and loving midwife, and vertical postures inducing another level of consciousness are major components. In other words, a positive material and human environment is especially important when the labor or birth might be difficult or dangerous, for example, in the case of a previous cesarean birth, a breech delivery, or a mother who is not accompanied by a support person.

To help the woman in labor, it is first necessary to help her to reach a level of consciousness that is on a par with a reduced adrenergic secretion and an optimum secretion of oxytocin and probably of endorphins, and that is also on a par with the capacity to find spontaneously the most physiological postures. In our own practice a homelike environment is always possible and beneficial (except at the time of a cesarean birth). The best way to reduce the risks is first to make the labor easier.

An informed-consent form accepting the physiological disturbances induced by a conventional hospital atmosphere might be also signed!

M. Odent

The birth may be attended by either a member of the obstetrical staff or a member of the family practice or nurse-midwifery staff with backup from an attending obstetrician. One-to-one nursing care is provided throughout the labor and birth and for 4 hours after birth by a special group of obstetrical nurses who are committed to supporting this type of maternity care. The nurses frequently monitor the infant's heartbeat with a Doptone, counting for 15-second intervals following a contraction to detect any abnormalities in fetal heart rate. The obstetrical staff are present but unobtrusive in their involvement with the family. The mother moves about and labors in a position of comfort with support from her family and staff (Fig. 2-21). At the time of birth a simple pack is opened, and the mother delivers her infant with the assistance of the physician or midwife. The mother's legs are held by one of her support persons rather than by stirrups. The infant is immediately dried and placed on the mother's chest with a warm blanket over him and is assessed by the birth center nurse.

COMMENT: Why not, in some cases, use a more physiological posture? For example, rather than supporting a recumbent mother's legs, why not support the shoulders of a squatting mother? When the mother is vertical, for example, resting on the floor after giving birth in a squatting position, one need not place the baby on the mother's chest, but the mother takes the baby in her arms. The skin-to-skin and eye-to-eye contacts are much richer.

M. Odent

CRITERIA FOR IMMEDIATE ROOMING-IN

The criteria for immediate rooming-in follow:
1. Apgar score at 5 minutes greater than 7
2. Weight over 5 pounds, but under 9.5 pounds
3. Heart rate between 110 and 170 beats/min; respiratory rate 37 to 70 breaths/min
4. Color normal
5. Nasal passages open; infant able to breathe without difficulty

If the infant meets these criteria, all further examinations and assessments are done in the room by the pediatricians. At 4 hours hematocrit and Dextrostix tests are done; if there are no problems and the mother and infant meet the early discharge criteria shown below, discharge is permitted as early as 6 hours after the birth.

MOTHER
1. No signs or symptoms of complications requiring close supervision (hemorrhage, signs of infection, etc.)

2. Length of labor:
   Under 30 hours for primiparous mother
   Under 24 hours for multiparous mother
3. Membranes ruptured less than 24 hours prior to birth
4. Episiotomy or laceration sutured without extension to anus; no vaginal or cervical lacerations and no severe bruising
5. Blood loss under 500 ml
6. Spontaneous vaginal delivery; early discharge permitted with low-forceps delivery
7. No mother who has had spinal, caudal, epidural, or general anesthesia may go home in less than 24 hours
8. Vital signs normal
9. Fundus firm with no excessive bleeding
10. Hematocrit over 32% and/or hemoglobin over 10.5 gm/100 ml
11. Ability to urinate without difficulty
12. If Rh-negative mother, Rho-Gam eligibility determined and plan for administration developed
13. Ability to walk easily and care for self and baby
14. Plan for assistance at home for at least 2 days

INFANT

1. At least 6 hours old
2. Birth weight over 5 pounds, under 9.5 pounds
3. Vital signs normal
4. Physical examination by pediatrician normal
5. Hematocrit between 45% and 65%; Dextrostix over 45 mg/dl
6. If Rh-negative mother, cord blood shows no signs of incompatibility
7. No complications requiring additional observation
8. At least one feeding observed by birth center nurse
9. Mother able to demonstrate she can handle and care for infant
10. Birth certificate complete
11. Home care record understood*

When early discharge occurs, nursing staff from the birth center make home visits at 24 and 72 hours, and any abnormalities of the mother or infant are reported to the obstetrician or pediatrician, respectively. All patients are visited at 72 hours to assure their well-being and to obtain the state-required phenylketonuria (PKU) sample. If indicated, a bilirubin determination is also done.

---

*In the home care record the parents make notes of first urination (notify if not within 24 hours), first meconium stool (notify if not by 36 hours), feedings, and any changes in infant.

ISSUES

1. *Safety*. Of the first 800 women to be admitted to the birth center at Mount Zion, 607 actually gave birth in the center (76%) (Ballard et al., 1980). Of the 193 women who were moved from the birth center, 68 (8.5%) required a cesarean birth (the majority for cephalopelvic disproportion); 15 women were removed for elective anesthesia, 37 for failure to progress, and 51 for prolonged rupture of the membranes of whom 31 returned to the birth center for delivery after a regular labor pattern was established. There were 53 women with either a fetal or maternal complication, such as heavy meconium staining or fetal heart rate abnormalities, transferred to the regular labor and delivery suite.

Seventy-four of the 800 infants (9.25%) required admission to the nursery. More than one third of these admissions were for dilutional exchange transfusion for venous hematocrit greater than 65%. Twenty-three percent were observed in the nursery for delivery through meconium. There was one infant death. This infant had a high meningomyelocele, and the family and staff decided against surgery. There have been no maternal deaths.

The safety of the center has been compared with outcome in 200 women giving birth in the regular labor and delivery suite at the time of the opening of the birth center in 1976. These women met the medical criteria for delivery in the center, but either they or their obstetricians chose the traditional service. The lower use of anesthesia and analgesia by mothers in the birth center was notable. The outcome for the infants with regard to the need for resuscitation, or admission to the nursery was also favorable when compared with that of infants born in the regular labor and delivery suite.

Emergency situations arose in 1.5% of births in the alternative birth center in which there would have been significant morbidity or mortality in either the mother or infant had the birth occurred in the home; for example, the necessity of endotracheal intubation for resuscitation of the infant (thick meconium discovered too late to move the mother), an infant with congenital heart disease, and mothers with significant postpartum hemorrhage. Infection has not been a problem in the birth center. Siblings who attend the birth or visit soon after are screened by nursing personnel for infection. Questionnaires returned by the first 500 women giving birth in the birth center reported eight infants who developed superficial *Staphylococcus aureus* skin lesions. On review, all of these infants had required admission to the regular nursery for some period of time after birth. There were 43 infants in whom some type of upper respiratory tract infection was reported within the first 4 months of life. All except two of the first 800 infants have been breastfed.

COMMENT: A practical point I found in one of the three alternative birth centers I visited in the United States was a labor care program or contract for each mother. This was developed during

pregnancy between parents and caregiver and gave clear details of the parents' wishes. This approach impressed me greatly and is something that could be implemented anywhere.
D. Henschel

2. *Sibling presence at birth.* The presence of siblings at births was a major issue among families interested in the development of our birth center. They felt that inclusion of siblings was an important part of a viable alternative to home-birth experiences. At the same time, questions were raised by pediatricians and mental health professionals about the impact on the siblings of such inclusion. Therefore we have had an ongoing study of several issues around this feature of the program.

The first issue involved the motivation of the parents. We interviewed a group of families before and after the birth. Children and parents were interviewed separately by our research social worker and psychologist. Reasons for wanting to include siblings at birth fell into three main categories: (1) opposition to traditional exclusion of children from birth; (2) concerns about a more natural transition for older siblings; and (3) concerns about sibling rivalry.

Many families choosing a birth center would have preferred home birth if the physical safety of the infant and mother could have been guaranteed. A considerable number of families, however, came from the other end of the spectrum. These families preferred a hospital setting but considered the technological emphasis in most obstetrical services too intrusive into their birth experience. This group of families generally viewed that including siblings was a part of humanizing the experience. The traditional exclusion of children from any part of the hospital experience did not make sense to them. Some mothers felt more comfortable having their child or children present than leaving them at a relative's or friend's house. In these families children had often assumed they *would* be present and expressed surprise when asked by parents if they *wanted* to be present. In general, this first group of families could be characterized as "against hospitalism." Acting from this perspective, a number of families came to the birth center orientation session prepared to *demand* sibling participation; occasionally, when they found the policies provided for this, they no longer felt compelled to have their children present for the birth.

The second group of parents might be characterized as "for families." They demonstrated a strong emphasis on family togetherness. Parental and child roles were well defined, and cohesion was stressed throughout the family relationship. In some of these families, all siblings slept in the same room, even though other bedrooms were available in the home. These families were most concerned with integrating the new infant into the existing family structure in a smooth and controlled way for the siblings. One mother in this group whose infant had just been born, when handed her baby, gave him to the father and went to talk quietly with her 4-year-old child, whom she sensed was worried about something. The movitation for sibling inclusion at the birth for these families appeared to be a strengthening of the family unit.

Although all parents surely give thought to problems of sibling rivalry, a small number of families in our study believed this to be the most important reason for including other children in the birth of a sibling. They thought that sibling rivalry would be diminished if children participated in the experience of a new sibling's birth and that the children would become so attached to the new infant that they would live in harmony. This notion, unfortunately, overlooks the fact that even parents sometimes fail to live in continuous harmony with their children. Conflict is unavoidable in parent-child and sibling-sibling relationships and serves the purpose, hopefully, of furthering ego development and social maturation.

A second part of our study focused on observing the behavior of children present at births, using a behavior checklist and affect-rating scale completed by the nurse attending the birth. This part of the study has been reported in detail previously by Leonard and associates (1979). Our purpose was to monitor whether children displayed signs of distress by noting children's activity during five stages of the birth center experience: early labor, late labor, birth of the infant, delivery of the placenta, and episiotomy repair (if necessary).

A natural progression in the children's behavior was evident. Initially, most children played or talked with the mother. Some children timed contractions. During late labor, when the mother was generally unavailable, the children tended to withdraw. They moved back in the room and watched. At this point two active children were removed by the father or a support person who felt the children were too distracting to the mother. In another family a nurse asked the support person to take a child who seemed upset outside the room.

Most children watched the birth and afterwards moved toward the mother and newborn infant. There was great interest in the infant and only a few children noticed delivery of the placenta.

Some parts of labor and birth were somewhat distressing to some of the children. Although different children responded differently during the various stages of the experience, sounds made by the mother often were worrisome to the children unless they had been prepared specifically to expect unusual sounds and could interpret them as signs of labor progressing. Children who watched the episiotomy repair frequently had many questions, and one child cried. Support persons were most helpful when a child showed signs of overt distress; however, they varied in their ability to sense subtle signs of stressful responses.

Our preliminary observations have sometimes been construed by others as advocation of sibling participation at birth as a uniformly positive experience. We do believe that the effects of inclusion in the birth of a sibling are largely dependent on the quality of the family life and relationships and to some extent are dependent on the developmental level of the child. We respect a family's wish to find a propitious way of introducing a new sibling and have endeavored to accommodate them. We do not necessarily, however, believe that sibling presence for the entire birth experience is either the only or the best way to make this transition.

COMMENT: Sibling involvement in a birth must remain a big question mark! Even when long-term effects have been obtained, they will not alter the fact that the presence of a child during the birth process must be a very careful individual decision, for which the long-term effects cannot be assessed in advance.
D. Henschel

We have developed the following guidelines that have proved helpful in planning and managing sibling participation in the birth center.

a. Discourage children under 4 years of age. They are less likely to ask questions about what they do not understand, and they are still dependent on their mothers for emotional support. If a child under 4 years is part of a larger sibling group and his or her absence would be notable, this must be taken into consideration.

b. Provide a sibling orientation program.

c. Screen children for infection.

d. Provide a support person for the child who knows him or her well. Select someone who will remember to focus on the child during the time of the birth.

e. Provide an ancillary room for the child with toys and food.

f. Give age-appropriate information. Children being prepared for attendance at a birth are often overloaded with information. Some books and films may be too explicit. Children should be informed that their mothers may make distressing sounds during the labor and birth.

g. Discuss all *routine* details. Drawing blood for laboratory work from the mother, for example, may scarcely be noticed by adults but may be frightening to a child.

h. Respect each child's way of handling the situation. A "sleepy" child may be trying to maintain some distance. Although the child may miss the actual birth, the sense that the family wanted him to share an important experience will be remembered.

We are also interested in the long-term impact on these children of being present at a sibling's birth. One thing that is clear to us is that the involvement of the sibling in the period immediately after the birth, minimizing separation of the family and including the older child in a very happy experience, has been a positive and well-accepted event for both the families and the staff (Fig. 2-22).

COMMENT: In regard to siblings, the questions are put in only one direction: What is the impact on the siblings? The questions must be put also in the other direction: Does the sibling's presence affect the process of labor? Our own experience suggests that the sibling presence seems to be often negative in this point of view, as if creating an inhibition, as if preventing the would-be mother

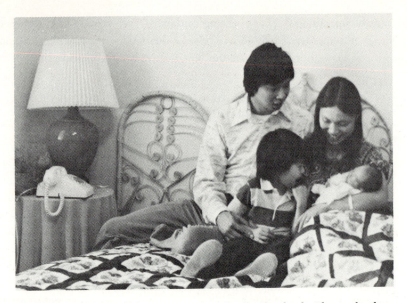

Fig. 2-22. Sibling joins the parents and new infant shortly after birth. This is clearly a positive experience for all.

from reducing the control by the upper brain, from "regressing," that is, preventing her from becoming more instinctive. More generally speaking, there are usually too many people watching the woman in labor. It is fundamental to disclose which person is negative—sometimes the obstetrician sometimes the baby's father, or exceptionally the midwife if she is not an experienced female and not ready to engage herself effectively.
M. Odent

3. *Relevance of the alternative birth center to other kinds of maternity care.* Can the positive aspects of maternity services as provided in a birth center be translated to other facets of perinatal care? It is our feeling that the development of the alternative birth center rooms, per se, was more necessary in 1976 for changing staff attitudes than for providing care for the families involved. We believe that separate birth center rooms will ultimately be considered to have been a fad in making the transition to providing a style of maternity care that is identified with sensitivity to humanistic concerns. We think that the need for such sensitivity will be recognized for all women, whether they are classified high risk or low risk, and whether or not they desire anesthesia or analgesia. Certainly, staff throughout our perinatal program have come to place greater emphasis on the emotional and supportive aspects of care and to include families in decision-making processes to a greater extent than previously.

From questionnaires sent to families who have used the birth center, we have learned that the most significant thing for them about this experience is not having been separated from family and friends during an important time in their lives. The second significant aspect of the program for these families is the supportive staff, who allowed them to have control over their experiences and demonstrated flexibility within the hospital situation. The room is considered to be a nicety but is definitely less important than other issues with which the alternative birth center movement has been concerned.

4. *Can an alternative birth center improve parenting for the socially "high risk?"* What is the relevance of this type of care for the single, the poor, and the teenage mother? We do not know the answer to this question because, to date, the birth center continues to be sought out by a primarily middle-class, highly educated group of families. However, in viewing the uniformly positive impact of this experience on these families, it is hard to imagine that it would not be wise to provide at least the humanistic qualities of the birth center experience for all mothers. As mentioned earlier, we have seen positive changes in staff-patient relationships throughout our perinatal services as a result of staff participation in the birth center. The qualities sought by the families have included a measure of control, flexibility, and support. Surely, women whose social circumstances are consonant with great stress must benefit from extension of these aspects of care to all women experiencing childbirth.

5. *Is the alternative birth center a true alternative to home birth?* The question remains whether parents will choose hospital or home births. Our experience has indicated increasingly that the answer to this question will be hospital births *if* birth center programs are based on attitudes that admit flexibility and are not regimented. The parents considering home births who are deeply concerned about their children's welfare, we believe, will choose a hospital setting that offers choice, control, and keeping the family together.

SUMMARY

The experience described here has been our program's attempt to respond to what we have seen as important and legitimate concerns for maternity care services. Our alternative birth center has been a rewarding and exciting effort that has had a positive impact on staff attitudes and understanding of humanistic aspects of maternity care in terms of services provided to families throughout the perinatal program and on the training of obstetrical and pediatric house officers. We feel that the accomplishments realized in changing maternity care in the birth center represent only the beginning of a general recognition by all health professionals of the need to respond to the human as well as the technical requirements of medical care.

CHAPTER 3

CARE OF THE SIBLING

MARY ANNE TRAUSE and NANCY A. IRVIN

The little child does not necessarily love his brothers and sisters, and is often quite frank
about it. It is unquestionable that in them he sees and hates his rivals.
Sigmund Freud

Toddlers and preschoolers love to explore their world and discover the delights of mastering new experiences. When confident about the whereabouts of their loved ones and the security they provide, children can venture away with only occasional returns for refueling. However, when young children encounter stressful events, the balance between exploration and security tips, and the need for support and reassurance takes priority. Events that upset children's familiar routines are especially difficult, since routines provide the framework within which new experiences become manageable.

For some children the experience of having and becoming a sibling is likely to be among the most stressful of early childhood (Legg and co-workers, 1974). With the arrival of a new baby, both familiar routines and familiar relationships begin to take on unexpected dimensions. Mommy's lap and Daddy's attention may not be as available after the new baby's birth, even though they may be needed more than ever. To many children the new baby seems to replace the old one. As Stein (1974a, p. 6) says, "And why would a mother want a new baby, unless the old one were not good enough?" Some clinicians even go so far as to compare the birth of a sibling to the death of a parent in terms of its potential significance for later personality development (Moore and Ucko, 1961).

BASIC CONSIDERATIONS
Responses to the birth of a sibling

The most common reactions to the birth of a sibling described in the literature include hostility or aggression directed toward the baby or mother, regression in some areas of functioning, and increased efforts to gain attention. At the same time, investigators report that children often show spurts in mastery or independence once they have become older brothers or sisters.

110

When discussing the stressful nature of the experience, Legg and co-workers (1974) refer to Henchie's (1963) study of the reactions of 66 young children to the birth of a sibling: 15% were extremely negative and 27% slightly so. The younger the child at the time of the birth the more likely disturbances were to occur. Distinctly negative reactions were found in 89% of the children under 3 years of age but in only 11% of those over 6 years. The sex of the newborn also affected sibling reactions, with male babies causing more difficulty. For boys, a new brother evoked more negative reactions than did a new sister. For girls, a new brother was more likely than a new sister to cause disturbances in their relationships with their mothers. Henchie (1963) also reported that the older siblings' reactions worsened as the infants grew into play-disrupting toddlers.

Sostek and Read's (1979) recent work supports a number of Henchie's findings. Based on questionnaires completed by mothers when their infants were 2 months old and again when they were 9 to 10 months, Sostek investigated the reactions of firstborns between 1 and 6 years of age to the birth of a sibling. Eighty-five mothers returned completed questionnaires at 2 months and 61 again when their baby was 9 to 10 months. The results indicated that attention-seeking behavior toward the mother and affectionate behavior toward the infant were generally more frequent than regression or hostility. However, as the infants grew toward toddlerhood, attention seeking and affection diminished as hostility toward the baby increased. Younger children (less than 3 years old) showed regression in eating and using pacifiers. No regression was noted in toileting behavior. Increases in sleep disturbances became more prevalent as the infants grew older.

Sostek and Read, like Henchie, found the sex of the newborn to influence older siblings' reactions, although these influences varied with both the sex and age of infants. When new babies were female, siblings, especially boys, showed increased attention-seeking behavior. Hostility, on the other hand, was greater toward 2-month-old male infants and toward 10-month-old female infants. Most hostility at 10 months was shown by siblings who were male and/or younger than 3 years old.

In a study designed, in part, to assess the reactions to becoming siblings of 37 firstborn children who were 1 to 3$^{1}/_{2}$ years old, members of our group observed mother-child interaction and asked mothers to complete questionnaires a few weeks before and again after their second child's arrival (Trause et al., 1977). The sample of children as a whole showed significantly more problems in daily routines after the sibling birth. Ninety-two percent of the children showed an increase of at least one problem; 54% showed an increase of three or more problems. The largest increase in problems occurred in sleeping patterns, with 73% of the children showing more sleep disturbances after the birth of their sibling. Significant increases also occurred in behavior problems, such as temper tantrums and excessive activity, with girls showing greater increases than boys in this area. Children were observed to stay near their mothers more after the sibling's birth, with children younger than

1¹/₂ years of age showing the greatest increase. In terms of improvements in behavior, the children showed fewer problems in eating after the younger sibling's arrival (Trause, 1978; Trause et al., 1977).

Anderson (1979) interviewed the parents of 43 children present at the births of their siblings to determine the children's reactions in the months following birth. She also found evidence of some difficult adjustments. Regression was shown by 19% of the children in the forms of increased wetting, thumb sucking, stuttering, and baby talk. Aggression toward the baby or parents was seen in 16% of the children. As in Henchie's and Sostek's findings, hostility toward the infant increased as the infant became mobile. On the positive side, 42 of the 43 children wanted to participate in the infant's care, and all parents perceived the siblings as having loving relationships in the first weeks.

These studies offer empirical support for the frequent observation that the appearance of a sibling is troublesome for many young children and strains their capacity to adjust. Yet research barely begins to clarify the factors involved in making this experience so trying. From the toddler or preschooler's point of view, the most salient attributes of the experience are likely to be the separation from the mother associated with a hospital birth and the appearance of a new baby. Examining these factors may help health professionals to modify their health care policies for families who are attempting to cope with the stresses of a new sibling.

Maternal separation

In three of the four studies cited earlier (Henchie, 1963; Sostek and Read, 1979; Trause, 1978) in which significant numbers of children displayed distress reactions after the births of younger siblings, the mothers had given birth in hospitals. Our study (Trause, 1978) suggests that separation played a role in causing children's distress. In addition to assessing children's behavior before and after sibling birth, we filmed the reunions of children and mothers at the time of hospital discharge. Approximately one half of the children had visited during their mothers' four- to six-day hospital stay and one half had not visited. During the filmed reunion, children who had not visited were much more likely to avoid contact with their mothers than the children who had seen their mothers in the hospital. Children who had not visited usually looked up only momentarily as their mothers entered the room, then deliberately looked away, keeping their gazes averted as much as possible. If mothers attempted to embrace them, the children either stiffened or turned away. They neither smiled nor verbally greeted their mothers, and they kept their interest glued to the toys that were present. Mothers often responded to these rebuffs with comments like, "I'm your mother!" or "She doesn't even care." One said afterward that her 16-month-old had looked right through her.

Children who had visited, on the other hand, often ran to meet their mothers, exclaiming, "There's Mommy!" with a smile and ready hug. During these reunions children who had visited were also more likely to hug or kiss their mothers and to say they liked the new baby. The emotional distance shown by nonvisiting children suggests that being separated from their mothers without the benefits of even one short visit was distressing for them. Surprisingly, even one short visit seemed to allay some of their anxieties. Among the 21 families Legg and co-workers (1974) interviewed about the reactions of preschoolers to the births of siblings, the contact helped the children (especially toddlers) remember that "out of sight" did not mean "out of mind" in every case where the children visited their mothers in the hospital.

Robertson and Robertson's (1971) work presents detailed descriptions of the behavior of four children whom they fostered and of one child who was placed in a residential nursery while their mothers were hospitalized for childbirth. The children were 17 to 29 months old, and separations lasted from nine to 27 days. Although all the children showed distress while separated from their parents, only John, who spent nine days in a residential nursery, was devastated by the experience. In nine days he changed from an easy, undemanding, lively 17-month-old to a despairing child who alternated between convulsive sobbing and impassive apathy. The description of his reunion with his mother suggests the intensity of his disappointment at being abandoned by her to strangers in an unfamiliar setting that was utterly out of tune with his particular needs.

> At the sight of his mother John was galvanized into action. He threw himself about crying loudly, and after stealing a glance at his mother looked away from her. Several times he looked, then turned away over the nurse's shoulder with loud cries and a distraught expression.
>
> After a few minutes the mother took him on her knee, but John continued to struggle and scream, arching his back away from his mother, and eventually got down and ran crying desperately to the observer (Joyce Robertson). She calmed him down, gave him a drink, and passed him back to his mother. He lay cuddled into her, clutching his wooly blanket but not looking at her.*

John's first month back home was extremely rocky, with frequent temper tantrums and severe deterioration in eating and sleeping patterns. For several weeks his behavior toward his mother alternated between rejection and clinginglike behavior. Although John seemed to have a much better relationship with his mother after a month, at $4^{1}/_{2}$ years of age he was still fearful of losing her and became upset if she was not where he thought she would be.

The four children for whom the Robertsons provided consistent sensitive care clearly missed their mothers and were under stress, but they did not exhibit John's desperate unhappiness. Rather than breaking down right away, the children were

---

*From Robertson, J., and Robertson, J.: Young children in brief separation: a fresh look, Psychoanal. Study Child **26:**293, 1971.

active and cheerful for the first few days of separation. In some cases the Robertsons felt this cheerfulness was a result of the children's attempts to defend against their anxiety. These initial reactions often gave way to more turbulent behavior, including sadness, anger, lowered frustration tolerance, restlessness, increased thumb sucking, poorer sleeping, outbursts of aggression, and pretending to be a baby. Thomas, the child who seemed to manage the separation best, was 28 months old and the most mature child in the sample. Since he was able to express his anxieties verbally, the foster parents could help him maintain an understanding of the situation.

Three of these four children showed changes in behavior after separation that suggested how difficult it had been for them. The problems included restless sleeping, bedwetting, increased crying and demand for bottles, increased defiance, aggression, and deliberate disobedience. Although under considerable strain, these children developed relationships with the foster mother that were sufficient to sustain them and keep their anxiety manageable. In the words of the Robertsons (1971) they ". . . functioned and related well, learned new skills and new words, and greeted their mothers warmly. The separations had not been traumatic. The children had not been overwhelmed."

How detrimental are separations from the mother for the young child's subsequent development? There is some controversy about this issue. Many of the early observations of hospitalized children's reactions were made by James Robertson while he was a researcher at the Tavistock Clinic in London (Robertson, 1953, 1958). In 1953 he delineated the phases of Protest, Despair, and Denial (later called Detachment). John Bowlby, a leading theoretician on infant-to-mother attachment, has summarized these observations.

Whenever a young child who has had the opportunity to develop an attachment to a mother figure is separated from her unwillingly he shows distress; and should he also be placed in a strange environment and cared for by a succession of strange people such distress is likely to be intense. The way he behaves follows a typical sequence. At first he *protests* vigorously and tries by all means available to him to recover his mother. Later he seems to *despair* of recovering her but none the less remains preoccupied with her and vigilant for her return. Later still he seems to lose his interest in his mother and to become emotionally *detached* from her. Nevertheless, provided the period of separation is not too prolonged a child does not remain detached indefinitely. Sooner or later after being reunited with his mother his attachment to her emerges afresh. Thenceforward, for days or weeks, and sometimes for much longer, he insists on staying close to her. Furthermore, whenever he suspects he will lose her again he exhibits acute anxiety.*

---

*From Bowlby, J.: The making and breaking of affectional bonds, Br. J. Psychiatr. **130:**421-431, 1977.

Few would disagree that prolonged separation in a strange environment with multiple caregivers, like the one experienced by John (Robertson and Robertson, 1971), leads to the protest-despair-detachment syndrome. However, in a number of recent works, various clinicians and researchers, including the Robertsons (1971), Rutter (1979), Dunn (1977), and Legg and co-workers (1974), have questioned the universality of these reactions during brief separations. They feel that the impact of separations varies tremendously, depending on the reasons for the separation and the child's preparation, how long the separation lasts, with whom and where the child is left, and the child's age and level of maturity. Legg and co-workers (1974) concluded that children could tolerate the temporary separation from their mothers well if they were solidly prepared beforehand, if they stayed at home with a familiar person, if their fathers were actively involved, and if visits to their mothers were possible. Rutter (1979) has gone further in suggesting that beyond being merely tolerable, some separations may even be beneficial. In recent studies Emde and Robinson (in press) have demonstrated the importance of the emotional availability of the mother. Children whose mothers were present but not responsive because they were preoccupied with thoughts or feelings (e.g., busy reading a newspaper) stayed close to their mothers, were fearful, and did almost no exploring. This may have relevance for some mothers who are overtired and burdened in the first weeks after returning home with the new baby. (See section of this chapter on Changes in the mother-child relationship.)

Thus separations from the mother are potentially traumatic for the toddler or preschooler. Yet with careful planning and consideration of the child's needs, the stressfulness of the experience can be largely diminished. Hospital policies, such as sibling visiting and early discharge, can be designed to minimize the potential hazards of separation.

Children present at birth

Largely in response to the separations inherent in traditional hospital births—separation of mother and father, mother and older children, parents and newborn, and newborn and siblings—increasing numbers of couples are choosing to give birth at home or in maternity centers or hospitals that allow the family to stay together throughout the birth experience. Home births tripled between 1973 and 1978. Hospitals countered with "birthing rooms" or "alternative birth centers," which numbered over 1000 by 1979. The practice of sibling participation in hospital births began as a California phenomenon in about 1976 (Goodell, 1980). A nationwide survey by the American College of Obstetricians and Gynecologists in 1979 found that in a sample of 78 alternative birth centers, 53% allowed children in the labor facilities and 44% at the births. It has been estimated that 50 to 100 hospitals allow children to attend births at the present time (Goodell, 1980).

Yet little is known about how attending a birth affects young children. The existing empirical studies primarily describe the behavior of participating children during labor and birth. One observational study of 40 children, 1 to 14 years of age, who attended the births of their siblings at the Mt. Zion Hospital Alternative Birth Center in San Francisco, reports that the children's behavior varied according to the mother's stage of labor or birth (Leonard et al., 1979). During early labor children typically interacted with their mothers by asking questions, timing contractions, and acting solicitously. As the mother became less accessible during late labor, children generally drew back and observed. The investigators noted that there was often an increase in the intensity of the children's natural coping style during this period: quiet children became even more quiet, and active children became restless and distracting to others. Most children watched during the birth, although a few watched only intermittently. By the time the placenta was delivered, most children were involved with the newborn infant. The behavior of children whose mothers needed repairs for episiotomies or lacerations varied during this stage. Although one child seemed distressed, most ignored the surgery, asked questions, or watched intermittently without apparent distress. After birth the children's excitement quickly subsided, and they usually resumed their normal activities soon thereafter. The investigators concluded that "no child displayed extreme distress while present at the birth of a sibling, but some parts of labor and delivery did seem to be somewhat distressing to some children." A recommendation was made that children under 4 years of age not be present unless part of a larger sibling group because they are less likely to ask questions about what they do not understand and they are still fairly dependent on their mothers for emotional support (Leonard et al., 1979).

According to parental reports, children present during the births of their siblings at home behaved similarly to those described in the Leonard study (Anderson, 1979; Mehl et al., 1977). Children usually entered and left their mother's room of their own accord, with older children staying for longer periods. They usually interacted with mothers early, then became increasingly observant as labor progressed. Mehl and colleagues (1977) found that children were concerned about their mothers after birth and needed an acknowledgement from her before shifting their attention to the baby. Anderson (1979) found that in 17 of 25 cases, parents reported their children spontaneously reached out to touch the baby soon after birth. Both studies of children present at home births reported the experience to be positive for most children (Anderson, 1979; Mehl et al., 1977). Mehl and colleagues found that seeing blood seemed to be especially worrisome for 6- to 10-year-olds. Leonard and co-workers (1979) reported that in the hospital children especially noticed their mother's labor sounds, which were sometimes upsetting.

Unfortunately, no study either compares children's behavior and concerns before and after participation in birth or presents data on children's reactions to becoming a sibling in the days and weeks after birth as a function of the level of participation in the birth. Mehl and colleagues (1977) did examine children's notions of where babies come from in relation to their experience of sibling birth. Children from 2 to 14 years of age who attended births were reported to have accurate notions as to how babies were born, whereas children not present "seemed mystified and found the idea of birth puzzling and inconceivable."

Anderson (1979) who gathered data cited earlier on responses in the weeks following birth for 43 children present at the birth of a sibling, attempted to collect data on a control group. This was not possible, however, because there were too many differences between groups to allow meaningful comparisons. An illustration of this can be found in the work of Mehl and colleagues (1977), who compared the sexual attitudes of parents who chose to have their children present at birth with those of parents who chose to exclude them. The attitudes of the two sets of parents were notably different, suggesting a wide diversity in the ways the two sets of children were raised. Thus, as surmised by Anderson, parents who presently choose to include their children in childbirth are likely to represent populations different from those who choose otherwise. At present we simply do not know how attending the birth of a sibling affects children. Their short- and long-term emotional and behavioral responses are likely to be result of a variety of factors, such as the family's attitudes and interaction patterns before and after birth, the birth experience itself, and the age, maturity, and temperament of the child.

CLINICAL CONSIDERATIONS

At first glance, the birth of a sibling suggests one change in a young child's life: the addition of a new brother or sister. In fact, the birth of a sibling ushers in a host of changes. Alterations in routines and family interactions begin for the toddler or preschooler even before the new baby arrives. During pregnancy the mother's familiar body changes, as may her moods and level of energy. As Stein (1974) described it, "Before the new baby was born, there was already no lap for Charles." And this is just the beginning. A new brother or sister is also likely to cause rearrangements in living space, to alter existing family relationships, and to create new ones.

Changes in the physical environment

Because more living space is often needed as the size of the family grows, many families move shortly before or after a child is born. Legg and co-workers (1974) found that a move to a new home soon after the birth of a sibling was such a stressful event that regression, separation anxiety, and problems with aggression could all be manifested in response to it. As an illustration, they described the case of a girl who was 14 months older than her new sibling and who accepted her new sister very well, continuing to be an open and active toddler. Four months later, when the family moved and the sisters began sharing a room, the older sibling became extremely withdrawn, regressed in her ability to dress herself, developed sleep disturbances, and did not achieve toilet training at the expected time. The investigators concluded that a move which removes the security of a child's known environment provides a type of stress which may trigger maladaptive reactions when coinciding with a sibling's birth.

Legg and co-workers (1974) also highlight the potential stressfulness of changes in sleeping arrangements coinciding with the birth of a sibling. Many children in their sample responded adversely when the new baby slept in the parents' room. Jealousy, sleep disturbances, and regression often appeared as manifestations of the older child's feelings of exclusion. The situation was intensified when the older child was accustomed to sleeping with the parents. The introduction of a new "big" bed also frequently accompanies the arrival of a new sibling. Legg and co-workers suggest that young children can best manage these changes in sleeping arrangements when they occur well before the new baby arrives and when they are associated with a sense of achievement rather than the necessity of making room for the new sibling. Many parents who were interviewed used successful techniques for helping their children accept these changes.

> **COMMENT:** A new baby plus a separation is a time of crisis for any very young child, when his resources are stretched to meet the stress. We agree that it is advisable to avoid moves of home and changes of sleeping quarters. However, the child of under about $2^{1}/_{2}$ years of age, because he is still a baby himself, cannot be adequately prepared for events by explanations. We suggest therefore that entrance to nursery school, toilet training, or weaning from bottle and comforters should be added to the list of potential stresses to be avoided at this time so that all the child's resources are available to deal with the separation and the new baby.
> **James and Joyce Robertson**

Changes in the mother-child relationship

The mother-child relationship is likely to become strained as the mother finds herself meeting the demands of a newborn. We found mothers using more stern or angry commands with their firstborns two to four weeks after the births of younger siblings than they used before childbirth (Trause, 1978). Taylor and Kogan (1973) reported a consistent decrease in the expression of warmth and an increase in the emotional flatness of both mothers and children after the births of new siblings. The postpartum mothers were observed to be fatigued and appeared to react to their firstborn $2^{1}/_{2}$- to $3^{1}/_{2}$-year-old youngsters with more effort during videotaped sessions one to two months after childbirth (Taylor and Kogan, 1973). Mothers reported less time for everything as the number of small children increased.

Aside from behavioral changes on the mother's part, she is likely to feel both guilty and sad about the diminished time she has for her older child, yet resentful of the intrusions he makes on her time with the newborn. Many mothers have commented that breastfeeding a second baby can be a trial because the older child quickly discovers that nursing is the opportune time to act out frustrations. One toddler routinely turned all the lights out when the mother was breastfeeding at night and turned them all on whenever she breastfed during the day. How mothers handle these bids for attention—whether with increased nurturance or increased discipline—is likely to affect greatly how the older child manages his distress.

Changes in the father-child relationship

Becoming a father for the first time involves a number of adjustments for most men. First-time fathers-to-be are known to experience concerns about such issues as the health and well-being of their wives and newborns, the added financial responsibilities of a child, how their relationships with their wives will change, and how well they will cope with being fathers (McNall, 1976). Much less is known about the concerns of men becoming fathers for the second, third, or fourth time. One can imagine, however, that a number of the same concerns appear during each pregnancy. For example, second-time fathers probably worry about the health of their wives and expected babies, how to father more than one, how an additional child will affect established family interaction patterns, and how the family will manage the added expenses. They also may wonder how their first children will cope with the prospective changes and how they can divide the strong feelings of love that have been focused on the older child. In short, fathers, like mothers and children, are likely to experience some inner turmoil as their families grow. In addition, they are likely to have to cope with added responsibilities as they serve as liaisons between hospitalized mothers and children at home, fill in for busier-than-usual mothers, and juggle demands from work and home. The more adequately fathers can cope with these conflicts and pressures the better they will be able to help their first children master the stresses of becoming and having siblings.

> **COMMENT:** Fathers also miss the interest and attention of their wives as the second child and the first child require and dilute the availability of the mother.
> **A. Solnit**

Legg and co-workers (1974) have highlighted the importance of the father's role in the older child's experience, especially if the mother gives birth in a hospital. The investigators concluded that "the prior and contemporary involvement of father in the older child's life seems to relate directly to the level of adjustment made by the child to the temporary separation from mother and to the degree of acceptance shown to the new sibling." If the mother is physically absent during birth and emotionally distant after birth, the father can provide continuity in his children's emotional lives. The five case studies described by the Robertsons (1971) showed that the children keenly missed their fathers while living away from home. The children typically looked forward to their fathers' visits and showed increasingly intense sadness and anger on their fathers' repeated departures. Both physical and emotional separations from the father are likely to be especially difficult when children are already undergoing the stressfulness of their mothers' absence. Even in home births, Anderson (1979) reported that one fourth of the participating children were unusually close to their fathers after the births of their siblings.

When a special problem occurs

As difficult as it may be for children to adjust to the birth of a healthy full-term sibling, they can usually lean on understanding parents for help with their feelings. With the birth of a sibling who is premature or born with a serious problem, however, children must contend with added burdens. Their parents' happy anticipation of the new baby's birth is likely to have suddenly changed to sadness and worry. The children are probably aware that something is wrong but with only a dim understanding of what that is. Often they will lose the attention of their parents, who are preoccupied by their own shock and grief. Even more than attention, the parents' time may suddenly be filled with hospital visits, unexpected errands, and extra telephone calls from worried family and friends. At a time when young children need their parents the most, they may experience parental busyness, depression, and withdrawal. The toddler or preschool child is likely to become the forgotten family member. Health care professionals can play an important role by helping parents find ways to summon their resources to be available to their children in spite of their personal turmoil.

Sometimes during a crisis the first impulse of parents is to try to protect their children from the sadness and confusion by sending them away to stay with relatives or friends. Parents feel that the stable atmosphere of someone else's home would be better than their own unpredictable surroundings. Experience has shown, however, that this is not likely to help children cope with and master the difficulties associated with the birth of a small or sick sibling. Children manage better when they remain part of the household and experience the family's reality along with their parents.

This conclusion is based on three factors. First, as previously discussed, children are likely to be distressed by being separated from their parents. Their distress will be intensified in a crisis when the separation is likely to be unexpected and surrounded by the aura of emergency.

Second, most children, like adults, suffer more from their fantasies of what has gone wrong than from their firsthand experience with the real problem. When children are sent away from their families, their imaginations evoke fantasies far more frightening than the reality. Away from home, children have few opportunities to correct their fantasies and few trusted adults with whom to share their worries. Since children's suffering is so painful to acknowledge, adults may unwittingly overlook the cues children give to signal their concerns. Unfortunately, children interpret being sent away to mean that what they have to say and what they feel are too burdensome for adults to bear. This leaves them feeling confused and isolated.

Third, children need reassurance from their parents that they were not responsible for the baby's problems. When someone close to us suffers a misfortune, we feel guilty because of the angry feelings we may have had toward this person from time to time. Children often have ambivalent and negative reactions to the prospect of a new baby moving into their lives. Sometimes they even wish the baby would never come. To children these feelings seem enough to have caused the baby's problems, reason enough for the problems to be their fault. Within this context being sent away may be construed as punishment for their evil wishes. Children need to be reassured, perhaps repeatedly, that what happened was completely beyond their control. Parents can say something like, "None of us expected Susie to come early and have to stay in the hospital. Some babies just do that. Nothing you thought or said could have caused it. The doctors and nurses didn't expect her to be early either, but they know how to take good care of her until she grows bigger."

Beyond merely keeping children at home, parents must attempt to discuss what is happening with them. In discussing a newborn's problems with siblings, two issues must be considered: (1) what is wrong with the baby, and (2) how the parents are feeling and why. Even an 18-month-old will know that something is wrong and would profit by parents talking about it. Although the depth and content of discussions will vary with the children's ages, parents should be advised to keep explanations simple, be truthful, take one question at a time, and check to be sure children understand what they have been told (Bittman and Rosenberg, 1978).

COMMENT: The authors are clearly aware of the significance of age and level of development, but in a number of places they appear not to give sufficient weight to this factor.

In our experience children under about 2¹/₂ years of age are unlikely to verbalize their fantasies and are unlikely to be verbally reassured. In our films *Jane* and *Lucy* (17 and 21 months, respectively) we see vividly the impossibility of verbal reassurance at this early level of development. Even in the films *Thomas* and *Kate* (2.4 and 2.5 years of age), although these two older children sometimes show through play what is worrying them, verbal reassurance has only limited value and is liable to cause confusion (Robertson and Robertson, 1967, 1968, 1971, 1973). The 2¹/₂-year-old may be able to repeat what he has been told, but that is no guarantee he understands or will remember the explanations.
James and Joyce Robertson

If a baby is born prematurely, toddlers and preschoolers can be told something like, "Baby Peter came too early and he is too small to come home yet. He needs special care in the hospital until he grows bigger. Mommy and Daddy are sad because we miss him just like we miss you when you are not with us." A baby who is born with a congenital anomaly like Down's syndrome may seem perfect to the siblings. Nonetheless, parents are likely to be terribly upset, and so the children must be told why. Parents might say something like, "Lisa is a special kind of baby. We can take her home and take care of her just like any baby. She can look around and eat and sleep and soon she'll smile at us. But Mommy and Daddy are sad because when Lisa is 2 years old, she won't be able to do what you could do when you were 2, and when she's 5, she won't be able to do all that you will be able to do when you are 5 years old. Sometimes grown-ups worry about things like that."

If a baby has a congenital anomaly like a cleft lip or palate, the particular defect can be simply explained. Sometimes the problem will seem much less apparent to a child than to adults, who worry about the ramifications of the anomaly. Nurses often report that children first notice a new baby's hands or feet or curly hair. One 5-year-old who was visiting the hospital to see her new brother for the first time, exlaimed, "He looks just like me when I was a baby!" She did not seem to focus on his unilateral cleft lip at all.

In discussing any problems with the siblings, it is important to be reassuring that the baby's problem or illness will not happen to them or to their parents. Children often worry about this, even if they cannot express their fears. The ramifications of why the problem happened to this particular infant or family may continue as issues in the future. The older siblings may wonder for a long time why it happened, and sometimes they begin feeling guilty that they are normal. If an infant's congenital anomaly is one which will continue past infancy, counseling for the family may be helpful in avoiding future problems (Trenino, 1979). Counseling at the time of the crisis can provide support and set the stage for future short interventions.

If the newborn has to stay in an intensive care nursery, visits to see the baby would help siblings both to understand where the baby is and to participate in the family experience. If the visit is very early in the infant's hospitalization, children should be accompanied by their parents and another adult. This will allow the parents to attend to their own needs to assimilate their baby's status and at the same time provide the children with help in understanding and coping with the experience. For some children a sad experience can be so overwhelming that they need to remove themselves from it temporarily, usually by suddenly asking to go somewhere like the cafeteria or by engaging in silly behavior. If someone besides the parents is with the children, this "time out" is easier to provide. If a visit to the intensive care nursery occurs once the newborn's course is stable and parents have made their initial adjustments to having a premature or sick baby, an extra adult may not be needed. Health care professionals can be helpful by offering age-appropriate explanations of the complexities of the intensive care nursery.

Children's reactions to the intensive care nursery are variable and likely to be related to their ages.

COMMENT: There is good reason to question the desirability of toddlers being brought to an intensive care nursery to see their younger sibling. The parents' apprehension or sadness may set the emotional tone for the visit, and the toddler's ability to comprehend the plight of the infant in an isolette with tubes going into the infant's body may be more frightening than reassuring.
A. Solnit

Most children will relate what they see directly to themselves and their own bodies. Thus seeing an infant lying naked in an isolette with monitors and intravenous tubing attached to his body may cause concern. Children are likely to identify with the baby and imagine how they would feel. Depending on their comments and questions, they may need to be reassured that the infant will be protected from most pain. Since children are struggling to attain independence, they may have difficulty relating to an infant who is so completely dependent. Adults can emphasize what the baby can do—see, hear, and hold his big brother's or sister's finger as soon as he comes home.

When the baby dies

A poignant situation occurs if the infant dies. If this occurs before the newborn goes home and the siblings' contact with the baby has been limited, their major reactions are likely to be to the emotional loss felt by their parents. The parents are likely to have a keener sense of loss, having experienced pregnancy and the anticipated birth. Grief is likely to produce an extremely solemn household. Children will feel abandoned if parents do not say what is wrong. As described earlier, parents should discuss both what happened to the baby and how they are feeling.

As much as individuals try to avoid death because they fear it, children should be told honestly that the baby died (or is dead). Using terms like "went to heaven" or "passed away" will be confusing, since children find the permanence of death difficult to comprehend. The truth should be said—that the baby no longer sees or feels or moves. It is only the children and grown-ups who are alive who will feel lonely for the baby they wanted (Stein, 1974*b*). Parents who find talking about the baby's death too difficult at first should tell their children how they feel and reassure their children they will talk more as soon as they are able. It is tremendously important for parents to share their grief and tears with their children. Children are far more able to deal with their parents' sadness than with their parents' emotional withdrawal. However, chronic sorrow or grief would be unduly burdensome for children. Thus parents need to allow themselves to mourn so the family can move on to new experiences.

Even if the older children had limited contact with the baby, they will probably be disappointed and sad not to have a new brother or sister. They may also harbor worries that they are responsible for the death and concerns that they themselves or their parents will also die. A parent or a favorite relative should take time to listen to the children in order to understand and help clarify their confusion.

Many young children of about 3 years of age or older could be included in the funeral or memorial services. Being with the family is better for them than being left with a babysitter.

COMMENT: It depends on how the parents feel and who the babysitter is. A babysitter with an ongoing relationship to the young child can provide adequate supportive care when parents feel they will be unable to provide the care for a young child at a funeral that they feel will be more than they can bear without losing control of their feelings. It is urgent that we enable parents to have options which allow them to make choices as parents which can be useful to their children, to themselves, and above all to the child-parent relationship.
A. Solnit

When children are not included, the message is either that the death of their baby brother or sister is of no concern to them or that they are too little to share in important family experiences. Exclusion may also be interpreted to mean that death is too dangerous or secret for them to know about.

However, children are not likely to behave in the way adults expect at the funeral. They may be alternately serious and restless, solemn and giddy. They may need to get away briefly. Anticipating such a possibility beforehand by asking an understanding and familiar adult besides the parents to stay near them will relieve the tension their restlessness might otherwise cause during the service. Participating in the rituals like the funeral with the family and talking about them afterward will help make the baby and his death real to the siblings. This, in turn, will help them complete their mourning.

Children's normal resilience can be enhanced by including them at a time of family crisis. While parents are coping with nearly all-encompassing shock and grief reactions, health care professionals can be alert to suggesting interventions to clarify confusing issues and to provide support for the whole family. Even though everyone would prefer to spare children from any tragedy, their growth can be enhanced by coping with and overcoming the difficult experience.

SUMMARY

Having and becoming a sibling is likely to introduce a number of changes in a young child's life. Change is not necessarily stressful for young children. In fact, a measure of novelty within the context of the familiar is exciting. However, too many changes at once or changes enforced without regard for the child's needs can be overwhelming. Legg and co-workers (1974) reported that the development of some children appeared to be enhanced after the birth of a younger sibling. The mothers who reported developmental gains, such as the rapid achievement of toilet training or the increased ability to play independently, were the mothers who offered a variety of supportive influences for their children. These included early preparation for the birth, successful introduction of any alteration in sleeping arrangements, contact with the mother during the period of her hospital stay, and the active involvement of the father. When the baby is born prematurely or with a problem, other important supportive measures include the creation of many opportunities for discussing what is wrong with the baby and how the parents are feeling, in addition to reassurances that the older children are not responsible for the problem and that nothing similar is likely to happen to them or their parents.

Even the most sensitive planning, however, will not prevent all adjustment problems. Having a new sibling will be difficult for most children, at least some of the time. Jealousy and rivalry are likely to appear. As Stein (1974a) so aptly stated, "Sibling rivalry is not a disease." It is part of life, and the family may be the safest place for children to learn how to deal with the jealousy and anger they will sometimes feel. Our first task as health care providers is to help parents understand the stresses and opportunities their children will be experiencing so that they can keep change within bounds and provide the supports children need so that they may thrive. Our second task is to understand the stresses and joys the family will be experiencing at the time of childbirth so we can make our health care practices and institutions responsive to their needs and preferences.

RECOMMENDATIONS FOR CARE

1. *Educating parents*. Nurses, midwives, and physicians who see mothers during pregnancy should help them to assess and plan for the changes a new sibling will introduce into family routines and interaction. Options that minimize stress should be discussed.

2. *Sleeping arrangements*. Any changes in sleeping arrangements that involve the older children should be planned and carried out well before the new baby's arrival.

3. *Moves*. When possible, moves to new residences should not coincide with the birth of a sibling.

4. *Caregiving during mother's hospital stay*. Parents should arrange for the best care possible for the older children during the mother's absence for childbirth. Ideally, a well-known, trusted relative (father or grandparent) or friend should care for the children in their own home. The second choice would be a well-known, trusted relative or friend caring for the children in a different home. The third choice would be a stranger who became acquainted with the sibling before the birth in the children's own home. The fourth choice is one no parents should *have to* make: a stranger in an unfamiliar place (Solnit in Stein, 1974a).

5. *Preparing for mother's absence*. Visits to the maternity hospital before the mother is admitted will help young children understand where she will be while she is away. Brochures from the hospital with pictures might be taken home so that children can see where the mothers and babies will stay. A mother might help children to cook and freeze meals to eat while she is gone. They might make a calendar together to mark off the few days until she returns. The hospital's telephone number where the mother can be reached can be written in large numbers on a sign and taped near the phone. If the child is not accustomed to talking to the

mother on the phone, a few calls should be made in the weeks before she is gone so her voice will be familiar. A large picture of the mother and a possession of hers (a piece of clothing or jewelry) could be left with the sibling.

6. *Fathers*. Fathers provide the secure base while mothers are away. When fathers are with young children throughout the perinatal and early postpartum period, this will help the children tremendously in their efforts to adapt. Having another person do errands, housework, cooking, and so on might help relieve pressure on fathers who are pulled in opposite directions by work, household tasks, older children, wife, and new baby.

7. *Sibling visits*. Four studies (Jordan, 1973; Legg et al., 1974; Robertson and Robertson, 1971; Trause, 1978) suggest that visits to the mother during her hospital stay help children to manage being separated from her. The visits also help mothers to overcome their loneliness and concern for their children at home. Most children enjoy the visits and do not get too upset at having to leave. Some children, however, do cry in protest when they must depart. The anticipation of this reaction is often an important factor in the prohibition of visits by hospital policy. Some staff members, and mothers too, believe that children manage better without visits. Although this may occasionally be true, we generally believe that young children are likely to miss their mothers intensely while separated. Sometimes, however, children only feel secure enough to express their longing when they are with their mothers. Yet expressing distress and being reassured is likely to be much healthier for children in the long run than *coping with* their worried feelings. Usually by the second or third visit children understand the visiting routine. Even those who protested as they departed after the first visit may no longer do so. It helps children to have the same person take them to visit each day. The primary purpose of the visits is to see the mother, not the baby.

COMMENT: Referring to recommendations 5 and 7, when writing about "young children," it is essential to make clear the age and level of development being discussed. A 5-year-old is very different from a 3-year-old, and a 3-year-old is very different from an 18-months-old. It is usually not appropriate to write of them as if they were a psychological homogeneous group, yet in many papers on the under-5s the reader could infer that the under-3s have the same attributes as the 3- to 5-year-olds.

For instance, there are many ways of helping a 3- or 4-year-old over a brief separation by using explanations and preparation, telephone calls, letters, parcels, visits, and mother-linked objects as the authors suggest; between visits, talking with the child about the absent mother, answering questions, and making plans to receive her back help relieve the child's anxieties.

After the visit to the hospital, a doll family is extremely useful in helping the child to express feelings about events and to ill-treat the family if that is how the child feels about the situation—as Kate does in our film of that name. We found that through the dolls the foster mother could help the child remember the reality of the mother's love instead of being overtaken by fantasies of being abandoned. But we found that children under 2 years of age cannot profit from these measures, that for instance they are unable to use the dolls as family, and that it is important to understand this in planning the substitute care of the under 2-year-olds. Their language and comprehension, their ability to reason and to understand explanations, and their memory structure are all immature, which makes preparation and explanation unprofitable.

A few well-placed words—and we emphasize *few*—such as, "Mummy gone, Mummy come back" and games of a peek-a-boo type using a photograph of the mother, as the foster mother did in our films *Jane* and *Lucy* (Robertson and Robertson 1968, 1973) will be of some help.

Frequent visiting several times a day is essential, coupled with responsive substitute care. These are the children at greatest risk—too young to understand or to accept visits without upset; if they stop showing overt upset, they are undesirably distancing themselves from the mother.
James and Joyce Robertson

8. *Visiting hours*. Care should be taken that visiting hours not be limited to times when children are likely to be tired and/or hungry. Children often enjoy being able to eat with their mothers and fathers. Hospitals might allow families to order meals to be eaten together in the mothers' rooms. Some maternity units have reported that giving each visiting child a name tag saying, "Hi! I'm _____, Baby _____'s big sister (or brother)" makes the children feel important and helps staff to identify them if necessary.

9. *Hands free*. At the time of hospital discharge, fathers or nurses should hold babies so that mothers have their hands free while greeting their older children.

10. *If the child will be present at the birth*. Show the child colored pictures in books, slides, films, and videotapes to acquaint the child with the sights and sounds of labor and birth. Specific attention should be given to the blood, which will be noticed on the mother and baby and also to the sound of work and/or pain emitted by the mother in the process of birthing the baby (Anderson, 1979). Also prepare the child for the unavailability of the mother.

WE (M.H.K. AND J.H.K.) DO NOT RECOMMEND THAT SIBLINGS BE PRESENT AT BIRTH. LONG-TERM EFFECTS ARE UNCERTAIN.

COMMENT: We share the authors' disapproval of having young children present at birth and think it unnecessary to await research findings. Research in this area could even be open to abuse. There are enough potential risks to the children's emotional development to make it prudent not to approve the practice.
James and Joyce Robertson

11. *If the child will be present at the birth*. Discuss with the child the appearance of the newborn with special attention given to the umbilical cord and the placenta. The child should realize that the cord will be cut and that this will not be painful to the mother or baby.

COMMENT: The presumption should be against this plan. Under certain circumstances the presumption could be changed.
A. Solnit

12. *If the child will be present at the birth*. Carefully plan for a caregiver to be present who will have sole responsibility for the child during labor and birth. This person should be known and trusted by the child. The caregiver should be there to support the child, answer questions, and anticipate the child's concerns and needs (including food and sleep). The caregiver should also feel confident in making decisions about what is best for the child's and parent's well-being. If parents need

more privacy than they had expected or the parent or child needs or wants the child to leave the birthing room, the caregiver can babysit somewhere else. No child should be forced to stay in the room where the mother is laboring and giving birth. In fact, the caregiver and everyone else in the room should make it easy and acceptable for the child to depart at any time.

13. *Help in the postpartum period.* Most mothers, and especially multiparous mothers, find that having someone stay at home for a few days after the birth helps them to adjust to the new demands they must meet.

> COMMENT: We think that the mother, whether multiparous or uniparous, needs as much help as possible in the first month to relieve her of some of the domestic chores so that she can devote herself to her new role as mother of one or more children. She needs help that does not bring problems—a home aide who keeps out of the way, a grandmother who does not try to take over the baby, and a husband who stays home for a week or two to give emotional support and be an extra pair of hands to fetch and carry.
> James and Joyce Robertson

14. *Breastfeeding.* Mothers who have successfully breastfed a later-born baby say the most important fact to remember is that the older children's acting out is not because of nursing. The bids for attention occur regardless of how mothers feed the new babies. When the child who has been weaned asks to nurse again, many mothers find it is helpful to allow the child to try.

> COMMENT: This often is upsetting to the child and indicates an absence of reassuring limits.
> A. Solnit

Usually, once given permission, the child refuses the breast. Yet the mother has given the important message that the child still has access to her. If the child does remember how to suck and does get milk, he is usually surprised by the taste and warm temperature. One try is often enough to curb the desire for nursing. The wish to be cuddled and held close, however, will probably not go away. If mothers do not wish to wean an older child, there is no need to do so (Lawrence, 1980). Some mothers "tandem nurse." The La Leche League and other breastfeeding support groups can help mothers with questions about breastfeeding.

15. *When the baby is born prematurely or with a problem.* If at all possible, children should be kept at home with their parents even when an unexpected birth crisis throws the family into turmoil. Young children especially need the security of their parents when routines and expectations are disrupted. However, trusted relatives and friends can "spell" parents by taking older children out for an afternoon or babysitting when parents go to the hospital.

16. *Talking to the sibling about the problems.* Parents should talk to their children about (1) what is wrong with the baby and (2) how the parents are feeling and why. Although explanations will vary with the age of the child, even an 18-month-old will know something is wrong and should be told what is happening. In general, parents should keep the explanations simple, be truthful, take one issue or question at a time, and check to see how well the children understand what has been said.

17. *When the sibling visits the nursery*. If the baby must be kept in the hospital, children would profit by visiting. This will both help make the baby real to the children and help them to feel part of the family. Health care professionals can help parents to explain the puzzling and sometimes frightening aspects of what is being done for the baby. Asking children to draw the nursery later and tell parents about the pictures may serve as a vehicle for adults to understand what was most salient for the children. Their confusions and concerns can then be better discussed.

18. *When the baby must stay in the hospital*. Children might feel closer to their new baby brother or sister if they could bring a small toy to be put in the isolette or a special shirt to be worn. Big brothers and sisters will feel very important if they can bring a photograph of themselves or a picture they have drawn to be taped to the isolette for the baby to see.

19. *When the baby is born with a problem*. The normal siblings of a baby with a problem should be observed for potential adverse reactions due to the trauma the family has suffered. If the baby's problems are chronic, the likelihood of future difficulties in adjustment for the sibling is increased.

20. *If the baby dies*. Parents should again discuss what has happened and how they are feeling with the other children. Honestly saying the baby died, rather than "passed away," "went to sleep," or "went to heaven," will help children realize the permanence of the baby's death. They must understand that the baby will not come back before they can complete their mourning. If parents can share their sadness and tears, children will have an avenue for expressing their own disappointment, sadness, and anxieties.

21. *The funeral*. Many children of about 3 years of age and older would profit by accompanying their parents and other relatives to the funeral or memorial service. Participating in rituals like funerals will help the baby's death seem real, even if the children only stay 5 or 10 minutes. Other signs of the baby's reality, like naming him or having a photograph of him, will help the whole family later when they want to share their memories and sadness about the baby they expected but never got to know very well.

22. *Films*. The authors have found the following films especially helpful in teaching parents and professionals about this subject:

Robertson, J., and Robertson, J.: Young children in brief separation. A series of five films.

> *Kate*, 2.5 years, in foster care for 27 days (1967)
> *Jane*, 17 months, in foster care for 10 days (1968)
> *John*, 17 months, in a residential nursery for 9 days (1969)
> *Thomas*, 2.4 years in foster care for 10 days (1971)
> *Lucy*, 21 months, in foster care for 17 days (1973)

New York Film Library, Britain, Concord Films Council.

CHAPTER 4

MATERNAL BEHAVIOR IN MAMMALS

MARY ANNE TRAUSE, MARSHALL H. KLAUS, and JOHN H. KENNELL

It is only through a real understanding of the ways in which chimpanzees
and man show similarities in behavior that we can reflect with meaning
on the way in which men and chimpanzees differ. And only then can we
really begin to appreciate, in a biological and spiritual manner, the full
extent of man's uniqueness.

Jane van Lawick-Goodall

Just as the neonatologist who is interested in the respiratory changes occurring
at birth has used the models of the fetal lamb and monkey, scientists attempting to
understand maternal behavior in humans find it valuable to study maternal behavior in a wide range of other animal species. This is done not to explain human
behavior but rather to view human beings within the context of evolutionary development. The requirements of air breathing resulted in similar morphological
structures in both human and nonhuman primates; the requirements of caring for
the young have led to the evolution of similar patterns of maternal behavior in
humans and other animals. The study of human parental attachment has been
partly aided by observation of animal mothers. However, Schneirla (1946) reminded us, "While . . . analogy has an important place in scientific theory, its
usefulness must be considered introductory to a comparative study in which differences may well be discovered that require a reinterpretation of the similarities first
noted."

Kaufman (1970) has described the evolutionary importance of certain reproductive changes in mammals (internal fertilization, the development of the amniote
egg, and the development of the placenta) and states the following:

> Of at least equal significance, mammals also evolved a *behavioral* program of reproduc-
> tive economy, namely, a higher order of *parental care* of the young after birth, without
> the consequence of which it is impossible to visualize the development of man. Care of
> the very young was already evolved in fish, reptiles, and especially birds, but what made
> possible the tremendous advance in mammals was the system of feeding the infant,
> through special glands, a substance, milk, which contains everything needed for growth
> and development. The improved feeding arrangement keeps the young physically close

130

to the mother and thus safer from harm. . . . Finally, and very importantly, the close physical relationship and the shared personal experience provided to the infant and mother by the feeding from her body constitute a degree of contact and intimacy which creates a new kind of bond, with durable characteristics.*

In lower primates the infant clings to the mother; in higher primates such as the gorilla and human being, the infant is unable to cling, and the mother must carry him. In these more advanced species, therefore, the mother plays a more important role in maintaining contact with the infant, and his survival hinges on the mother's attachment to him to a greater extent.

COMMENT: Patterns of maternal behavior among mammals appear to be adapted mainly to the altricial (i.e., immature) or precocial (i.e., more mature) status of the newborn. Species with altricial young are usually nest builders or live in burrows or caves, whereas species with precocial young are generally surface-living, migratory animals that live in herds or social groups. In the former group there is an extended period of intense maternal care, then a tapering off as weaning begins, and the young soon leave the mother. In the latter group there is a shorter period of intense maternal care but a more extended weaning period, during which the young are integrated into the social group alongside the mother, and they may never really leave their original social group.

Primates share features of both patterns, since the young are altricial in certain ways but in other ways they are precocial.

J.S. Rosenblatt

SPECIES-SPECIFIC BEHAVIOR

Detailed observations of parturition in a large number of species have illuminated the evolution of species-specific patterns of parturitive behavior that serve the needs of the newborn young. For example, parturition is similar in the domestic cat all over the world: toward the end of her pregnancy the female is less agile than usual, and her activity greatly decreases. For a birth site she selects a sheltered, dark place, preferably with a soft surface. The degree of seclusion varies, and in home pets it depends on the closeness of her relationship with her human owners. Although pet cats have been known to bear their young in the bed of a sleeping person, more often they find a secluded spot, such as the back of a closet or the space under a stairway.

During parturition the female cat usually licks herself, the neonates, and the floor of the birth site. She licks the posterior part of her body, especially the vaginal area, and immediately after birth this leads her to lick the kitten. Typically she lifts one leg during labor to aid in expulsion of the fetuses.

After the birth of the last kitten and eating of the last placenta, the female generally lies down, encircling her kittens, and rests with them for about 12 hours. This encircling is the earliest direct adaptation she makes to her young after birth.

---

*From Kaufman, C.: In Anthony, E.J., and Benedek, T., editors: Parenthood: psychology and psychopathology, Boston, 1970, Little, Brown & Co.

She "presents" by lying down around her kittens with her ventral surface arched toward them and with her front and rear legs extended to enclose them. While lying with the kittens, she licks them, stimulating them to nurse. This may begin as early as a half hour after birth and typically before the end of the 12-hour resting period. For the first few days the mother stays with her litter at the birth site, leaving them only once every couple of hours to feed. If the kittens wander away from the home site, they usually begin to vocalize and the mother responds by retrieving them, becoming more skillful with practice.

The mother initiates nursing during the first 20 days after parturition. For the next 10 to 15 days either mother or kitten may initiate feeding, but after the thirty-fifth day the kitten is more likely to seek out the mother for feeding (Schneirla et al., 1963).

Another mammal for which the sequence of mothering behavior at the time of birth has been meticulously described is the rhesus monkey. During the last five days of pregnancy the female manually explores her genitals, then looks at, smells, and licks her hands. She removes the mucous plug from her vaginal opening with her hands just prior to the birth. When the fetus's face appears, she squats and pulls it forward, helping to deliver the trunk and legs. Although the infant rhesus sometimes vocalizes during parturition, the mother does not. As soon as its hands are free, the infant clutches the mother's fur, and the mother in turn holds her infant to her chest and alternately cleans herself and the infant, licking it thoroughly from head to toe. When the delivery of the placenta begins, she temporarily ignores her infant while she eats the placenta. Grooming and retrieving of the infant increase during the first month, as does restraining it from leaving her. During this period the mother spends much time holding the infant close or cradling it loosely in her arms (Brandt and Mitchell, 1971).

> **COMMENT:** There is no doubt that parturition is important in the formation of the behavioral bond between the mother and her offspring. In rats, disturbance of mothers during parturition not only has immediate effects on delaying deliveries but also has long-term effects on the young, very likely through an altered mother-young relationship. These long-term effects on the mother can also be seen when mothers are either permitted or not permitted to lick their young during parturition. Those which lick them can have them removed, and 25 days later they are more responsive to pups than those which have not licked them (Bridges, 1975, 1977). It is also true, however, that the hormonal stimulation which underlies the mother's responsiveness to pups at parturition continues to act for some time after parturition in the rat. Therefore the mother will still accept pups that she has not licked during parturition, either because they were removed as they were born or she was delivered by cesarean section.
> **J.S. Rosenblatt**

Although two species may be closely related taxonomically, they have not necessarily evolved exactly the same responses to similar environmental demands. For example, although the North Indian langur mother is closely related to the rhesus mother, and her behavior around the time of delivery is similar in many ways, she

Animal	Preparation for birth	Birth site	Birth	Protection of young	Nursing	Stimulation of young	Other observations
Domestic cat	Genital licking	Warm, dark place	Licks self, young, and floor of birth site; eats placenta	Retrieves vocalizing young	Initiates by presenting; begins $1/2$ to 12 hr postpartum	Licking (Schneirla et al., 1963)	
Laboratory rat	Builds nest; anogenital licking	Birth nest (Rosenblatt and Lehrman, 1963)	Eats placenta	Nests; retrieves; attacks intruders	Mother drapes herself over litter	Licking (Rosenblatt, 1969)	At first somewhat afraid of young (Rosenblatt, 1970)
Goats	Separate from herd	Secluded	Self-licking; licks newborn all over	Butts away all intruders; moves toward vocalizing kids	Adjusts position; accepts only own young	Licking	Attempts to steal other young before birth (Ewer, 1968; Hersher et al., 1963a)
Sheep	Separate from herd	Domestic: indoor shelter. Big horn: inaccessible mountain area	Licks anal area; licks newborn all over	Moves toward bleating lamb (Hersher et al., 1963a)	Adjusts position; accepts only own young	Licking	
Primates North Indian langur				Keeps to herself for first hours		Licking, grooming, manipulating, stroking	Allows other females to hold in first day (Dolhinow, 1972)
Rhesus monkey	Explores genitals; removes mucus manually	Floor of cage or metal bar	Squats; pulls fetus forward; eats placenta; licks young	Holds young close, cradles, avoids others for a long time; retrieves and restrains		Grooming (Brandt and Mitchell, 1971)	
Chimpanzee	Moves away from herd		Carries placenta by umbilical cord	Stays away from group for several days; 5 months before allows others to touch (Kaufman, 1970)			Other behaviors similar to rhesus monkey

will allow as many as eight other females to handle her infant after the first few hours, whereas the rhesus mother jealously holds her newborn close and avoids the approach of other animals.

Two related species that show widely differing postparturition behavior are pigtail and bonnet macaques. Normally bonnet adults tend to stay close to each other, whereas pigtail adults make few contacts with other animals in their group. Likewise, after parturition the bonnet mother rejoins her peers, whereas the pigtail mother remains isolated with her infant (Rosenblum and Kaufman, 1967). These examples dramatically illustrate the caution necessary in drawing conclusions about the behaviors of even closely related species.

Table 4-1 summarizes observations of maternal care in a number of mammalian species. All mammals prepare for the birth of their young, establish a birth site, and during parturition lick their bodies. After birth they display a profound interest in the protection of their young, ensuring their warmth, maintaining control over visitors, warding off intruders, keeping an eye on the young, and in some species retrieving those which stray. In addition, most mammalian mothers clean and arouse their infants by licking and grooming them.

The universal needs of young mammals are met in a variety of specific ways by different species. Each species has specific patterns of organized behavior that it has evolved in relation to its environment to ensure its survival. Individualized, enduring bonds develop between mother and infant in species such as primates, in which the young are particularly helpless, and in species such as ungulates, in which the young are part of a moving group and can easily be lost.

SEPARATION

In view of the foregoing it is significant that a human newborn is immediately separated from his mother if he is born prematurely or becomes sick after a normal term birth. Does this early separation affect subsequent maternal-infant attachment? In our search for clues as to whether the effects of early separation on maternal behavior in the human would be a fruitful area to study, we have looked at the effects of separations in a wide variety of animal species. Especially relevant to our inquiry is the point at which separation occurs, the length of separation, the mother's behavior on reunion with her infant, and species-specific differences in the effects of separation. It is necessary to emphasize that our principal interest is the effect of separation on the mother's behavior rather than on the infant. Which aspects of separation interfere with the emergence of maternal behavior?

Laboratory rats

In attempting to answer this question, Rosenblatt and Lehrman (1963) studied the effects of mother-infant sparation on maternal behavior in laboratory rats. An important characteristic of the maternal female is that she will act maternally to pups other than her own young: Under certain conditions alien pups elicit her maternal care. This permitted experimentation in reeliciting maternal behavior by introducing new pups ("test pups") for short periods to observe the reactions of mothers separated from pups for various lengths of time.

Table 4-2 presents the findings of Rosenblatt and Lehrman (1963) and reveals that, in the laboratory rat, separation of mother and infant is debilitating, especially if it occurs immediately after each pup of the litter is born. Mothers without pups from then until the fifth day postpartum did not respond to foster pups that were given to them to rear, and all of the pups died. Even when the separation lasted two days, one half of the pups given to the mothers died within the first five days. Moreover, lactation was affected and after a four-day separation from the pups, it had ceased. Therefore, although foster pups eventually elicited nursing, nest-building, and retrieving behavior, the pups could only survive for a short time, and as they weakened the mother stopped exhibiting maternal behavior.

The amount of *contact* with pups necessary for the establishment of maternal behavior has been more precisely defined by Bridges (1975, 1977). He found that if pups were left with newly delivered mothers for 4 to 6 hours after birth, the mothers would behave maternally within one day after test pups were introduced, even after a 25-day separation. Furthermore, he found that contact with only half the litter throughout parturition (rather than each pup's immediate removal after birth) was equally effective (Fig. 4-1).

On the other hand, removal of the pups before the female had the opportunity to lick them or delivering pups by cesarean section resulted, 25 days later, in a level of responsiveness to foster pups that was no higher than that of completely inexperienced females exposed to pups for the first time.

Among hamsters, too, early removal of the pups after parturition results in a loss of maternal behavior. If hamsters are permitted only 1 hour of postpartum contact with their pups and are offered pups each day thereafter (different groups of females being tested each day with fresh pups), they no longer respond maternally after the fourth day. If they are allowed 24 hours of postpartum contact, this period of responsiveness is extended by one day, but if they are allowed 48 hours of postpartum contac with their pups, they remain maternal even though they are without pups for 11 more days (Siegel and Greenwald, 1978).

Sheep and goats

Mother-infant separation affects maternal behavior among sheep and goats even more significantly than in the rat, since maternal responsiveness wanes more rapidly among these species.

Among sheep, Poindron and Le Neindre (1979, 1980) have found that if separation begins at birth and lasts for 4 hours, 50% of the ewes are still willing to accept lambs. However, when a separation beginning at birth lasts for 12 to 24

Table 4-2. Effects of separation on maternal behavior in rats*

Beginning of separation	Length of separation	Tested (with 5- to 10-day old foster pups)	Effects
At birth	Permanent	Weekly for 4 weeks after birth	Decline in maternal responsiveness at end of first week; nursing and retrieving by only an occasional female and nest building absent
After female cleaned pup and ate placenta	Experimental: permanent	Beginning of third day	Nursing; retrieving; nest building decreased
	Control: no separation	Third day	Increase in maternal behavior
At birth	2 days, then foster pups left with mothers for 9 days	Tested on either the third or fifth day, then left with pups and tested daily	Behavior increased after introduction of foster pups, then decreased to level of mothers with no pups; behavior decreased after separation, more for mothers with 4-day separation
	4 days, then foster pups left with mothers for 1 day		
At birth	4 days	After separation	No maternal behavior
3 days after birth 9 days after birth 14 days after birth	4 days	After separation	Maternal behavior returned; 60% to 75% of mothers nursed
Ninth day after birth	Permanent	Every other day after separation	Maternal behavior declined earlier and to lower levels than controls
Fourteenth day after birth	Permanent	Every other day after separation	Decline in maternal behavior did not decrease—had already begun naturally

*Data from Rosenblatt, J.S., and Lehrman, D.: In Rheingold, H.R., editor: Maternal behavior in mammals, New York, 1963, John Wiley & Sons, Inc.

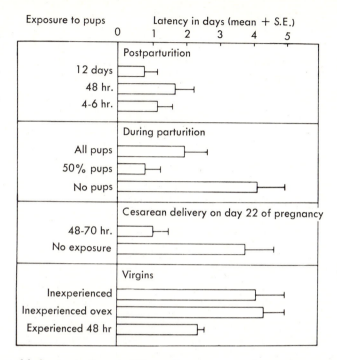

Fig. 4-1. Maternal behavior in the rat. Effects of parturition and postparturition contact with pups on latencies for induction of maternal behavior 25 days later. Period of exposure to pups shown on ordinate and latencies on the upper abscissa. Cesarean section–delivered females and virgins shown for comparison. (From Bridges, R.S.: Physiol. Behav. **18:**487-490, 1977.)

hours, the percentage of ewes who accept lambs drops to 25%. In contrast with this, if a 24-hour separation begins two to four days after parturition, all ewes will reaccept their lambs.

Although studies of maternal responsiveness in the goat are less definitive than studies in sheep, they suggest that maternal responsiveness wanes more rapidly after parturition in goats than in sheep (Rosenblatt and Siegel, in press). Collias (1956) and Klopfer (1971) have found that dams will not accept their own young after the kids have been removed at birth for more than 2 hours. However, if allowed 5 minutes of contact with their kids immediately after parturition, virtually all the young are reaccepted even after 3 hours of separation.

The study of the effects of separation on maternal behavior among sheep and goats is complicated by the fact that ewes and dams develop individualized bonds to their young. Earlier studies suggested that once these individualized bonds were formed among goats, mothers would butt away any alien young animals. Thus animals other than the mother's own species could not be easily introduced for test purposes. Recent work by Gubernick and colleagues (1979) suggests that this rejection is only partially because the mother has formed an individualized bond to her own young. Gubernick found that whether or not the test young had spent any length of time with their own mothers before being used for testing determined whether or not they were accepted or rejected by a mother rearing her own kid. Gubernick has suggested that each mother marks her young in several possible ways during the first 24 hours (e.g., through licking and the kid's milk intake), and mothers reject young with the marking of other mothers. Rosenblatt and Siegel (in press) conclude that the waning of maternal responsiveness does not coincide with the establishment of a specific bond in the goat. Dams are capable of responding maternally to kids other than their own even after they have developed a bond to their own, provided the alien kid has not been marked by another female.

Monkeys

A series of experiments by Sackett and Ruppenthal (1974) suggests that mother-infant separation may also affect monkey mothers. Because mothering behavior per se was not their focus, these studies are not strictly comparable with those involving goats or rats. Here the behavior measured was maternal motivation, defined as the preference to be near neonates as opposed to monkeys of other ages. These authors used a choice situation consisting of one central compartment surrounded by six others to which other cages containing stimulus animals could be attached. The female monkey was placed in the central compartment, and the cages of two stimulus animals were randomly hooked to two of the six outer compartments. Plexiglas dividers allowed the subject animal to have a clear view of the stimulus animals. The number of seconds spent near a given stimulus provided a measure of relative preference for that stimulus animal. Table 4-3 presents the relevant results of these experiments. Mothers separated from their infants for 1 hour after birth showed a preference for neonates. However, if this separation lasted for 24 hours, the mothers' preference for neonates seemed to disappear.*

Separation of a newborn or young animal from its mother during the formation of the maternal bond therefore significantly alters maternal behavior. The sooner after birth the separation occurs the stronger are the effects. For each species there seems to be a specific length of separation that can be endured. If separation extends beyond this sensitive period, the effects on mothering behavior during this breeding cycle are often drastic and irreversible.

---

*Sackett and Ruppenthal (1974) suggest an explanation for the different behaviors exhibited by feral- and laboratory-reared monkeys. The latter as a rule are "motherless monkeys" who were reared in cages without their own mothers. Feral monkeys, on the other hand, were typically captured after having been reared by their own mothers. So, in a sense, one is seeing the second generation effects of inadequate mothering in laboratory monkeys, whose maternal behavior is more easily extinguished under stress.

Table 4-3. Maternal motivation in pigtail macaque mothers separated
from their young*

Separation began	Length of separation	Preference (neonate or adult female macaque)
At birth	1 hour	Neonate
2 weeks after birth	1 hour	Neonate
1 month	1 hour	Neonate
2 months	1 hour	Equal preference
6 months	1 hour	Adult
Controls (had not been pregnant or lived with infants)		Adult
At birth	24 hours	Adult
2 weeks	24 hours	Neonate
1 month	24 hours	Neonate
2 months	24 hours	Equal preference
6 months	24 hours	Adult
Controls		Adult
At birth	7 days	Adult
2 weeks	7 days	Neonate
1 month	7 days	Adult
2 months	7 days	Adult
6 months	7 days	Adult
Controls		Adult

*Data from Sackett, G.P., and Ruppenthal, G.C.: In Lewis M., and Rosenblum, L.A., editors: The effect of the infant on its caregiver, New York, 1974. John Wiley & Sons, Inc.

ADOPTION

Separation studies are concerned with the stimuli that support maternal behavior, the removal of which causes it to decline in parturient females. Adoption studies, on the other hand, deal with the conditions that promote maternal behavior in nonparturient females toward infants that are not their own. We are interested in whether there is a particularly sensitive period during which a new infant can be introduced, how long a period of time is required for successful adoption,* whether certain environmental conditions are necessary for successful adoption, and species-specific differences in adoption behavior.

COMMENT: The situation most parallel to the human phenomenon of adoption in which a non-maternal woman is required to carry out maternal care of an infant is found in several animal species in which nonmaternal females are either presented with newborn young or are exposed to them in a social group. The response of the female in this situation varies greatly in different species: Mice, both female and male, respond almost immediately with maternal behavior, whereas

*"Successful adoption" is the situation in which the female performs the behaviors necessary for the survival of the adopted young.

among rats the response develops slowly over five to seven days but can be speeded to two days by forcing the female into close contact with the young. In rhesus monkeys the phenomenon of "aunts" exists, in which young females try to gain access to newborns and exhibit the preliminary forms of maternal behavior when permitted to do so. Among certain species of primates, males are capable of exhibiting maternal care to young, but this is frequently obscured by the greater initiative of females when both are together.
J.S. Rosenblatt

Grota's (1968) experiment with laboratory rats demonstrates that certain conditions facilitate adoption. Pups introduced to a female who has been lactating for one day have a greater chance for survival and rapid growth than pups introduced to a female who has been lactating for 10 days. Thus the closer the introduction of new pups is to the female's date of delivery the more successful the adoption will be. When the new pups were introduced after one day, females successfully adopted as many as 10 pups. However, when 10 alien pups were given to a mother who had been lactating for 10 days, significantly fewer survived than when only four pups were introduced.

> **COMMENT:** The problem being discussed comes under the broad heading of synchrony between the mother and her offspring. Normally synchrony develops from early beginnings at birth and becomes refined (in some mother-young groups) as the two interact in the days that follow. Synchrony exists with regard to many functions, both behavioral and physiological, including lactation and nursing. The greater the discrepancy between the mother's condition and the developmental status of the young the more difficult it is for the two to become synchronized, and of course the greatest discrepancy exists when the female is nonmaternal and the young are in need of maternal care.
> **J.S. Rosenblatt**

Schneirla and colleagues (1963) found that litter size also affects adoptive maternal behavior in the female cat. Although one new kitten was accepted and nursed whether introduced on the seventh, twelfth, or fifteenth day after birth to a female whose own pups were removed at birth, a litter of three new kittens was only encircled if introduced before the fifteenth day. After 15 days the introduction of three kittens caused attacking and avoidance behaviors in the mother. It is interesting to note the differences in the time periods during which cats and rats will accept alien young. If a female rat's own pups are taken from her at birth, alien pups are incapable of eliciting maternal behavior four days later; however, if a cat is separated from her kittens at birth, an alien kitten can elicit maternal behavior 12 and sometimes 15 days afterward.

Under normal conditions dams butt away alien young. However, Hersher's group at the Cornell Behavior Farm in Ithaca, New York, demonstrated that goats can be induced to adopt alien young, provided that the mother and kid are isolated from others but left in close proximity to each other and that the dam is prevented from butting the kid. Once bonding occurs under these conditions, no differences may be observed between dams with foster young and dams with natural young. It is also possible to foster cross-species, adoptions, but cross-species mothers often seem more "anxious" (Hersher et al., 1963*b*).

Hersher speculates that the agitation often appearing in cross-species foster mothers may largely result because the young animal maintains the behavior characteristic of its own species, to which the mother is incapable of adjusting. For example, kids wander away from their flocks more than lambs, thus ewes raising kids spend much more time away from the flock and are more often anxious than ewes raising adopted lambs (Hersher et al., 1963*b*).

The following principles may be derived from the work just described:

1. There appears to be a sensitive period after birth, distinct for each species, during which females will adopt alien young.
2. In some species, such as goats and sheep, adoption will not take place after the sensitive period without specific conditions (i.e., close contact, isolation, and adequate length of time).
3. Environmental conditions, such as the number of young introduced, influence the success of adoptions.
4. Unusual behavior on the part of the infant may interfere with successful adoption.

MECHANISMS

Our final task is to attempt to understand the mechanisms underlying the reasons why female animals behave the way they do before, during, and after the birth of their young. Why do pregnant females prepare for birth? Why is it that the closer to the time of parturition that alien young are introduced the greater is the probability of their acceptance? Why is the length of separation of a mother from her young such an important factor in whether she will again behave maternally when they are returned? The studies of both Klopfer (1971) and Rosenblatt (1963-1975) have been designed to answer these questions. Each has asked: Is maternal behavior elicited by characteristics of the young or is it primarily triggered by hormonal changes within the female's body? Each has attempted to answer this question by observing the effects of one variable at a time in a carefully controlled series of studies.

Cosnier (1963), Cosnier and Couturier (1966), and Rosenblatt (1967) first established that maternal behavior in rats may be exhibited by nonmothers. Both virgin female and male rats, even those who were gonadectomized or hypophysectomized, responded to 5- to 10-day-old pups after 5 to 6 days with the maternal behaviors of retrieving, crouching, nest building, and licking.

More recent work by members of Rosenblatt's laboratory on the ontogeny of maternal behavior showed that unweaned juvenile pups, 18 to 22 days of age, actively sought contact when exposed to pups younger than 10 days of age (Mayer and Rosenblatt, 1979). They exhibited sniffing, approach, licking, forepaw manipulation, and lying in contact with pups, the latter two behaviors resembling the contact of maternal adult rats. When the daily exposure to pups was extended from 15 minutes to 22 hours (allowing the preweanlings 2 hours per day suckling with their own mothers), the 22-day-old young also exhibited retrieving, nest building, and lying in contact with pups, often draped over the pups as in nursing. About 50% of the pups showed these maternal behaviors, with an average latency of one day.

When juveniles were 24 days of age, however, their interest in the young pups declined sharply and the juveniles began actively to avoid contact with them (Mayer and Rosenblatt, 1979). This avoidance has been shown to grow stronger with age and is present in most adults at their initial exposure to a litter of pups. As a result of their own observations and those of other investigators of the behavior of 20- to 30-day-old rats in a number of situations, Mayer and Rosenblatt have attributed the appearance of pup avoidance to the rapid maturation of the young rat's defensiveness to external threats during this time. It is the odor of the pups that appears to become aversive (Mayer et al, 1979). The timidity can be overcome, however, by continuous exposure (Mayer and Rosenblatt, 1979; Mayer et al, 1979; Rosenblatt, 1967).

These studies demonstrate that maternal behavior is not completely dependent on hormonal changes and in part may arise ontogenetically from the gregarious behavior of young rats. Yet the fact that new mothers exhibit maternal behavior immediately after delivery suggests that hormonal factors during pregnancy and parturition play an important role in its natural onset.

> **COMMENT:** Pup odors that cause females to avoid or perhaps fear the pups at first appear to prevent virgin rats from responding to pups immediately. If virgin rats are prevented from smelling the pups, they act maternally after less than a day of contact, and sometimes immediately. Of course when females give birth, they do not avoid pup odors. This indicates that an important part of the initial attachment involves overcoming avoidance or fear of pups, and this may be one role of hormones or perhaps may be based on experience with similar odors during pregnancy.
> **J.S. Rosenblatt**

To determine whether pregnant rats behave more like virgin rats or more like newly delivered mothers, Rosenblatt and Siegel (1975) compared the latencies of maternal behavior for rats whose pregnancies were terminated at various stages. They found that rats which delivered before the eleventh day of pregnancy did not behave significantly differently from nonpregnant females, whereas rats delivered by cesarean section on the sixteenth or nineteenth days of pregnancy responded to pups almost immediately. Similar results were found when pregnancies were terminated by hysterectomies: Rosenblatt (1971) again found that the latency was shorter for females further along in their pregnancies. This clearly demonstrated that during the course of pregnancy, changes occur within the female which affect her responsiveness to young pups.

After several colleagues had failed to isolate hormones that might account for these phenomena, Terkel and Rosenblatt (1968) attempted to establish whether the humoral substance regulating maternal behavior is carred in the blood plasma. They injected virgin rats with 3 to 4 ml of plasma taken from mother rats within 48 hours of parturition or plasma from donors who had not delivered or with a saline solution. Virgin rats injected with plasma from maternal rats showed maternal behavior significantly earlier than did rats in the other groups. This experiment confirmed the existence of a plasma-carried substance that influences maternal behavior.

To supplement these findings, Terkel and Rosenblatt (1972) developed a technique for transferring larger amounts of blood between two rats while both rats moved about freely. By continuously cross-transfusing, they were able to achieve about a 50% mix of the rats' blood. With this method they studied the effects of transferring blood from female rats at different times centering around parturition.

They concluded that "Only blood transfused during a limited time at parturition induces maternal behavior. . . . Blood from pregnant females twenty-four hours before expected delivery did not yet have the capacity of inducing maternal behavior in a significant proportion of virgins, while blood transferred in the same amount and for the same duration from mothers twenty-four hours after parturition had already lost this capacity." The authors caution that these are not necessarily the precise limits within which the humoral basis for maternal behavior is established, since they sampled only three intervals and achieved only a 50% blood mix. Nevertheless, this study definitely highlights the importance of the period surrounding parturition. Physiological mechanisms seem to heighten the mother's sensitivity to infants at parturition. This suggests that maternal behavior can be supported by hormones, but only for a brief period. Other evidence suggests that after this the presence of the pup is necessary to ensure the continuation of maternal behaviors.

COMMENT: We have come to interpret these findings differently because at the time we did not know that female rats really become maternal within the 24 hours that precede parturition. That is, the mother herself is not stimulated to maternal behavior by the hormones circulating after parturition but probably by a hormone (estrogen) that was secreted 48 hours earlier. This study therefore showed that the hormone was still present in the mother in sufficient concentration to induce maternal behavior in a virgin rat during at least 6 hours after parturition but not 24 hours later.
J.S. Rosenblatt

Rosenblatt and associates have further isolated the hormonal substance involved in stimulating maternal behavior. They had earlier found that ovariectomized and hysterectomized pregnant female rats do not show a decreased latency for maternal behavior, whereas female rats that are only hysterectomized on the sixteenth day of pregnancy and later do show such latency. Therefore they hypothesized that the ovaries play a crucial role in the onset of maternal behavior. To test this hypothesis directly, Rosenblatt and Siegel (1975) ovariectomized and hysterectomized rats at various stages of the second half of pregnancy. They found that removal of the ovaries at the time of hysterectomy did in fact result in a significantly longer latency than hysterectomy alone.

In a subsequent study they attempted to restore short-latency maternal behavior in hysterectomized-ovariectomized females (Siegel and Rosenblatt, 1975). At the time of surgery the females were injected with estradiol benzoate. One group also received progesterone 44 hours later. Estradiol benzoate in either a high or low dose restored short-latency maternal behavior typical of females hysterectomized at the same stage of pregnancy. Progesterone did not affect the action of estradiol benzoate.

COMMENT: Progesterone at 44 hours did not adversely affect the action of estradiol benzoate but in later studies it was shown that progesterone given at 24 hours after estrogen could inhibit maternal behavior almost entirely. Recent studies reviewed by Rosenblatt and associates (1979) suggest also that the rapid decline in circulating levels of progesterone which occurs at about 30 hours prepartum may facilitate the appearance of maternal behavior. Progesterone therefore has both an inhibiting action on maternal behavior when present and a facilitating action when it is withdrawn.

Recent studies on sheep by a group of French investigators (Poindron and Le Neindre, 1979, 1980) have established that in sheep, estrogen appears to be the principal hormone which stimulates maternal behavior. Moreover, they have shown that there is a transition period in the shift from hormonal to nonhormonal control of maternal behavior in this species also. They have investigated the stimuli from the lamb that are responsible for the maintenance of maternal behavior and for some features of the individual bond between the mother and her own offspring.

The hormonal basis of maternal behavior in sheep was studied by these investigators using ovariectomized ewes that were given a single injection of either estradiol or progesterone and tested with young lambs at 6, 10, and 24 hours after treatment. At 24 hours more than 80% of the estradiol-treated females were maternal toward lambs, whereas only 45% of the progesterone-treated females became maternal. Untreated females (30%) also became maternal in response to lamb stimulation alone. Later studies ruled out prolactin as a possible stimulus for maternal behavior.

To study the transition period, ewes were separated from their lambs at parturition, and at intervals during the first 24 hours they were tested for their maternal responsiveness. As shown in Fig. 4-2, females with the normally low levels of estrogen declined in responsiveness over the first 12 hours, and only 25% responded to lambs at 12 hours. With elevated estrogen levels, 50% of ewes accepted lambs, indicating that the normal decline was based on the waning of hormonal stimulation. The age of the test lambs was an important factor: At 12 hours ewes were more responsive to newborn lambs than to their own 12-hour-old lambs from which they had been separated at birth.

Fig. 4-2 also shows the period, frequently called the "critical period," for the formation of an individual bond between the mother and her own offspring. During the first 2 hours, mothers rearing their own lambs accepted alien young less and less, and at the end of 2 hours no alien young were accepted. However, lambs older than the mother's own were rejected after 30 minutes of contact with her own lamb, whereas newborn lambs were accepted for 1½ hours before they began to be rejected. One thing which emerges from this study is that the formation of the individual bond between the mother and her lamb is *not* a good measure of the hormonal influence on maternal behavior, which lasts for about 12 hours compared with the 2 hours required for an individual bond to be formed.

In a second experiment Poindron and Le Neindre (1979, 1980) studied the lamb stimuli that are necessary to maintain maternal behavior during the first 12 hours postpartum and those which promote individual attachment between the mother and lamb. As shown in Fig. 4-3, as long as the

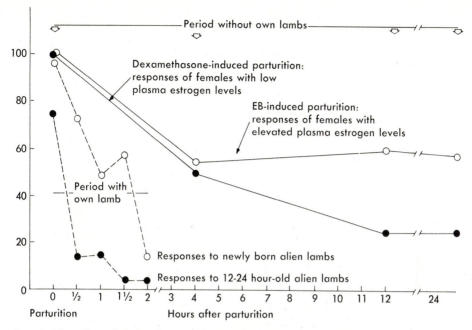

Fig. 4-2. The effect of elevated estrogens *(EB)* on maternal responsiveness for 24 hours post-partum in ewes without their own lambs. At 12 hours 60% of females with elevated estrogen were still responsive as opposed to only 25% of ewes with low levels of estrogen (dexameth-asone-induced parturition). For comparison, the maternal responsiveness levels of ewes kept with their own lambs are shown at lower left.

mother could smell and touch her lamb *(1,2,3)* she remained maternal at 12 hours, but if she could barely smell it or it was completely out of olfactory range or absent, she lost a good deal of her responsiveness. Those stimuli which maintained her maternal behavior also provided a basis for an individual relationship to grow between the mother and her lamb and these mothers rejected alien lambs, whereas those stimuli which were less able to maintain maternal behavior resulted in a weaker individual relationship and acceptance of alien lambs at only a slightly lower rate than acceptance of the mothers' own lambs. Fig. 4-3 shows again that estrogen-treated groups (EB) were more responsive at 12 hours postpartum than untreated females (DEX); in this instance the "critical period" for acceptance of young was extended from the usual 1/2 to 2 hours to 12 hours in one half of the females. The critical period is therefore not a fixed period but may be altered by hormones or by lamb stimulation.
J.S. Rosenblatt

Siegel and Rosenblatt's (1978) recent work in rats on the latency and duration of estrogen effects showed that estrogen requires 48 hours to have its maximal effect on maternal behavior. Furthermore, nonpregnant rats required a much higher dose of estrogen to stimulate maternal behavior than did pregnancy-termi-nated rats, suggesting that pregnancy and surgical termination result in an in-creased sensitivity to estrogen. The presence of pups also seemed to have sensitized rats to estrogen effects.

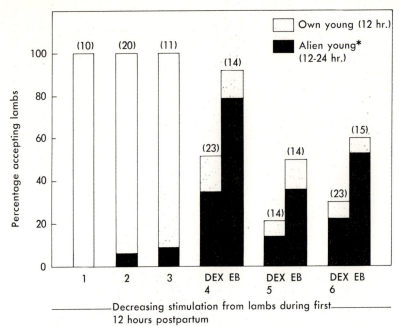

*Only ewes accepting own lambs were tested with alien lambs

Fig. 4-3. The stimuli necessary to maintain maternal behavior during the first 12 hours postpartum and those which promote individual attachment between the mother and lamb in six separate studies. In studies *1, 2,* and *3* the mothers could smell and touch their lambs for 12 hours. In studies *4, 5,* and *6* estrogen-treated ewes *(EB)* were more responsive than untreated females *(DEX)*. All ewes were tested 12 hours after delivery.

Zarrow and co-workers (1971) showed that blocking the release of prolactin during the last six to seven days of pregnancy did not interfere with the onset of maternal behavior at parturition. Therefore the effect of estradiol cannot be accounted for by the fact that estrogen releases prolactin.

In an effort to determine whether estradiol was the hormonal stimulant of maternal behavior, Rosenblatt and Siegel (1975) studied whether maternal behavior began before parturition, as would be predicted by Shaikh's (1971) finding that serum concentration of estradiol rises rapidly just before parturition. By testing pregnant females with young pups at 2-hour intervals starting 40 hours before parturition, they found that nest building does in fact begin 34 hours prepartum and retrieving begins 24 hours prepartum. Interestingly, significant falls in progesterone and rises in estradiol have been noted by Turnbull and associates (1974) in the five weeks preceding labor in the human female (Fig. 4-4).

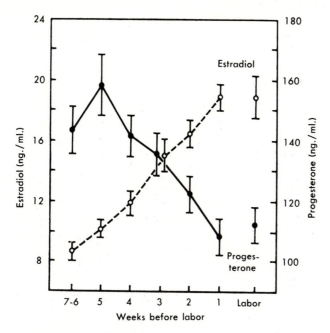

Fig. 4-4. Plasma progesterone and estradiol in human mothers near the time of delivery. (From Turnbull, A.C., Patten, P.T., Flint, A.P.F., Keirse, M.J.N.C., Jeremy, J.Y., and Anderson, A.: Lancet **1**:101-103, 1974.)

In summary, virgin and male rats will show maternal behavior if left with pups for a sufficient length of time, but latencies are relatively long. The latency for maternal behavior in female rats decreases after the eleventh day of pregnancy. The finding that a plasma-carried substance stimulates maternal behavior near the time of parturition, coupled with the demonstration of the importance of estradiol, clearly shows that physiological mechanisms are partly responsible for the occurrence of maternal behavior prepartum.

After parturition the presence of pups seems to be necessary to maintain rat maternal behavior. If each pup is taken away immediately after its birth and no new pups are introduced for four days, maternal behavior is completely extinguished. If, however, at least one half of the litter is left with the mother for the entire period of parturition, she will show maternal behavior in approximately one day of pup exposure, even after a 14- to 25-day separation. Thus there appears to be a period soon after birth when a transition occurs from internal (i.e., hormonal) stimulation of maternal responsiveness to primarily external support through the presence of pups. If the pups are removed before this transition occurs, the maternal behavior fades as the estrogen effects subside. Once established on a nonhormonal basis, the maternal behavior can be reelicited even after relatively long separations. Although the mechanism for this transition is not yet fully understood, Rosenblatt and co-workers have stated:

> Our studies on the neural basis of maternal behavior suggest a neural site at which both hormonal and sensory stimuli act to elicit maternal behavior. Implanting estrogen at this site stimulates maternal behavior, and destroying this site prevents sensitization of non-pregnant females and interrupts ongoing maternal behavior in postpartum females. The successive interaction of hormonal and sensory stimuli at this site may account for the effect that sensory stimuli have in maintaining maternal behavior postpartum once it has been initiated under the influence of estrogen in the prepartum period.*

Once the transition occurs, the behavioral interactions of mother and young appear to maintain maternal behavior. An example of a pup characteristic that elicits a variety of maternal behaviors is odor, which is instrumental in triggering the release of maternal prolactin, maternal licking of the pup's perineal region, and maternal retrieving, especially when paired with the pup's ultrasonic calls. Other characteristics that may serve to attract and maintain the female's interest include the young pup's warmth, activity, vocalizations, and anogenital secretions (Rosenblatt et al., 1979).

Klopfer (1971) focused on the characteristics of the young animal that evoke maternal responses in the goat. To examine the effects of visual cues emanating from the kid, he compared the behavior of females which were blindfolded during parturition and the first minutes of contact with their kids with that of females which were not. He found that after a period of separation all goats, whether blindfolded or not, reaccepted their own kids and butted away aliens. Therefore it appeared that visual cues do not trigger maternal behavior in the goat.

He also compared the behavior of goats whose kids had vocalized during parturition with that of goats whose kids had not. Again he found no differences after a period of separation; all females showed maternal behavior when reunited with their kids and all rejected aliens. Auditory cues do not seem to play a crucial role in eliciting maternal behavior.

In a third experiment Klopfer tested the importance of olfactory cues by cocainizing the nostrils of female goats either at the time of parturition or at the time of the acceptance test after separation. Females cocainized at parturition did not reject their young, as would be expected if olfactory cues elicited maternal behavior. Instead, eight of the nine female goats accepted their own young, but six also accepted alien young. Those cocainized at the time of the acceptance test rejected their own young as often as they accepted them. Klopfer (1971) therefore modified

---

*From Rosenblatt, J.S., Siegel, H.I., and Mayer, A.D.: In Rosenblatt, J.S., et al., editors: Advances in the study of behavior, New York, 1979, Academic Press, Inc., Vol. 10, p. 126.

his original theory that sensory cues, particularly olfaction, give rise to maternal behavior. He hypothesized instead that olfactory cues must aid the mother's recognition of her young but that "events that transform a female from a rejecting to a motherly animal, events which must be exploited within five or so minutes after parturition (for the goat), must presumably be sought elsewhere than in some kind of external 'releasor.' "

This shift of focus from external releasors to factors endogenous to the female led to a final study. Klopfer reasoned that if endogenous factors are primarily responsible for the appearance of maternal behaviors, females should be receptive to any kid presented immediately at parturition. The results of his study confirmed his expectation. Of five female goats presented with an alien kid for 5 minutes immediately after parturition, all five accepted that alien after a separation of up to 3 hours. Five of the six goats that were presented with their own and alien kids at birth reaccepted both after separation. However, no female accepted an alien other than the one with which she had first been presented at parturition.

Klopfer (1971) concludes that "Something happens in the space of a few minutes after parturition which makes her ready, then and only then, to attach herself to a kid. Once she is attached, she displays many of the human signs of distress on the removal of the kid. Spared the attachment, the removal leaves her as nonchalant as any virgin, despite the fact that she may be lactating heavily." Klopfer suggests a model in which hormonal changes during the final stages of labor cause a temporarily heightened responsiveness to infants.

Poindron and colleagues' (1978) work on maternal behavior in the sheep supports this model. They found the onset and length of the initial period of maternal responsiveness is related to the rise in estrogen, and perhaps prolactin as well, before parturition. When mothers were treated with estrogen at the time of delivery, 60% accepted the lambs after a 24-hour separation. Without estrogen only 10% accepted them (Poindron et al., 1979). Thus the duration of estrogen effects determines the length of time during which ewes will act maternally on first contact with a lamb. Once the estrogen effects have subsided, the maintenance of maternal behavior is based on nonhormonal factors.

Rosenblatt (1963-1975) and Klopfer (1971) both present models in which biological mechanisms are primarily responsible for a mother's receptivity to young at the time of birth but quickly subside afterward. Within the sensitive period, maternal behavior quickly disappears if young are not present to elicit and maintain it. However, if young are present, a smooth transition takes place. Because of her physiological state after parturition, a mother is sensitized to the behavioral cues of her newborn and begins to respond to them. The infant, in turn, responds to maternal behavior, and patterns of interaction quickly develop that establish the bond between the mother and her infant, preventing her from abandoning him. Relatively flexible behavioral mechanisms soon replace more rigid biological mechanisms. From an evolutionary perspective such a model is reasonable, since it provides for the survival of the species in the face of changing and potentially destructive environmental conditions.

> **COMMENT:** I think your statement of the concept of transition between hormonal and nonhormal mechanisms regulating maternal behavior is a good one, accurate and spelled out. I think it is a matter of philosophy if one wants to call that period a "critical period" for the formation of the mother-young attachment. I tend to think in terms of developmental stages rather than critical periods. Therefore transitions from one developmental stage (even in mothers) to the following one involve all the events of preceding stages, not just the events occurring during the transition. It may be of practical value to emphasize a critical part of the transition, as you have done, but in the long run I believe it is better to keep in mind that important factors outside the critical period affect the success or failure of transition from one developmental stage to another.
> **J.S. Rosenblatt**

CHAPTER 5

CARING FOR THE PARENTS OF PREMATURE OR SICK INFANTS

JOHN H. KENNELL and MARSHALL H. KLAUS

It is better by far to put the little one in an incubator by its mother's bedside, the supervision which she exercises is not to be lightly estimated.
Pierre Budin

The tribulations and struggles of parents of premature infants in learning to cope with their infants provided the stimulus to explore how normal parents develop a close attachment to their infants. As investigators began to study the ways in which the parent of a premature infant manages to meet the needs of this immature, sleepy, unpredictable, fragile infant, they noted many common adaptations, problems, and detours. During the last 10 to 15 years, research on parent-infant attachment has mainly focused on the parents of full-term infants. However, in recent years a number of investigators have looked closely at the complex and confusing ecology parents encounter when the birth of a premature or sick infant brings them into an intensive care nursery. This chapter attempts to place in perspective the creative work of the investigators who have ventured into this strange arena. Research in this area is not easy or straightforward but, rather, is frequently confounded by harassed, overworked nurses and physicians, overwhelmed parents, and critically sick infants. Recent observations based on the completed studies suggest a number of interventions that appear to have merit and deserve further investigation in the traditional hospital environment. A few brave investigators have been refreshingly innovative and have broken down the walls of the intensive care unit to create a new and more positive environment for parents of sick infants. In this chapter we will attempt to integrate these studies into a general framework from which we will develop some clinical recommendations.

HISTORY

Had we read closely the first text of neonatology by Budin (1907), we could have foreseen and perhaps avoided the tragic problems that became associated with

151

the care of premature or sick infants. In his book *The Nursling* he wrote, "Unfortunately . . . a certain number of mothers abandon the babies whose needs they have not had to meet, and in whom they have lost all interest. The life of the little one has been saved, it is true, but at the cost of the mother." He recommended that mothers should be encouraged to breastfeed their own premature infants in addition to another full-term infant to increase the mother's milk production. He designed and promoted the use of the glass-walled incubator that allowed the mother to look at her infant easily, and he permitted mothers to visit and care for their infants. Because of the introduction of these changes, mothers became and remained attentive to their infants' needs, even though the infants were in hospitals for a prolonged period.

Martin Couney, a young pupil of Budin, was sent by his teacher to demonstrate the new techniques to German physicians at the Berlin Exposition of 1896, where his *Kinderbrutanstalt* ("child hatchery"), which specialized in caring for premature infants, was successful commercially (Silverman, 1979). Since premature infants were not expected to live, German physicians gave them to Couney. He exhibited the infants at fairs in England (Covent Garden) and came to the United States in 1902 for the Pan American Exposition in Buffalo, after which he went on to Omaha, Nebraska, in 1904. From there he traveled throughout the United States. Couney finally settled on Coney Island, successfully caring for more than 5000 premature infants during the next four decades. He exhibited the infants in many major fairs and expositions (Fig. 5-1) from 1902 until the New York World's Fair of 1940. As late as 1932, Couney took infants from the Michael Reese Hospital to be exhibited at the Chicago World's Fair. The receipts they brought in were second only to those of Sally Rand, the fan dancer (Liebling, 1939).

Couney followed all the precepts of his teacher, Professor Budin, with one major exception. Mothers were not permitted to help take care of their infants at Couney's exhibits, although they were given free passes. Significantly, but perhaps not surprisingly, he observed that he could not make a living if he only collected an admission fee from the mothers. It is also revealing that on some occasions he experienced great difficulty in persuading mothers to take their babies back once they had grown to 5 pounds. As premature nurseries were established in hospitals in the United States, the staffs adopted many of Couney's methods of newborn care. Ironically, it was Budin's initial desire to have his methods demonstrated in Germany that finally and sadly resulted in the practice of excluding mothers from nurseries.

The first hospital center for premature care in the United States was established at the Sarah Morris Hospital in Chicago in 1923. Following the precepts of Budin, the director encouraged the production of breast milk at home. However, the mother's assistance in actually caring for the premature infant was not stressed.

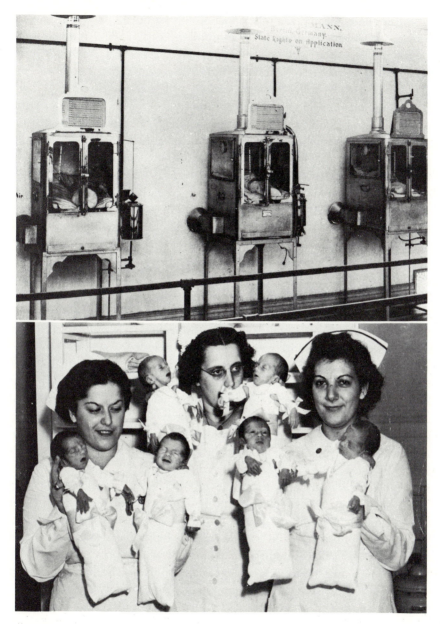

Fig. 5-1. *Top,* Interior of Couney's exhibit. *Bottom,* Nurses holding six exhibition babies. Couney's daughter Hildegarde is the nurse in the center.

Premature units created after the Sarah Morris Hospital followed a standard set of regulations, which remained in effect until the early 1960s. Textbooks on the care of the newborn from 1945 to 1960 continued to reflect the traditions and fears of the early 1900s, recommending only the most essential handling of the infants and a policy of strict isolation from any visitors, including the parents.

Across the Atlantic in Newcastle-on-Tyne, F.J.W. Miller, working with Sir James Spence, was studying the nursing of prematurely born infants in the home. In a comparison of home versus hospital nursing in 1945 to 1947, he found that both were equally favorable for premature infants weighing more than 3½ pounds at birth. However, he concluded that home care was safer from the standpoint of infection, more economical, and it served the essential purpose of unifying the infant's family. Miller (1948) stressed that each family member should have assigned duties so that "everyone interested is involved and all have a sense of achievement, which gives the child a good start and is far better than if he were taken away to a hospital and returned a month or six weeks later, an unknown infant, feared and strange."

Home care of premature infants did not spread to the United States but remained confined to England and Europe. The first observations of the parents of premature and sick infants in the United States in the 1950s and early 1960s were made at a time when parents were still totally excluded from the nursery. The reactions of mothers described by the pioneering investigators at that time may have been extreme because of the total separation from their infants. It is important to keep in mind that regulations for pediatric hospitals in the early 1950s limited parental visiting to only 30 to 60 minutes once or twice a week for older children. However, Blake and co-workers (1975), in spite of the gradual acceptance of more relaxed visiting regulations, report that the general pattern of parents' reactions appears to be the same today.

Although revolutionary changes in the approach to the diagnosis and management of other infants and children in the hospital were made during the period between 1945 and 1960, the premature infant in the nursery remained untouched and unaffected. For example, the scientific approach of Gamble and Darrow to fluid and electrolytes, which required the measurement of a number of blood constituents, had no effect on the care of the premature infant. The premature nursery remained a fortress, protected from innovations, investigations, and parents.

BASIC CONSIDERATIONS

In the last decade remarkable strides have been made in improving both the survival rate and quality of the survivors of neonatal intensive care units. Stewart and associates (1977) revealed that if all the modern techniques, which include early fluid administration and close and detailed monitoring of oxygen, environmental temperature, pH, respiration, and heart rate, are employed in treating the premature infant, he has only a slightly greater chance than a full-term infant of being disabled (Carter, 1978).

OUTCOME—SHORT TERM AND LONG TERM

There has been intense interest in the later abilities and characteristics of graduates of premature nurseries and their interaction with their families. Advances in obstetrical and neonatal care and technology have gradually led to a measurable improvement in quality of survival for even the smallest of low birth-weight infants. In the last eight to 10 years in an optimal clinical setting, approximately 90% of surviving infants below 1500 grams will be found free from significant mental or physical handicap (Fig. 5-2). Those nurses and physicians who had experience with damaged and handicapped premature infants born during the 1940s, 1950s, and 1960s often find it difficult to accept fully either these statistics or the optimistic predictions of the present-day neonatal intensive care nursery staff. Neonatologists and the other members of the staff of neonatal intensive care units now assume that with meticulous attention to the baby's well-being before, during, and after birth, the premature infant will be able to survive intact. This attitude contrasts sharply with the former policy of minimal treatment and a pessimistic attitude.

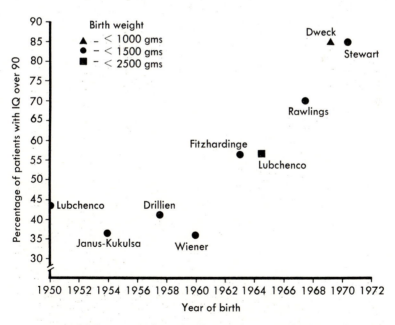

Fig. 5-2. A summary of follow-up studies of infants with varying birth weights. (From Horwitz, S.J., and Amiel-Tison, C.: Neurologic problems. In Klaus, M.H., and Faranoff, A.A.: Care of the high-risk neonate, Philadelphia, 1979, The W.B. Saunders Co.)

> **COMMENT:** A study by our group of survivors of respiratory distress syndrome in 1975 versus survivors of 1970 in fact suggests significantly better performance on developmental scales at 4 years of age among the more recent survivors. However, along with changes in intensive care unit technology during that time span, there were also changes in nursery practices such as the encouragement of parent visiting and the provision of a special room for breastfeeding mothers, all of which may have contributed to improved outcomes.
> **T. Field**

With a larger number of premature or sick babies who weigh less than 1000 grams and have extremely difficult, prolonged, and complicated courses and are transported to regional centers, we will have to wait several years before we know the abilities and outcomes for these babies and their parents.

After a lengthy review of studies exploring the later effects of perinatal factors on the development of children, Sameroff and Chandler (1975) were forced to conclude that "even if one continues to believe that a continuum of reproductive casualty exists, it's importance pales in comparison to the massive influence of socioeconomic factors on both prenatal and postnatal development."

Bakeman and Brown's (1980) three-year data support the conclusion that prematurely born babies from a disadvantaged population were more at risk for cognitive deficits than babies from a middle-class population. Bakeman and Brown's studies showed that cognitive ability was predicted by their status at birth and their mother's education. This is in agreement with the ground-breaking work of Drillien (1966,1967) in Scotland 30 years ago.

Many of the more recent observations on infant and family outcome are encouraging. However, it is necessary to stress that all reported studies of parenting disorders reveal a twofold to fourfold increase in the incidence of nonorganic failure to thrive and child battering among infants separated from their mothers because of prematurity or early neonatal illness.

> **COMMENT:** A more frequent problem than failure to thrive and child battering appears to be behavior problems, such as limited attention span, inability to sit still, and general symptoms of the "spoiled child" syndrome.
> **T. Field**

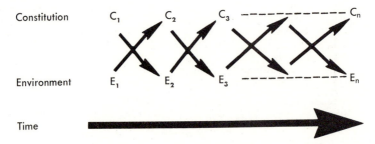

Fig. 5-3. Continuum of environmental casualty transactional model. (From Sameroff, A.J., and Chandler, M.J.: In Horowitz, F.D., et al., editors: Review of child development research, Chicago, 1975, University of Chicago Press, vol. 4. © 1975 by The University of Chicago.)

Although we agree that a transactional model in which the constitution and environment are continually interacting with each other over time, as pictured in Fig. 5-3, is a valid and extremely helpful concept, there is evidence that present care practices for infants and parents must be reviewed and studied further.

PARENTAL REACTIONS TO THE BIRTH OF A PREMATURE INFANT

In the era before parents were permitted to enter the premature nursery, Prugh (1953) made a series of sensitive and insightful observations of the mothers of premature infants. He reported that during the first months of the baby's life the mother is forced into a supporting, peripheral position. Because of having to assume this involuntary role, the mother "often finds herself the prey of disturbing, and at times strongly conflicting, feelings," particularly if this is her first child.

Anxiety and guilt were the two most evident emotions in the mother during this period. She was understandably apprehensive about her infant's survival during the early period of hospitalization. However, persistent anxiety often indicated other stresses. Her feelings of guilt heightened her feelings of anxiety. She feared that something which she did or did not do during pregnancy affected the baby and produced the prematurity.

Prugh (1953) noted that the mother may have also felt guilty after birth because she could not care for the baby as skillfully as the nurse. Although the mother was grateful to the nurse and physician, she resented the necessity for intervention by a substitute mother. He commented that "a mother often became jealous of the capable nurse and this led to an unconscious attempt to handle such unacceptable feelings by projecting the jealous resentment onto the nurse, leading to suspicion and hostility." Although the nurse was the object of resentment, she could serve as a valuable support to the mother during the difficult period of the infant's hospitalization. The mother must be allowed to proceed emotionally at her own pace. In Prugh's (1953) words, "It is important for the nurse to accept her as she finds her, without judgment or criticism."

> **COMMENT:** This is an extremely common syndrome even among mothers of normal infants, for example, leaving the infant with the more experienced grandmother or infant nursery school teacher. It is particularly a problem in the intensive care nursery because the nurse has highly technical knowledge and skills, all of which are more mysterious to the mother, who has been provided with very little information.
> **T. Field**

Prugh also stressed that it is essential for the mother to see the premature baby as soon as possible after birth to help "minimize the frightening fantasies which she may develop and help her to begin the process of handling any 'emotional lag.'" He described "emotional lag" as an alienation of feeling that any new mother experiences during her early relationship with her baby. The "difficulty in experiencing the warm, maternal feelings which she expected" is not confined to mothers of premature infants but may be equally intense anytime mothers are denied close contact with their full-term infants (Prugh, 1953).

Kaplan and Mason (1960) viewed the reactions of mothers to the birth of a premature infant in the context of an acute reaction to trauma rather than in the context of an ongoing pathological process. Their approach is in tune with the crisis theory concepts of Caplan (1960, 1964, 1965). He defines crises as "time-limited periods of disequilibrium or behavioral and subjective upsets which are precipitated by an inescapable demand or burden to which the person is temporarily unable to respond adequately. During this period of tension the person grapples with the problem and develops novel resources, both by calling upon internal reserves and making use of the help of others. Those resources are then used to handle the precipitating factor and the person achieves once more a steady state." Following this definition of crisis, Kaplan and Mason (1960) recognized that the reactions to a stressful event, such as the birth of a premature infant, could be heavily conditioned by previously existing personality factors. However, they emphasized that hospital practices and the role of health agencies can exert a positive influence on these factors. They also outlined four psychological tasks that the mother of a premature infant must master to establish a "healthy mother-child relationship."

1. At the time of birth the mother must prepare for the possible loss of the child whose life is in jeopardy. This "anticipatory grief" involves a withdrawal from the relationship previously established to the child in her uterus. She hopes the baby will survive but simultaneously prepares for his death.
2. The mother must face and acknowledge her maternal failure to give birth to a normal full-term baby.
3. The mother must resume the process, which has been interrupted, of relating to the baby. She has previously prepared herself for a loss, but as the baby improves, she must now respond to the change with hope and anticipation.

COMMENT: To see the special needs and growth patterns, the parents must be educated. Some intensive care nurseries provide this in the form of visiting ex-parents and their former ICU children and others in the form of films tracking the development of ICU graduates. In other nurseries only reassuring words are given, which cannot be as reassuring as true-life examples. Unfortunately, little research has been conducted on the forms of intervention provided parents of ICU babies.
T. Field

4. The mother must come to understand how a premature baby differs from a normal baby in terms of special needs and growth patterns. To provide the extra amount of care and protection, the mother must see the baby as a premature with special needs and characteristics. It is, however, equally important for her to see that these needs are temporary and will yield in time to normal patterns.*

---

*From Kaplan, D.M., and Mason, E.A.: Maternal reactions to premature birth viewed as an acute emotional disorder, Am. J. Orthopsychiatry **30:**539-552, 1960. Copyright 1960, The American Orthopsychiatric Association, Inc. Reproduced by permission.

COMMENT: The mother may invariably prepare for the possible loss even if she is given extra support and early contact. Preparation for loss may continue until the very moment she takes the baby home. An intensive care nursery, after all, is an intensive care nursery, which denotes a place of treatment for life and death conditions.
T. Field

We believe that the tasks outlined by Kaplan and his group are, in part, the result of the earlier care practices and the more traditional hospital setting. It is our impression that a mother need not start to prepare for the death if she is given extra support and early contact with her infant in the first hour of life. We believe that she will have a different set of tasks if the physical arrangements in the hospital are altered and her contacts with nurses and physicians are focused on providing both the mother and her infant with the special attention that the situation demands.

COMMENT: Although the mother may be helped to realize that the baby will probably live, she still must face the loss of not having had a full-term infant. Therefore the emotional response as outlined in these four points, although being less profound, will probably still be in evidence, even if the mother has early contact with the infant.
K. Barnard

COMMENT: We must also realize that Kaplan and Mason's four psychological tasks are based on a very traditional concept of womanhood. Thus contemporary thinking does not automatically associate the birth of a premature infant with a maternal failure and consequently many women do not feel this any more. In addition, fathers also have to face similar issues.
K. Minde

E.A. Mason (1963) reported a study in which he predicted the quality of the early mother-child relationship from information gathered during interviews with mothers of premature infants during the lying-in period. By utilizing the interview technique once again, an independent judge evaluated the mother-child relationship between six and 10 weeks after the baby was discharged. A good outcome was defined as one in which the mother was moderately successful in meeting the baby's physical and emotional needs, the baby gained weight, or the family seemed pleased with the baby. In the cases judged to have a poor outcome, the mother was hostile or irritable and impatient, the baby was neglected and either lethargic or in poor health, and the family was severely disrupted. The predictions agreed with the outcome ratings in 90% of the cases (17 of 19 cases; $p<.01$).

Mason found that certain aspects of the mother's coping mechanism were extremely valuable in predicting the nature of her subsequent relationship with her child. The interviewers predicted a good outcome if the mother expressed a fairly high level of anxiety, actively sought information about the condition of her baby, and showed strong maternal feelings for the baby, even when she had not yet seen or held him. Strong support by the father and a previous successful experience with a premature child also indicated a favorable outcome.

If the mother showed a low level of anxiety and activity, chances were that her relationship with her child would be poor. These mothers often denied that they were anxious and focused their concern on matters other than the infant's condition. They often lacked support from husbands and relatives and evidenced little maternal feeling. Mason (1963) concluded that efforts to prevent poor outcomes for mothers and their premature infants should be directed toward increasing "the interaction between the mother and her premature baby."

> **COMMENT:** The mother who demonstrates a low level of anxiety about the child may simply be overwhelmed by other circumstances of her life. For example, in a recent study, when sample mothers of premature babies were asked what their primary concerns were at one month postpartum, about 65% of the mothers had concerns that related to the child or parenting; 35% of the mothers did not. In looking at circumstances within these 35% of the mothers, major circumstances of financial constraint or family problems were their primary concern. The answer may not always be to increase interaction between the mother and her premature baby; circumstances may require investigation of what may be blocking the mother from having the capacity to interact with her baby.
>
> **K. Barnard**

During the same year Blau and associates (1963) examined the possible psychogenic etiology of premature births. They compared the results of psychiatric and psychological tests administered one to three days after birth to 30 women who delivered prematurely and 30 matched control mothers of full-term infants. They did find clinical differences between the two groups. The mother of a premature infant tended to be more immature, was uncertain about her role as a woman and mother, and needed more outside emotional support during pregnancy. Blau and associates noted that "though ambivalence is undoubtedly common to all pregnancies, the premature mother has less, in that she tends to become more definitely negative to the pregnancy and hostile to the fetus. She harbors more destructive fantasies about the outcome to herself and to the baby, and is more apprehensive regarding difficulties in labor and delivery." However, it should be remembered that these intriguing observations were made after birth, not before.

In recent years when parental visiting in the intensive care nursery has been permitted, studies of Harper and colleagues (1976), Benfield and associates (1976), Minde and colleagues (1975, 1978, 1980*a*), and Newman (1980) have continued to reveal that most parents are under severe emotional distress.

Harper and colleagues (1976) found that even when parents were permitted to have close contact with their infants, they experienced prolonged stress. However, they reported that parents believe that the opportunity to have this contact with their infant in the neonatal intensive care unit is valuable, in spite of their anxiety. Ninety percent of the parents questioned would have been opposed to restricted contact with their infants; 85% believed that holding their infants made the infant feel more loved and secure; and 44% thought that the quality and quantity of care rendered improved when they were present. Harper and colleagues state that although "frequent parental-infant contact may build long term relationships, the emotional price tag is high."

Benfield and associates (1976) studied 101 mother-father pairs who had premature infants and noted that most parents experienced grief reactions similar to those whose infants had died. The level of their response was unrelated to the severity of the baby's problem. (This recalls the comments of Kaplan and Mason regarding the first task, p. 158.)

Newman (1980) raises a series of questions that are highly relevant now that parents are permitted into special care nursery units. What does being in the special care nursery mean to parents? While the baby is undergoing intensive care of a therapeutic nature he will receive sufficient other care from the professional staff. What is the role of parents whose infant is cared for entirely by others? In the professionals' work place, with all the stresses of intensive care, how do these parents cope with the presumed or potential tragedies of the infants surrounding them and the unknown destiny of their own child?

Using anthropological techniques, in a small sample from the intensive care nursery, Newman noted individual variations between families and even within families that reflected individual coping styles and personal adaptations to the stress of a premature birth. "Coping through commitment" was the label given for an intense, yet variable, involvement in the care of a low birth-weight infant. "Coping through distance" defined a slower acquaintance process, where the parents relied on the care provided by experts and expressed fear, anxiety, and at times denial before they accepted the surviving infant.

Green (1979) graphically described the plight of the families of premature infants. "For the parents time seems both to slip away yet remain frozen in place. Geographically displaced, their work and lives disrupted, their biological rhythms in disarray, bewildered, anxious, and terribly tired, parents in the delirium of crisis are simply unable to comprehend what is happening."

OBSERVATIONS AFTER DISCHARGE

Minde and colleagues (1978, 1980*a*), in a series of creative studies done both in the hospital and the home during the first three months after birth, observed that the interaction of 32 mothers and their very low birth-weight infants could be divided into three groups relating to the level of interaction: high, medium, or low. Highly interacting mothers visit and telephone the nursery more while the infants are hospitalized and stimulate their infants more at home. Mothers who stimulate their infants little in the nursery also visit and telephone less frequently and stimulate them little at home. (Many investigators have noted that a severe illness or setback in a premature infant following a period of stability will often result in the mother fleeing the nursery and remaining away for a long period.) Strikingly, only psychological variables within the mother's background were found by Minde to relate significantly to the maternal activity pattern. The most important of these variables were her relationships with her own mother, her relationship with the father of the infant, and whether or not the mother had a previous abortion.

Minde and colleagues noted that mothers who touched and fondled their infants more in the nursery had infants with increased eye opening. Minde and colleagues (1978) examined the contingency between infants' eyes being open and the mother's touching and also between gross motor stretches and the mother's smiling. Their study did not determine to what extent in these cases the sequence of touching and eye opening was an indication of the mother's primary contribution or the infant's. This work suggests that the infant primarily steers the course of the mother-infant interaction at a very early age.

In a detailed follow-up study of infants weighing 1500 grams or less, Blake and colleagues (1975) have noted that many English mothers go through three phases in the first six months after the baby's discharge from the hospital. At first there is a "honeymoon" phase. Excitement prevails, and the parents are usually euphoric at the time of the first visit to the clinic seven to 10 days after discharge. A period of exhaustion follows, when the euphoria has waned, and the mother has many minor complaints about the management of the baby, particularly about feeding. The mother not only looks exhausted but is exhausted. The feeding problems are often genuine. This phase will last until the time when the baby begins to smile and respond to his mother, which can take anywhere from a few days to several weeks.

COMMENT: Our experience with parents of ICU graduates is that when they most need outside supports, that is, after the honeymoon phase when the infant is difficult and the parents exhausted, they have the least support. Perhaps more of our resources should be invested in home visit programs.
T. Field

COMMENT: We find that mothers are physically tired and usually depressed at one month after discharge. The babies are often becoming more irritable. Parents need counseling about what to expect from the baby and also themselves. We have found it important to help them focus on the baby's nonverbal cues such as motor activity and sleeping pattern. The changes in motor activity can be used to modulate arousal level. They don't have to wait for potent negative cues such as crying; they can use the increasing of motor activity and certain of the disengagement postures to begin to relieve the baby's distress. The parents also need to know that the positive cues which say, "I like you," don't come as easily. Therefore eliciting smiling and mutual eye contact can be taught to the parents.
K. Barnard

Blake and colleagues (1975) observed a specific pattern of behavior among mothers during the first few weeks that their babies were home, suggesting that the emotional conflicts were not completely resolved until after the baby left the hospital. "These mothers are inefficient in recognizing signals from the baby immediately after the baby goes home, they are anxious and probably react indiscriminantly to everything, consequently becoming exhausted." This exhaustion leads to inefficiency in practical tasks, and then to resentment. And "then the mothers feel guilty at their resentment." In addition to previously having anticipated the baby's death, most of these mothers have also already suffered from feelings of guilt and failure. The birth of a small premature baby is enough to induce these emotions in the mother, but Blake and colleagues make the following observation:

> Previous infertility, pregnancy failure or termination, abnormalities of pregnancy, denial of pregnancy and unwanted pregnancy, particularly when there have been attempts to terminate it, all tend to intensify these feelings. In addition, many of the mothers experience horror and hate at the sight of their babies, which must lead to even more guilt, especially as our culture dictates that babies are "beautiful" and that mothers automatically love them on sight. The mothers, however, cannot rationalize sufficiently to explain their problems. Instead, they complain of physical difficulties in the baby, such as feeding, vomiting, or constipation.*

COMMENT: The physical difficulties in the baby, such as feeding, vomiting, or constipation are real. Our study on maternal stimulation during infant feeding suggested that preterm babies with medical complications are more difficult feeders even at four months postdischarge. Their mothers stimulate them more frequently in response to the babies' reluctance to feed.
T. Field

In disagreement with these remarks are the recent studies by Boyle and co-workers (1977) who suggest that from their observations there is no evidence that the experience of having a very low birth-weight child has a significant or continuing impact on the family. Bakeman and Brown (1980) note that their observations over a three-year period provide little support for the belief that the way in which a mother interacts with her baby during the first months of life has any consequences for later social or cognitive development. They had previously described distinct differences between the behavior of parents of premature and full-term infants during this early period.

COMMENT: Early interactions cannot be underrated. There are many other studies, for example, those of Parmelee and colleagues (1976), Sigman (1979), Field and associates (1979), which suggest that there are relationships between early interactions and later development. In the Bakeman and Brown (1980) study other more significant factors like very low socioeconomic conditions may have overpowered any effects of early interactions on later development.
T. Field

When discussing the effects of early separation on the later development of premature infants, we must detour slightly and note that, in a report from the British Perinatal Study with its superb follow-up, Douglas (1975, 1976) provided unexpected evidence that one admission to a hospital of more than a weeks' duration or repeated admissions before the age of 5 years were associated with an increased risk of behavior disturbances and reading disorders in adolescents. However, admissions before 6 months of age seemed to have minimal consequences. The prevalence of troublesome behavior, poor reading ability, and delinquency was at approximately the same level for children who had both long- and short-term

---

*From Blake, A., Stewart, A., and Turcan, D.: In Parent-infant interaction, Ciba Foundation Symposium 33, Amsterdam, 1975, Elsevier Publishing Co., p. 278.

periods of hospital admission in the first 6 months as was found in children not admitted. Unstable job patterns among those admitted for a week or less in the first 6 months of life were at the same level as those with no admissions but were increased among children who stayed longer than a week. Little is known about the extent to which these early infancy admissions, which included babies kept in the hospital after birth, involved separation from the mother. However, it is reasonable to assume that some degree of separation occurred for all these children while they were in the hospital. If this is the case, the data from that study do not completely support the view that there are significant long-term consequences of early separation.

INFANT STIMULATION AND MOTHER-INFANT INTERACTION

Recently a burst of studies of infant stimulation has appeared that provide a connection between the many studies of mothering and the future development of the infant (Barnard, 1975; Hasselmeyer, 1964; Katwinkel et al., 1975; Katz, 1971; Korner et al., 1975; Kramer and Pierpont, 1976; Leib et al., 1980; Scarr-Salapatek and Williams, 1973; Segall, 1972; Solkoff et al., 1969; Van den Daele, 1970). These studies reveal that if a small premature infant is either touched, rocked, fondled, or cuddled daily during his stay in the nursery, he has fewer apneic periods, increased weight gain, fewer stools, and an advance in some areas of higher central nervous system functioning, which persists for months after discharge from the hospital. As an example, Fig. 5-4 illustrates the effect of a pulsating waterbed on apnea (respiratory phase). With a shortage of personnel to give this care, it seems logical to allow parents to provide this special mothering, this additional stimulation that helps a small premature infant to thrive. However, the short- and long-term

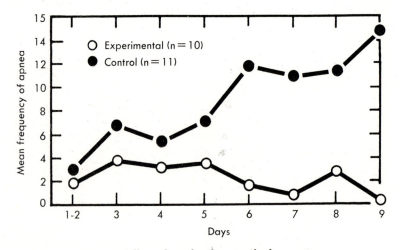

Fig. 5-4. Effect of a pulsating waterbed on apnea.

benefits of stimulation are now being questioned (see pp. 166-168 for a discussion of stimulation vs. imitation).

COMMENT: The whole business of stimulation should not be thought of as just providing additional or more stimulation to the premature infant. More thought should be given to the appropriate types of stimulation and its timing; in fact, many infants are bombarded with stimuli either in the hospital nursery or in the early home situation, when their capacity to deal with stimulus overload is less. They may even develop irritability and crying behavior because of stimulus overload, which then creates difficulty for the family.
K. Barnard

COMMENT: Stimulation outcome studies have traditionally concentrated almost exclusively on assisting the cognitive development of infants. They have failed to examine whether teaching a mother or a father to do things with their baby will also make these parents more sensitive to the infant's needs.
K. Minde

COMMENT: Professor Dobbing in England recently asked us to write a review of the supplemental stimulation programs in the United States because he was concerned that we had "willy-nilly" introduced lots of stimulation in our infant intensive care nurseries before all the data were in and he wanted to include our review as a cautionary note in his journal for the British readership. Our review of the literature did not reveal any negative consequences, but findings were certainly as mixed as the kinds of stimulation offered and the kinds of babies stimulated. Surprisingly, we found only one group who had documented the already-existing stimulation before introducing new stimulation (Lawson et al., 1977). The ICU sound level measurements they presented, sound levels comparable to the sound of a starting bus, suggest that we should be investigating the effects of the already-existing stimulation and possible modifications (e.g., dimmed lights, muffled monitor sounds, etc.) Introducing new stimulation prior to measuring the effects of existing stimulation does seem like "putting the cart before the horse."
T. Field

Several ingenious and detailed observations of mothers interacting with premature infants Brown and Bakeman, 1980;(DiVitto and Goldberg, 1979; Field, 1977, 1978) during feedings and in face-to-face play have shown quantitative and qualitative differences when compared with mothers' interactions with full-term infants. Premature infants tend to be unresponsive or hypoactive, whereas their mothers are typically hyperactive during interactions. However mothers from lower socio-economic groups and teenage mothers tend to be hypoactive (Field, 1978; Kilbride et al., 1977). The burden of maintaining the interactions appears to fall disproportionately on the mothers of the preterm infant (Brown and Bakeman, 1980).

Field has shown that there is a level of moderate maternal activity that results in optimal infant arousal and interaction. This is the level typically shown by mothers of full-term infants. Maternal activity that is excessive, or minimal, results in a "non-optimal interaction, probably as a function of its effects on infant arousal levels." In a two-year follow-up Field (1977) found that the mothers of premature infants who were overactive during early face-to-face interactions were overprotective and over-controlling during later interactions with their infants.

COMMENT: Field observed her mothers for only 3-minute periods, and while her results are obviously very important, other investigators have shown that mothers can behave very differently during the course of a day in different situations.
K. Minde

Brown and colleagues (1980) were unable to find any effects at discharge from the nursery or one year later when they compared (1) a group where the babies received extra stimulation to make them more active contributors to interactions with their mothers; (2) a group where the mothers received extra training to become more responsive to their babies' cries; (3) a group where infants received stimulation and mothers received training; and (4) a comparison group.

Although many studies of premature infants cared for in incubators have documented an effect of stimulation, our conceptual framework after discharge of the mother and infant must be drastically altered as a result of perceptive work by several investigators. We will now discuss three separate lines of evidence which suggest that the relationship between the mother and infant during their multiple interactions is not necessarily what might be deduced intuitively.

STIMULATION OR IMITATION—WHAT IS APPROPRIATE?

First, Winnicott (1971) described in a chapter entitled, "The Mirror Role of Mother and Family in Child Development" that what the baby observes in the caretaker's face in the early months helps him develop the concept of himself. He asked, "What does the baby see when he or she looks at the mother's face? I am suggesting that, ordinarily, what the baby sees is himself or herself. In other words the mother is looking at the baby and *what she looks like is related to what she sees there*. All this is too easily taken for granted. I am asking that this which is naturally done well by mothers who are caring for their babies shall not be taken for granted." At another point in the same chapter he notes, "Of course nothing can be said about the single occasions on which a mother could not respond. Many babies, however, do have to have a long experience of not getting back what they are giving. They look and they do not see themselves. There are consequences. First, their own creative capacity begins to atrophy, and in some way or other they look around for other ways of getting something of themselves back from the environment." He suggests that blind infants need to get themselves reflected through senses other than that of sight. The important implications of Winnicott's perceptive observations using pediatric and psychoanalytical observational techniques is that in the normal mother-infant dyads he cared for, the mother was often following or "imitating" the infant.

Second, Trevarthen (1977), observing mothers and infants using fast film techniques and detailed analysis, noted that mothers imitate their babies during spontaneous play. In a separate study he suggested that it is the mother's imitation of her infant's behavior rather than the reverse which sustains their interaction and communication. Detailed analysis of the periods when both are active reveals that the mother is studiously imitating the infant's expressions with a lag of between 0.1 and 0.2 second. Thus the infant is choosing the tune.

Third, Field (1977), in a series of creative experimental manipulations of infant-mother face-to-face interactions, noted that the mother and the normal full-term infant are each interacting about 70% of the time in their spontaneous play (Fig. 5-5). However, when the mother is asked to increase her attention-getting behavior, her activity increases to 80% of the time and, strikingly, the infant's gaze decreases to 50%. In the situation where the mother is told to imitate the movements of the infant, she moves at a much slower pace and the infant's gaze time greatly increases.

In observations of the high-risk premature infant, Field noted that in the spontaneous situation the mother is interacting up to 90% of the time, whereas the infant is only looking 30% of the time. If the mother is told to use attention-getting gestures her activity increases even above 90% of the time and the infant's gaze decreases further. If her interactions are decreased by asking her to imitate the baby's movements, there is then a striking increase in the infant's gaze.

Although generally the parents' activity is aimed at encouraging more activity or responsivity from the premature infant, the approach, if too vigorous, may be counterproductive, leading to less instead of more infant responsivity.

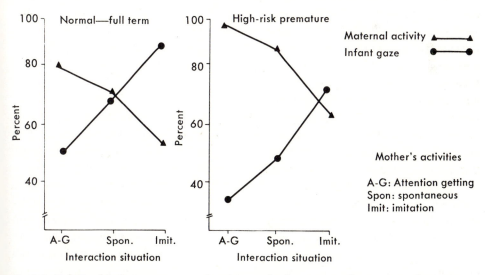

Fig. 5-5. Relationship between maternal activity and infant gaze in three maternal situations: (1) attempting to get the infant's attention, (2) spontaneous interaction, and (3) mother imitating the baby. (From Field, T.M.: Child Dev. **48:**763-771, 1977. Copyright The Society for Research in Child Development, Inc.)

Thus by three separate and different techniques, psychoanalysis, the detailed study of high-speed films, and experimental manipulations of infant-mother face-to-face interactions, it appears that mothers of normal infants follow or "mirror their infant's behavior" for significant periods of time. These agree with the work of Pawlby (1977), who finds that both the mother and infant imitate each other.

> **COMMENT:** In a recent analysis of our videotapes of fathers interacting with preterm infants with respiratory distress syndrome (at age 4 months), we found that although they too were overactive with these babies, they appeared less affected by their infants' lesser responsivity. When compared with the mothers, fathers smiled, laughed, and played infant games more frequently with their preterm babies. Fathers appeared to be less disturbed and to enjoy their interactions more than mothers. Perhaps fathers are less worried about the fragility and unresponsivity of their infants at this early age, or perhaps these fathers (who spent fewer hours with their babies on a daily basis) had experienced less exhaustion and frustration caring for them.
> **T. Field**

There may be many possible explanations for the mother's increase in activity in the interaction with her premature infant—she may have taken up the task of stimulation she observed in the premature nursery, she may be unhappy with the infant's responses and attempt to increase them, or she may develop this increased activity as a result of some natural intuitive compensatory reactions. There is still a great deal to be studied and defined about the mother's efforts to increase interaction with her premature infant, the timing and pacing of extra stimulation, how it should be provided, by whom, when, and its long-term significance.

At this point we would like to relate an observation of a special nurse, Louise, in our own nursery. We have always found her to be unusually perceptive and sensitive in picking out which infants will have problems in the first year or two of life. When premature infants who are often unresponsive are taken out of the incubator, she usually takes over their care. Then, with her handling over several days, we see the infants become bright, begin to look around, follow faces, and increase their activity. On close filming of Louise, we see little apparent activity. She holds the infant 8 to 10 inches from her face and seems to move imperceptibly. In reviewing the work of Winnicott, Trevarthen, and Field, it would appear that Louise may intuitively be following very slightly behind the movements of the premature infant and allowing the infant to begin to find himself.

It should be noted that once a person is a self-contained individual and has a well-integrated self, any imitation is an invasion of that indivdual's integrity. However, during the early months when the infant's self is incompletely formed, imitation of the infant's gestures appears to be a help in his finding himself. All these observations suggest that we should be careful about recommending increased stimulation for the premature infant. Instead, it would appear to be more appropriate to suggest that the mother attempt to move at her infant's pace. We hope that future studies will examine the effect of imitation on the premature infant's development.

COMMENT: In comparing mothers of preterm and full-term infants at 4 and 8 months of living age, we have found that mothers of preterm infants are less sensitive to the infant's behavioral cues. The preterm infants are also less clear in their cues and less responsive. We try to help the mother catch the cues the infant has. These cues are mainly in changes in level of motor activity and in postural orientations.
K. Barnard

INTERVENTIONS

To help parents to deal with the stressful situation of having a sick or small infant, a number of interventions have been introduced. In some cases they have involved the parents and infant together, whereas others have focused on either the parent or the infant. It should be noted that the ecology of the intensive care nursery is a difficult environment in which to make detailed and definitive assessments. Nurseries not only differ in their physical environment but differ also in patient population and physician interests, background, training, and sensitivity. In spite of this, there are sufficient data and measurements from several nurseries to enable us to begin to make recommendations. However, in assessing the potential value of any intervention, it may be inappropriate to generalize to a much wider population from a study carried out in one premature unit. The following interventions will be discussed in this chapter:

1. Opening the intensive care nursery to parents
2. Transporting the mother to be near her infant
3. Maternal day care for premature infants
4. Rooming-in for the parent of a premature infant
5. Nesting
6. Early discharge
7. Listening to parents (interviewing) during the infant's hospitalization
8. Parent groups
9. Programmed contact and reciprocal interaction
10. Transporting the healthy premature infant to the mother
11. Home-based intervention for young parents
12. Discussions with the parents after discharge

Opening the intensive care nursery to parents

The first study to investigate the feasibility of permitting parent into the premature nursery began in December, 1964, at Stanford University, California. Barnett and colleagues (1970) questioned whether parents of premature infants suffered from severe deprivation because of separation from their hospitalized infants. For a two-year period they studied the practicality of allowing mothers (44 in all) into the nursery soon after birth, first to handle and then to feed their infants while they were still in incubators. The mothers, because of state rules, wore masks and gowns, and the nurses in the unit instructed them in handwashing procedures.

Initially the nurses accompanied the mothers and stood by them while they handled their babies through the portholes of the incubators. On subsequent visits a nurse remained nearby to answer questions. When the babies were able to be fed easily by nipple, the mothers were encouraged to assume this task.

The threat of infection had been a formidable deterrent to permitting parents to enter the nursery. To evaluate the possibility that parents would bring pathogenic agents into the premature unit, cultures were taken weekly from the umbilicus, skin, and nares of each infant and from the nursery equipment for the entire period that mothers were allowed into the unit. These investigators observed that mothers washed more frequently and more thoroughly than both the nurses and house officers. The results of these cultures (Table 5-1) as well as the results of studies done by Williams and Oliver (1969), Silverman and Sinclair (1967), and Forfar and MacCabe (1958) showed no increase in potentially pathogenic organisms, as a result of mothers' presence in the nursery. In fact, at Stanford University the number of positive cultures actually declined between 1964 and 1965. It has been speculated that the infant may pick up nonpathogenic bacteria from his mother, which provide him with protection against pathogenic hospital organisms, and hence the number of positive cultures decreases. "A chart review showed no occurrence of staphylococcal, hemolytic streptococcal, or upper respiratory viral disease in the infants during the time when mothers went into the nursery. From these data it would appear that the presence of mothers in the nursery did not increase the risk or the occurrence of infection" (Barnett et al., 1970).

The investigators observed differences between the mothers allowed into the

Table 5-1. Culture results of infants and equipment by years*

Nursery population	1964	1965	1966
Number of infants in unit	38	48	49
Number and percent of mothers allowed to handle infants in incubators	2 (5%)	27 (56%)	12 (25%)
Infant data			
Total cultures of nares and umbilicus	680	718	694
Number of potential pathogens isolated and percent of positive cultures†	146 (21%)	102 (14%)	119 (17%)
Equipment data			
Total cultures of equipment‡	390	420	489
Number of potential pathogens isolated and percent of positive cultures†	44 (11%)	20 (5%)	24 (5%)

*From Barnett, C.R., Leiderman, P.H., Grobstein, R., and Klaus, M.H.: Neonatal separation: the maternal side of interactional deprivation, Pediatrics **45**:197-205, 1970.

†Includes coagulase-positive staphylococci, beta hemolytic streptococci, *Pseudomonas*, *Proteus*, pneumococcus, yeast, *Clostridium perfringens*.

‡Weekly cultures of incubator gaskets, water reservoirs, oxygen masks, suction bottles, and sink handles.

nursery and those who were excluded. Those who had entered the nursery showed increased commitment to the infant, more confidence in their mothering abilities, and greater stimulating and caretaking skills.

When mothers are first permitted to touch their premature babies, they typically begin by circling the incubator and touching the baby's extremities with the tips of their fingers (Klaus et al., 1970). These reactions are different from those of the parents of full-term infants who by the end of the first visit are stroking the infants' trunk with the palm of their hand. Mothers of full-term infants will align their head with their babies' heads in the *en face* position.

> **COMMENT:** *En face* is an important position for mothers and infants, since it is the one position assumed during caregiver-infant contact that increases the chances for social interaction between the mother or caregiver and the infant.
> **K. Barnard**

Fig. 5-6 compares the amount of time mothers of full-term infants spend in the *en face* position with the amount of time that mothers of premature infants spend in this position.

Two long-term studies on the effects of early mother-infant separation as a result of special care nursery policies, one at Stanford University and the other at Case Western Reserve University, Ohio, have been completed (Table 5-2). The hypothesis in each study was that if human mothers are affected by this period of separation, one might see altered maternal attachment and mothering behavior during

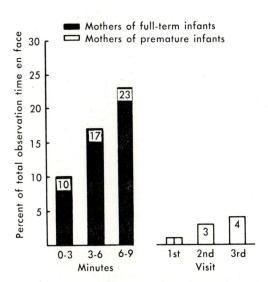

Fig. 5-6. The percentage of *en face* position recorded during the first visit of twelve mothers of full-term infants and the first three visits of nine mothers of premature infants. (From Klaus, M.H., Kennell, J.H., Plumb, N., and Zuehlke, S.: Pediatrics **46**:187-192, 1970.)

Table 5-2. Studies of early and late maternal contact in the premature nursery

	Stanford University*	Case Western Reserve University
Early contact	22†	27
		(1537 grams)‡
Late contact	22†	26
		(1428 grams)‡
Number of married mothers	44	42
Socioeconomic status	Middle class	Wide range
Hollingshead Index	3	1 to 5
Length of follow-up (months)	22	42

*Also included 24 full-term infants and mothers.
†Range of birth weights: 890 to 1899 grams.
‡Mean weight.

the first weeks and months of life in separated as opposed to nonseparated mothers and, as a consequence of this, differences in later infant development.

In the Stanford University study three groups of mothers from similar socioeconomic backgrounds were observed. One group of mothers was given "contact" with their premature infants in the intensive care unit in the first five days of life, a second group of mothers was "separated" from their premature infants with only visual contact for the first 21 days, and a third group of mothers of full-term infants had routine contact with their infants at feedings during a three-day hospitalization. When the separated infants reached 2100 grams, at ages ranging from 3 to 12 weeks, they were transferred to a discharge nursery where their mothers were allowed to be with them as much as they desired for the seven to 10 days until discharge at a weight of 2500 grams.

The interactions between the mothers of these three groups and their own infants were observed three times: just prior to discharge and a week and a month after discharge. The behavior of the mothers of full-term infants was not the same as that of the mothers of premature infants. The former group smiled at their infants more and had more ventral contact with their infants. No striking differences were found between the behaviors of the separated and contact mothers of premature infants. However, the primiparous mothers in the noncontact group showed significantly less self-confidence in their ability to care for their infants (Seashore et al., 1973). Sameroff (1975) interpreted this as suggesting the following:

> The previous successful childbirth experience of multiparous mothers seemed to insulate them from the debilitating effects of being separated from the premature offspring of their current pregnancy. In the group of mothers who were allowed to visit in the intensive care nursery, the initial deficits in self-confidence were reduced by the time the infant was ready to go home. Only one of the mothers in the separated group showed such a positive change. It would appear from this data that allowing mothers, especially

primipara, to be in contact with their premature infants reduces their feelings of inadequacy.*

COMMENT: Early contact may be more crucial for mothers who, because of their previous life circumstances, are at high risk for attachment, in addition to the prematurity.
K. Barnard

Leifer and associates (1972) also reported an important set of clinical findings that had not been anticipated. Only one of 22 mothers in the contact group became divorced during the period of the study, whereas five of 22 mothers in the separated group were divorced. It is worthy of note that a prerequisite for admission into the study was that the parents planned to keep and raise their babies. Surprisingly, in two cases in the separated group, neither parent wanted custody of their baby, and so the baby was given up for adoption.

In the Case Western Reserve University study 53 mothers of premature infants were assigned, on the basis of when the baby was born, to two groups, "early contact" and "late contact." Mothers in the early contact group were allowed to come into the premature nursery to handle and care for their premature infants one to five days after birth. The late contact group of mothers was not permitted to enter the nursery until 21 days after birth. For the first three weeks these mothers had only visual contact with their infants through the nursery windows.

Time-lapse movies of both groups of mothers feeding their infants were obtained just before discharge and one month later. Fig. 5-7 shows a posed mother illustrating four of the many behaviors that were analyzed from the 10-minute feeding films. In addition, to determine whether early contact influenced maternal behavior, which then affected infant development, Bayley developmental examinations were performed just before discharge and again at 9, 15, and 21 months of age, and a Stanford-Binet test was administered at 42 months of age.

The mothers who had early contact spent significantly more time looking at their infants during the first filmed feeding. Similarly, there was a correlation between the amount of time mothers looked at their babies during the second filmed feeding and the infants' IQ on the Stanford-Binet test at 42 months of age. That is, mothers who had early contact with their infants spent more time looking at them during feedings, and these children had significantly higher IQs ($r = .71$) with a mean of 99 for early contact children compared with a mean of 85 for late contact children ($p < .05$).

COMMENT: Mothers who in the hospital period and early first months of life look more at their infant generally tend to be more sensitive to the infant's cues and provide more appropriate stimulation to the infant than mothers who look less at their infant.
K. Barnard

*From Sameroff, A.: In Avery, G.B., editor: Neonatology, Philadelphia, 1975, J.B. Lippincott Co.

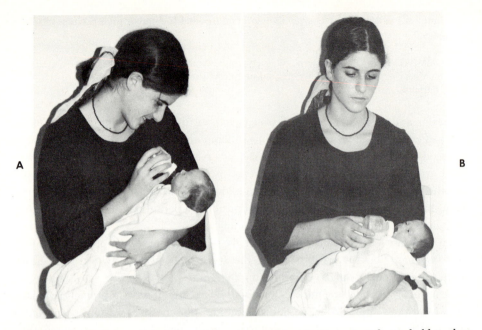

Fig. 5-7. A posed mother showing two different caretaking positions. **A,** Infant is held in close contact (mother's body touching infant's), mother is looking at infant *en face*, bottle is perpendicular to the mouth, and milk is in the tip of the nipple. **B,** Infant's trunk is held away from mother, mother is looking at infant but not *en face*, and bottle is not perpendicular to the mouth.

Interestingly, Bayley developmental scores for the two groups of infants were not significantly different for the first 21 months of life (Kennell et al., 1975).

Several problems associated with each of these studies should be mentioned. Both investigations were continued for two years, during which there were changes of procedure and personnel. Eighteen patients were lost from the Case Western Reserve University study during the long follow-up period. Had these patients been included in the testing, the final results may have been altered (Moss, 1965).

Studies of premature mother-infant dyads are especially difficult because of problems that occur during the long and stressful period of hospitalization, combined with the almost impossible task of obtaining a homogeneous population for both groups with respect to parity, sex of infant, birth weight, gestational age, religion, cultural background, and socioeconomic status. It is also difficult to control for the early life experiences of the mother, as well as for the stresses that occur at home. Neither group of investigators found it possible to run the early and late contact groups in the nursery simultaneously. Each study had a three-month period of late contact followed by a three-month period of early contact to prevent late contact mothers from observing early contact mothers in the nursery. Eventually both studies were discontinued because they were too painful for the nurses, who thought that it was unfair not to permit all mothers to have early contact with their infants.

As part of the Stanford University study, the parents were interviewed seven times before the infant was discharged. This tended to pull both the early and late contact mothers into the hospital, possibly increasing the number of visits the late contact mothers made to the hospital. It is surprising that in this study the early contact mothers visited only an average of once every six days.

There is evidence that early interaction may limit the advancement of anticipatory grief, which in turn would modify the first task of Kaplan and Mason (1960). Their studies were carried out 20 years ago, at a time when there was no parental visiting. Separation therefore was complete and prolonged, and the mother only handled her baby just before discharge.

Transporting the mother to be near her small infant

With the development of high-risk perinatal centers there have been an increasing number of mothers who are transported to the maternity division of hospitals with an intensive care nursery just prior to delivery or shortly after. This enables them to visit and care for their infants during the early postpartum period. We believe this trend is helpful for both parents, since the father is not distracted by having some members of his family in two hospitals and others at home. Data from several centers suggest that there is improved infant mortality when the mother is transported prior to giving birth, since facilities for the early care of the high-risk infant are often better in the hospital with intensive care facilities. If there is not sufficient time to arrange for her transport prior to giving birth, we strongly recommend that the mother be moved during her early postpartum period. Unfortunately at this time, studies on parenting after transportation of a mother, either before or following the birth, are not available. We look forward to investigations on this subject in the future.

Maternal day care for premature infants

In Russia the mothers take a limited part in the care of their premature infants. They live either at home or in the hospital. One of the authors (M.H.K.) had an opportunity to observe the care of premature infants in Russia. In one hospital there were 150 premature infants, and every day about 60 mothers came from home in the morning to spend the whole day with their babies. They showered, changed into clean smocks, had breakfast, and breastfed their babies. They were able to spend time with their babies, had a chance to talk with the physician, and believed that they were doing something positive to help their babies.

In the Leningrad Obstetrical Institute mothers were not discharged a few days after giving birth but stayed in the hospital until their premature babies were discharged—often as long as 60 to 90 days—and breastfed the entire time. Sadly, their husbands were unable to visit and could communicate only through letters.

These mothers appeared very depressed. In all the Russian hospitals visited, whether the mothers came in the morning to take care of their premature babies or lived in, they did nothing but breastfeed. The babies were brought to them wrapped, and mothers were not allowed to change the baby or participate in other caregiving tasks.

In an attempt to evaluate this practice, we tried to learn about the incidence of battering or failure-to-thrive syndrome among Russian infants. Russian physicians completely denied that battering occurred. Russian women are permitted unlimited abortions. If a woman has a child she does not want, she has the right to place him in an infant house, which will care for him on a 24-hour basis through the third year. Usually the mothers visited the infant house once or twice a week. It is the right of every Russian mother to admit her child to an infant house; however, only one out of every 150 infants is sent there.

In an effort to evaluate the effect of Russian obstetrical caretaking practices, one of the authors (M.H.K.) calculated the rate of admissions to infant houses for full-term and premature infants in several units and found that the percentage of infants in infant houses who are premature is eight to 10 times greater than would be accounted for by the overall prematurity rate in Russia of infants born prematurely. When the child is 3 years old, his mother must decide whether he is to be adopted or taken home. Interestingly, the Russian premature infants are given up for adoption twice as often as full-term infants. Thus Russians also have problems with maternal bonding in the case of infants born prematurely. From this brief look it would appear that simply permitting mothers to breastfeed will not eliminate or prevent these problems of attachment to premature infants.

Rooming-in for the parent of a premature infant

Special mention should be made here of the work of Tafari and Sterky (1974) and Tafari and Ross (1973) in Ethiopia. They were able to care for three times as many infants in their premature nursery compared with previous years, and the number of surviving infants increased 500% when they permitted mothers to live within the crowded unit 24 hours a day. The cost of care for the infants in the unit decreased from $120 in 1970 to $40 in 1972, since mother-infant pairs were discharged when the infants weighed an average of 1.7 kg. Also, most of the mothers breastfed. Previous to this most of the infants had gone home bottle feeding and often died of intercurrent respiratory and gastrointestinal infections. When the cost of prepared milk amounts to a high proportion of the parents' weekly income, policies in support of mothers rooming-in and breastfeeding in premature nurseries have a direct relation to infant mortality. We believe that Tafari's procedure is probably appropriate for 50% of the world.

Baragwanath Hospital in South Africa provides another model of successful premature infant caretaking. Mothers of premature infants live in a room adjoining the premature nursery, and at each feeding time they enter the nursery to feed and handle their babies. Dr. Kahn originally instituted this arrangement because of a shortage of nurses. However, his solution appears to have multiple benefits. It allows the mother to continue producing milk, permits her to take on the care of the infant more easily, greatly reduces the caretaker time required for these infants, and allows a group of mothers of premature infants to talk over their situation and gain from mutual discussion and support (Bell, 1960; Kahn et al., 1954).

Torres (1978), in a special care unit in the slums of San Diego, Chile, has also achieved an excellent, low perinatal mortality and morbidity by placing special care units for low birth-weight infants on the maternity unit and maintaining babies under professional observation for only as long as is necessary.

A new approach to helping parents adapt to a sick or premature infant has been developed by Donald Garrow at a district general hospital in High Wycombe, England. Opened in 1976, a new 20-bed special infant care unit can accommodate eight mothers at a time and 250 admissions each year. No matter how seriously ill they may be, some 70% of the babies have their mothers with them from the first few hours of life. Fig. 5-8, *A*, shows a diagram of the unit. Fathers may stay at night and young siblings may visit as frequently as desired each day. Six of the mothers' rooms open directly into the infant special care unit so the parents can easily see or care for their infants. Infection has not been introduced by the policy of allowing free entry to fathers, siblings, and grandparents. However, parents are told that children with diarrhea, fever, an upper respiratory tract infection, or any exposure to a contagious disease should stay home. Many mothers come to this special unit immediately after giving birth, and the nursery staff cares for both the mother and infant. Generally the mothers eat together, which allows time for sharing experiences and mutual support. When an infant death occurs, the mother involved usually remains on the unit for a day or so and the nurses and one or two other mothers are often able to help her begin her grief work. Fig. 5-8, *B*, illustrates a familiar scene in the unit.

It is the impression of the staff of the High Wycombe unit that the parents move more quickly to assume caretaking tasks, are less jealous of the staff, more chatty, and more readily adapt to the birth of a sick infant than previously, when mothers could not live in. Studies are now under way to evaluate the effectiveness of the unit.

Nesting

Other approaches have been taken in the hope of normalizing the interaction between parents and their premature infant. Crosse (1957) suggested, "Whenever possible the mother should be admitted for several days before the baby is discharged so that she can take over complete charge of her infant under supervision." She provided small rooms for mother-infant dyads so that the two would truly be-

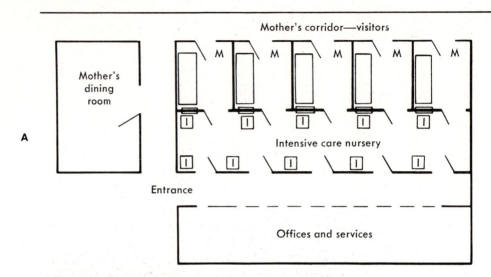

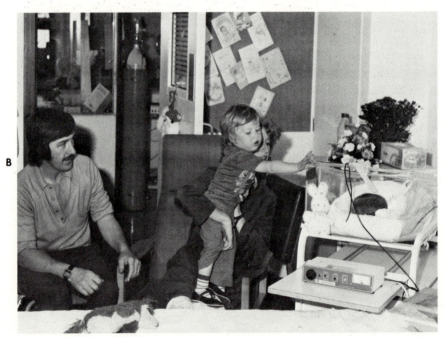

Fig. 5-8. A, Diagram of premature unit at High Wycombe, England. *M,* Mother's room; *I,* infant's bed. **B,** A familiar scene in this unit. Intensive care section is behind the father.

come acquainted before discharge. James (1969) described the successful introduction of a care-by-parent unit to provide a homelike caretaking experience. Nursing support was available for parents of premature infants prior to discharge if they needed it.

We have done a small feasibility study permitting mothers to live in with their infants before discharge, which we have termed "nesting". As soon as babies reached 1720 to 2110 grams, each mother, in a private room with her baby, provided all caregiving. Impressive changes in the behavior of these women were observed clinically. Even though the mothers had fed and cared for their infants in the intensive care nursery on many occasions prior to living-in, eight of the first nine mothers were unable to sleep during the first 24 hours. Most of the mothers closed the door to the room, completely shutting out any chance of observation, often to the consternation of the nurses, who felt a strong responsibility for the well-being of the infant. It was interesting to observe that the mothers rearranged the furniture, crib, and infant supplies, resembling in some ways the nesting behavior observed in animals. However, in the second 24-hour period the mothers' confidence and caretaking skills improved greatly. At this time, mothers began to discuss the proposed early discharge of their infants and, often for the first time, began to make preparations at home for his arrival. Several insisted on taking their babies home earlier than planned. The babies seemed to be quieter during this living-in period. In some mothers there were physical changes, such as increased breast swelling accompanied by some milk secretion. The mothers were not satisfied with the living-in nesting procedure until we established unlimited visiting privileges for the father and provided him with a comfortable chair and a cot (Kennell et al., 1973, 1975).

Initially we had difficulties in clearly defining the role of the nurse in the living-in or nesting unit. It soon became clear that the mother should be the responsible caretaker, and the nurse must function as a consultant. The role of the nurse and the mother must be clarified, or there will be resultant tussles over who makes the decisions, similar to those when more than one person writes orders for a single patient. Once the safety and feasibility of early discharge of premature infants has been fully confirmed, we suggest that early discharge, preceded by a period of isolation of the mother-infant dyad, may help to normalize mothering behavior in the intensive care nursery. Early discharge must be in conjunction with early parental visiting in the intensive care nursery. Encouraging the development of interaction and total caretaking may reduce the high incidence of mothering disorders among the mothers of small premature or sick infants.

COMMENT: The role of the hospital nurse in preparing the parents, particularly the mother, for caretaking is consistent with the traditional role that the community nurse has when she provides consultation to parents in home care.
K. Barnard

Early discharge

Some investigators have explored the effects of early discharge. Berg and associates (1971), Dillard and Korones (1973), and Davies and associates (1979) discharged premature infants when they weighed about 2 kilograms. Dillard found no deleterious effects associated with this early discharge. Actually, all of these authors followed Miller's (1948) suggestion about managing large premature infants in the home. However, they did not follow his additional recommendation that experienced personnel should visit the home to organize the families and supervise infant care. Recent studies of early discharge have not revealed any adverse effects on the physical health of the infants, but there have been no systematic observations of maternal behavior and anxiety or later infant development in these cases.

> **COMMENT:** Early discharge is appropriate as long as the parents are given the support they need. There should be someone to talk to about their questions and someone who can give them reassurance about the baby's condition and their parenting. Even though there are no apparent physical adverse effects of early discharge, the tremendous anxiety some parents experience when taking very young or relatively unstable babies home in terms of feeding, temperature, and respiratory status may have profound adverse effects on the parent-infant interaction and later developmental outcome.
> **K. Barnard**

Listening to parents (interviewing) during the infant's hospitalization

We are including vital information from a report by Dr. Bertrand Cramer* because it describes the reactions of mothers of premature infants in a nursery that has been a leader in the development and application of intensive care and because it is apparent that discussion and prolonged interviews are therapeutic for the parents. At the time of this study the nursery was beginning to allow mothers to enter and touch their premature infants. This was a psychological study of the reaction of mothers to the birth of a premature infant. It was conducted by a psychiatrist who was attempting to gather clinical information in the area of mother-infant attachment. The sample consisted of 13 mothers, each of whom was chosen if her infant was born prematurely, weighed less than 2500 grams, and was predicted to be in the premature unit for at least two weeks. The mothers were interviewed twice, once during the 10 days after the birth and then again approximately two months later. All the mothers were interviewed for 1½ hours each time. Discussions and prolonged interviews are also therapeutic. We would like to thank Dr. Cramer for submitting this manuscript to us.

---

*At the time of the study, Dr. Cramer was *medecin adjoint* at the University of Lausanne Pediatrics Department, Lausanne, Switzerland.

INTERVIEW WITH PARENTS OF PREMATURE INFANTS
BERTRAND CRAMER, M.D.

Self-esteem problems

The most frequent reaction among the mothers studied was a sense of failure. A typical comment by the mother was, "I am not even able to carry it through to the end like other mothers." Mothers explained their infant's premature birth on the basis of a personal defect, which they often believed to be a physical one. One mother thought that the prematurity was due to a hormonal deficiency; another requested an examination of her kidneys.

The separation of the infant from the mother only heightened this feeling of failure. To these women such an experience served as proof of their inadequacy as mothers. Having delivered prematurely, the mother now felt incapable of caring for her own infant.

The infant was a profound wound to the mother's self-pride. She saw the child, an extension of herself, as defective or of inferior quality because of his low birth weight, disappointing physical appearance, and frequently accompanying pathology.

Mrs. N. could hardly hide her disappointment: "I always hoped to have big babies weighing at least 3500 grams. If the baby had been that big, they would not have taken him away from me. I feel inferior to my girl friends. In my family they produce big babies. It was always the joy of my family to have big bundles. I told myself that the baby was not complete."

Insufficiency was a common theme for these mothers. The pregnancy was not complete, the baby was not complete, and so many of these women concluded irrationally, that they too were incomplete. As a further result of their initial feelings about their children's incompleteness, the mothers expressed concern for the future normality of their children, especially in the intellectual sphere. "Will he be like other kids?" "Will he be able to keep up in school?"

To understand the dynamics of these blows to the mother's self-esteem and the tremendous impact they can have on the evolution of the mother-child relationship, we have to borrow from the psychoanalytical concept of narcissism. Narcissism is the investment of love and interest in the self-image, the body and its contents. Although this form of love is centripetal, directed toward the self, other currents of love are centrifugal, directed toward people and the external world. This is object love.

In early pregnancy the embryo is enveloped by the mother's body, and hence the mother views her unborn infant as part of herself, incorporating it into her own narcissism. This total fusion, where the embryo is viewed merely as a content of the body, is disrupted at the first signs of quickening. The mother begins to perceive the fetus as a separate entity and therefore begins to invest it with increasing amounts of object love. By the time of birth the mother's transition from narcissistic to object love is more nearly complete. Now the mother is able to tolerate the

Continued.

INTERVIEW WITH PARENTS OF PREMATURE INFANTS—cont'd

anatomical separation and to consider her newborn as a complete person, well separated from herself. However, the infant remains encapsulated by his mother's narcissistic love, and it is only the slow development of the child into an adult that allows the mother to become increasingly aware of her child's separate existence.

However, in a premature birth there is an abrupt eviction of the fetus before the mother has been able to invest it with enough object love. We may therefore hypothesize that in a premature birth the fetus is the recipient of too much narcissistic love—as if it were still perceived as part of the mother's inner organs. The birth becomes an insult to the mother's bodily integrity. As one mother said when her child was taken from her at birth, "It was as if they ripped a piece of my guts out."

A clinical finding clearly illustrates the mother's inability to perceive the baby with enough object love because of premature eviction. The majority of the 13 mothers described a feeling of inability to believe that their child was real. The mothers made comments such as, "I just can't believe it, it is as if *nothing* had happened." "For me to believe it, I would have to see the child." This dreamlike unreality indicates that to the mother the child is still a part of her, not an independent real object. This feeling of unreality, heightened by the lack of object love, is strengthened by the enforced separation between the mother and her child. All the mothers thought that the real birth occurred weeks later, when they could touch and feed the child, and mainly when they could take him home.

None of the mothers had prepared a crib or clothing for her child. To these mothers their infants were not yet real, independent people who would need to be cared for once outside their protective body.

In veiw of these various findings, we propose the following hypothesis: The birth of a premature infant is a severe blow to the mother's self-esteem, mothering capabilities, and feminine role. It is conceived of as a loss of a body part, an insult to her bodily integrity, and a sign of inner inferiority. The premature birth enforces a feeling of unreality about the child, who is perceived as alien, thus more easily rejected.

Three mothers in Cramer's study did not have a self-esteem problem. Of these three, two started labor very soon after the death of a close relative (a mother, a brother). They explained that the newborn was called on to replace the lost relative. One of these two mothers said, "I had the little one for Mother. It will help me to cope with the loss of Mother. It fills up a void for my father too." The other mother, whose brother died in an automobile accident, said, "When the baby was born, my mother said, 'It is through your brother's death that we got the baby.'"

In these cases the premature child, far from revealing a defect, helped the mother to cope with another blow, the loss of a loved one.

The third mother previously had numerous spontaneous abortions, which had severely undermined her husband's respect for her. When she finally had a 1390-gram infant, it was experienced as a victory, despite his poor appearance. It was a great achievement, compensating for the severe blows dealt to her maternal pride by the previous miscarriages.

Guilt problems

Almost all the mothers of the premature infants expressed guilt feelings. They accused themselves of being bad mothers, of having exposed their child to great stress by forcing her out of the protective womb. "If she were still in me, she wouldn't have to suffer with all those needles and tubes."

To the mothers the premature birth was a punishment for some misdeed. When asked to explain the cause of the prematurity, they expressed varied irrational interpretations. Although there may have been some grain of reality in their explanations, the issue was blown out of proportion. For example, they attributed the prematurity to the following: engaging in sexual activity too frequently, drinking three glasses of cognac, smoking, enjoying a job, or feeling inadequate. Several mothers thought that they would never be able to forgive themselves if the child were to be damaged or to die. Some mothers were concerned that their child might later accuse them for having given birth prematurely. Often mothers attempted to transfer the guilt onto doctors, nurses, or their husbands—accusing them of some misdeed that caused the prematurity.

These feelings of guilt interfere, often severely, in three important areas:

1. In the establishment of a relationship with the child. The mother believes that she is dangerous and incapable of protecting the child. As a result, when finally in contact with the child, she does not dare to touch him unless given permission by the nurses. The greatest fear occurs when the child comes home. The mother is afraid to feed the baby by herself or to bathe him. "I am afraid he might choke to death." "He will slip out of my hands and drown." "I am afraid he might break in my hands." Considering themselves as potential dangers to the child, the mothers may not enter or even visit the premature unit.

Often mothers think that the nurses can offer better maternal care to their infant than they can. To them the premature unit is a surrogate womb, more successful in protecting the child than they are. These feelings of gratitude, however, are accompanied by a feeling of inferiority. The mother's feelings of maternal paralysis can be greatly increased when the staff considers the unit to be an air-tight, totally aseptic area where visiting mothers are essentially thought to be a bother and a source of infection.

2. Guilt feelings interfere with the mother's ability to ask the hospital staff medical questions. The mother's lack of information fosters the perpetuation of guilt-centered explanations and increases the mother's belief that she is a potential harm to her child. One mother clearly indicated that she did not want to know too much about the causes of the prematurity because she was afraid her "faults" would be revealed.

3. The mother's feelings of guilt determined whether the interview had positive or negative therapeutic results.

For several mothers the interview provided an opportunity to verbalize and neutralize their guilt feelings. When the mother was provided with a straightforward medical explanation and enabled to relocate the sense of guilt, she was able to neutralize her guilt feelings. For example, one mother was afraid of approaching her newborn until she was able to acknowledge her rejection feelings. She believed

Continued.

INTERVIEW WITH PARENTS OF PREMATURE INFANTS—cont'd

that she had rejected her son in the same way she had rejected all of her feminine functions. After the interview she "reestablished" the relationship with her son and said, "My maternal instinct has come back." She was grateful for the opportunity to express her negative, guilt-ridden feelings and have them "neutralized" by rational, medical explanations.

Mothers who could not cope with their guilt were cautious during the interviews and could not benefit from them. Just as the success of the interview depended on the mother's ability to tolerate guilt, it is probably the guilt factor that determines the outcome of the physician-parent relationship in cases of premature birth.

It was interesting to note that certain characteristics of the newborn influence the mother's ability to handle her guilt. One mother complained that her child did not respond to her—she did not smile, move, or vocalize. The mother interpreted the lack of feedback as a sign of her child's total defenselessness. The child would not be capable of protecting herself against the mother's possible wrongdoings. This made the mother feel dangerous, overpowering, and extremely anxious. The hypoactivity frequent in the premature infant is reminiscent of cases among animals, in which the mother will kill the offspring that show deviant behavior. Maternal behavior in humans might also depend on triggering stimuli stemming from the newborn.

Separation problems

The premature infant is quickly taken away from the mother in the moments following birth. Reactions to this separation are universal. The loss contributes to the process of anticipatory mourning described by Caplan and associates (1965).

Mothers experience a void, an amputation. They make remarks such as, "I never felt such a longing in my life." "It is as if they had taken out an organ." They express an intense wish to touch, to breastfeed the child. During this separation they imagine the worst possible outcome. They are positive that the truth is being kept from them and that the child is actually dying or is abnormal.

Parent groups

In recent years a number of neonatal intensive care units have formed groups of parents of prematures who meet together once a week, or more often, for 1- to 2-hour discussions. Documented clinical reports from these centers suggest that parents find both support and considerable relief from being able to talk with each other and to express and compare their inner feelings. All these parents had gone through a severe crisis after the birth of their small infant and expressed enormous relief at being able to talk about it (Erdman, 1977).

Minde and colleagues (1980*b*), in a controlled study of a self-help group, reported that parents who participated in the group visited their infants in the hospital significantly more often than did parents in the control group. The self-help

The anticipatory mourning can be so intense that the mothers refuse to contemplate their future relationship with the child. They avoid talking about the child with relatives. They rarely ask family members to visit the child. A typical remark is, "I don't want to think ahead until I'm sure." Only one mother sent birth announcements. None prepared a crib until the child made definite progress. There is a period of suspense, with an effort not to think about the child. This is in significant contrast to the total maternal preoccupation found in mothers with normal newborn infants.

The longer the waiting period persists the deeper will be the withdrawal of investment in the child. In some cases this withdrawal seems irreversible, with the possible results of deprivation syndromes (failure to thrive, battered child syndrome).

In favorable cases this break in the mother-child relationship begins to diminish at the first meeting between the mother and infant. It is only when the mother can handle her child, after he has made definite progress, that the relationship is revitalized and the mother allows herself to experience the typical gamut of maternal feelings.

In our study there was at least one case of totally irreversible rejection of a child. One of the mothers who had been most guarded in the first interview and refused to return for the follow-up had given birth to twins. The smaller of the two was kept in the premature unit for two months while the heavier one was taken home within the first month. When the smaller child finally went home, he developed a severe anorexia, which necessitated rehospitalization. After psychiatric consultation it was clear that the child who had been separated the longest from the mother had been totally rejected. Adoption by the grandmother was necessary.

Different sets of factors may be involved in explaining these defects in maternal functioning after separation. Maternal response needs to be stimulated by close neonatal interaction between the mother and child from the outset. It is as if separation—during this sensitive period when mothering is established—may unleash aggressive impulses in the mother toward her child, which cause her to refuse closeness and avoid the child.

parents also touched, talked, and looked at their infants in the *en face* position more and rated themselves as more competent on infant care measures. These mothers continued to show more involvement with their babies during feedings and were more concerned about their general development three months after their discharge from the nursery.

COMMENT: The ICU parents group in Toronto now operates by itself, successfully (according to Klaus Minde) under the leadership of parents of former ICU graduates. There seems to be a phenomenon of parents becoming experts on their child's problem once the crisis is over, and they then are rich resources for those in crisis. There are many examples of this, for example, in sudden infant death syndrome (SIDS) groups and in groups of parents of Down's syndrome children.
T. Field

COMMENT: We have found that parent-to-parent groups are extremely effective in helping parents deal with some of their questions, and they provide the support that helps them handle this crisis. Our experience suggests that contact both with other parents going through the crisis and with "graduate" parents who made it through are helpful. There seem to be three periods of time when a contact with another parent is important. The first is at birth or soon after, the second is when the parents are ready to take their baby home, and the third is when the infant is about 5 or 6 months old.
K. Barnard

Programmed contact and reciprocal interaction

The premature infant normally has prolonged sleep periods with only short intervals of wakefulness. This is disconcerting to the parents. Mothers often sit beside their babies' incubators for long periods waiting for them to awaken. Since the parents' affection and enthusiasm are stimulated and sustained by seeing the baby's open eyes, it is helpful to explain to them that as the premature baby develops, he will be awake for increasingly longer periods of time. Parents are often persistent and ingenious in arousing their babies to "send a message" to them. For example, parents will stroke or pat the baby who responds by opening his eyes. If the mother is able to stimulate and meet his special needs, the baby she takes home will be more responsive and closer in behavior to the full-term infant she had hoped for.

Over many years we have gained the impression that the earlier a mother comes to the premature unit and touches her baby the more rapidly her own physical recovery from the pregnancy and birth progresses. Interestingly, Budin (1907), the first neonatologist, commented that it is important to keep the mother involved with the care of her infant.

As a result of these observations and other experiences, we have studied the effect of a supplemental early intervention program to maximize the attachment of mothers and fathers to their premature infants. The study was designed to determine if mothers who (1) follow a pattern of stroking their infants, (2) are involved in caretaking such as feeding and changing diapers, and (3) are given special guidance on how to understand their infant's needs and responses will develop a closer attachment to their infants than will mothers who are not given these three experiences during the first two weeks of life. Mothers in both groups were allowed and encouraged to come into the nursery and were given a description and an explanation of all treatments such as monitors, catheters, and incubator hoods. Only the experimental group was given the special experiences during the first two weeks after the baby's birth. After the special program was ended, both the control and experimental groups received the same care.

There were three main differences in the experiences of the control and the experimental groups. First, the experimental mothers were encouraged to visit six times during the first two weeks after the birth of their babies. In the first hour of each visit they were asked to touch and stroke their babies four times for 5 minutes each time, with a 10-minute break between touching periods. Second, these mothers were encouraged to help with the care of the baby, for example, diaper changes for small babies, feeding and holding for larger ones. Third, after receiving special instruction about the capabilities of their babies, the experimental mothers were encouraged to develop an interchange with them, communicating by way of the infant's sensory systems. The bilirubin eye patches were removed and phototherapy was stopped during the mother's visit because seeing the baby's eyes is so important for most mothers. An initial pilot feasibility study was carried out with 10 mothers in each of the two groups. Analysis of a 15-minute standardized videotaped feeding at the time of discharge showed a significant difference between the two groups. The mothers in the experimental group kept their eyes on their babies significantly more than the mothers in the control group ($p < .02$).

After the pilot phase a larger number of mother-infant dyads were admitted to the early intervention and control groups. In the early period of the infant's hospitalization, after the first two weeks the mothers in the experimental group tended to visit the nursery more frequently (4.8 versus 3.5 visits per week) and to call less frequently (2.6 versus 3.3 phone calls per week).

However, as the length of stay increased beyond 1 month, these group differences in visiting rate disappeared. Suspecting that the experimental intervention might be affecting mothers of healthy and sick prematures differently, the sample was divided into babies who went home before one month and babies who stayed in the hospital for longer than one month. We then computed the visiting rates for *all* mothers during weeks 3 and 4 postpartum. There was no effect of the experimental intervention in those mothers whose babies ended up staying longer than one month. However, for the mothers whose infants were discharged home before one month, the experimental group visited significantly more often than the control group.

These findings suggested that the experimental intervention was effective when the baby was relatively healthy and would therefore often have a shorter stay in the hospital. As a result we examined the visiting rates again, this time separating the data according to the infant's birth weight. Similar results were obtained. The experimental intervention resulted in increased visiting only for mothers of heavier babies (birth weight > 1500 grams).

In her study of the parents' perceptions of their low birth-weight infants, Newman (1980) reported that the infants who were the sickest were visited less by their parents and the parents were in contact with them for shorter periods than infants with a less threatening course.

Minde (personal communication) has reported that "ill" infants were less active and less responsive during their medical illness but similar to well infants during later observations. Mothers of infants who were seriously ill for more than 30 days touched and smiled at their infants significantly less during and after the illness, and at home they looked at them and vocalized to them less than did the mothers of infants who were well initially and remained well during their hospital stay.

Mothers of infants who were seriously ill for less than 17 days showed an initial decrease in smiling and touching but then increased to the level of parents of well infants. Mothers' behaviors correlated with their personal perception of their infant's illness rather than the actual state of his health. Thus a mother who has an infant who was severely ill for a long period may not appreciate his improvement and may treat the infant as if he were still ill.

> **COMMENT:** In data from 24-hour videotaping of premature infants, we find that level of motor activity is significantly related to two-year mental and motor performance on the Bayley infant scales. The less active an infant is over 24 hours the lower will be the performance at 2 years of age. This supports Minde's observations of less activity in "ill" infants and the accompanying relationship of the pattern of effects on the interaction when this "illness" lasted over 30 days.
> **K. Barnard**

One month after the discharge of the baby in our study of programmed contact and reciprocal interaction, mothers in both groups behaved similarly during the physical examination. Their response to a questionnaire concerning their adjustment to the premature infant and their perception of the baby showed no significant differences between the two groups.

The findings in our study (and lack of them) have forced us to examine further the needs and problems faced by parents of premature infants. First, even the most sensitive interventions may fail if the parents view their infant as weak and unlikely to live. We belive the findings are consistent with this. Second, for years we had been thinking along one track when devising interventions for premature infants. We had been bringing parents into the intensive care nursery. However, the milieu in the nursery makes it difficult for parents to be confident about their infant's viability. Third, in our research we have tended to ignore the practical and emotional problems faced by parents when their premature infant, hospitalized for weeks or months, is finally ready to be discharged. With these factors in mind, we took a different approach in designing a new intervention for parents of premature infants. This is reported in the next section.

Transporting the healthy premature infant to the mother—a new intervention

Rather than bringing mothers into the tense environment of the neonatal intensive care unit with its frightening sounds, strange equipment, and unfamiliar faces, we are studying the effects of bringing the baby to the mother in her own room in the maternity division of the hospital. This contact is qualitatively different from that previously available to mothers of premature infants. In this way the mothers have an opportunity to become acquainted with their premature newborns under circumstances similar to those experienced by mothers of full-term infants. The results of studies of early maternal contact with healthy full-term infants served as a guide for the design of this intervention. Our pilot experiences strongly encouraged us to study this carefully.

For this study of early contact we asked mothers who gave birth to healthy premature infants to participate. We included infants whose birth weight was between 1500 and 2100 grams, whose gestational age was between 32 and 36 weeks, and whose medical status during the first day permitted the infant to stay with his mother, for example, no continuing respiratory distress or hypoglycemia.

The early contact consists of 1 hour of mother-infant contact on each of the first, second, and third days after birth. A research nurse brings the baby to the mother's room in a transport incubator. The baby, clothed only in a diaper, is placed in the mother's bed with a radiant heat panel overhead. The research nurse is present during the visit but seated out of the mother's view above the head of her bed. During the visit the nurse observes the infant's condition, particularly his color and respiration. Resuscitation equipment is carried on the transport incubator for use in the event of apnea. In addition, the nurse makes detailed observations of the mother's behavior during each of the three 1-hour visits as described below. Verbal interaction between the mother and nurse is limited to a standard statement and answers to the mother's questions.

It was an entirely new procedure when we started this study of early contact so there were many concerns about the health and well-being of the baby. We have monitored the babies' temperatures frequently and found that on a single occasion one baby had a temperature less than 36° C, but that was the only episode of hypothermia. Thus we have learned that with the use of a heat panel and transport incubator there have been no significant problems with temperature control. In addition, we have had no episodes of apnea, bradycardia, vomiting, or other unusual behavior. We appreciate that there may be times when difficulties with premature babies may occur, so the nurses continue to monitor them closely. So far it appears to be a safe precedure; however, one infant died with late streptococcal septicemia. We have found that this procedure is increasingly acceptable to the nurses caring for the premature infants.

The control group of mothers had the same care except that the baby was not present. We have discovered that a strong supportive relationship developed between the experimental mother and the nurse after 3 hours. Even though the nurse only answered direct questions, she provided more support and consistent information than often is available to the mother of a premature baby.

COMMENT: The permission an institution gives to staff to relate with patients is important. When a change in institutional policy occurs such as with this study, there will be a chance for timely, warm, and supportive relationships to develop between the nurse and parents or physician and parents. This type of relationship is significant, and we must change institutional structures to see that it happens. Parents, nurses, and physicians will all be better off. If you want to improve the lives of children, improve the situation of their caregivers.
K. Barnard

We have had a long-standing interest in the behavior of mothers at their first contact with their premature and full-term babies. Fig. 5-9 presents a summary of the behavior of mothers on the first and second visit of the premature infant in the early contact study compared with mothers visiting their preterm baby in incubators and mothers who have their undressed, full-term infants in their own beds on the maternity unit. The data in the early contact study are based on the behavioral observations of one nurse in the mother's hospital room after the infant is undressed and placed in the mother's bed. It can be noted that in the first and second visits there was far more touching activity than we have previously found in parents of premature infants. However, it should be noted that in our past research the infants were in isolettes in the premature nursery and the mothers walked to the incubator. At that time the total amount of touching during any observed period was 20% during the first visit and 36% during the second visit compared with more than 80% when the infant was in the mother's bed. Therefore bringing the infant to the

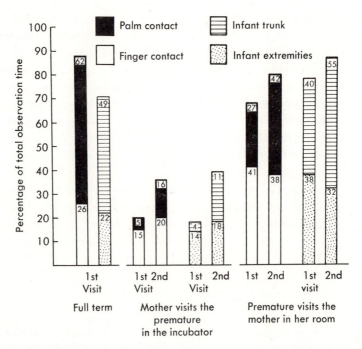

Fig. 5-9. Fingertip and palm contact on the trunk or extremities in three groups of mothers: (1) 12 mothers of full-term infants at their first visit, (2) 9 mothers who visited their premature infants in incubators in the ICU, and (3) 14 mothers whose premature infants were brought to their maternity rooms and placed in their beds.

mother significantly increased her physical contact with her infant, and touching the infant's trunk occurred more rapidly.

When the infants visited their mothers, the mothers did a striking amount of looking during the two visits—84% to 90% of the time. These results are of special interest, since in our study of premature infants several years ago there was a strong correlation between the amount of time a mother looked at her infant during a discharge feeding and the baby's development at 42 months.

In our earlier studies when the mothers visited their babies in isolettes in the intensive care nursery, we were greatly impressed by the observation that parents of premature infants rarely spoke to them. However, in the current study, vocalizations have occurred almost 40% of the time at the first and second visits. By the second visit 40% of the mothers (n = 14) were attempting to elicit a response from their infant and also moved the infant for close body contact.

Home-based intervention for young parents

Several studies, such as those by Field (1979), have noted that there are certain factors that place the preterm infant of the teenage mother in greater risk at birth despite equivalent prenatal care. Adolescent parents have less experience and knowledge of parenting and more unrealistic expectations regarding developmental milestones in their infants. They also have relatively punitive child-rearing attitudes. The preterm infants of teenage mothers who were in the home-based intervention group in Field's study showed more optimal growth, better Denver Developmental Screening Test scores, and high face-to-face interaction scores at 4 months of age. This intervention group of mothers rated their infants more optimally and expressed a more realistic understanding of developmental milestones and child-rearing attitudes. They also received higher rating on face-to-face interactions. At 8 months of age the intervention group had superior Bayley mental and Caldwell Home Stimulation Inventory and Carey Infant Temperament scores. However, the investigators have questioned whether this may be secondary to a Hawthorne effect. They wondered whether increased contact of any supportive nature would have a beneficial effect on teenage mothers.

COMMENT: The above-mentioned intervention group received parent training on a number of exercises during home visits every two weeks for the first four months and every month thereafter through the first year. A much less costly intervention was recently conducted by Sue Widmayer and me, with an equally effective outcome. Teenage mothers of preterm infants were simply given a demonstration of the Brazelton Neonatal Behavioral Assessment scale at birth just prior to discharge and again at one month in their homes. In addition, they were asked to rate their babies on an adaptation of the Brazelton scale once a week. At one year the developmental assessments of these infants were superior to those infants of the control group. It may be that even more than support, parents need a little of our knowledge, for example, pointing out that even preterm infants have impressive skills at the time of discharge.
T. Field

Discussions with the parents after discharge

We have found it extremely valuable to meet with a mother and father one month after the baby has been discharged, when the infant is gaining and well. We have asked the parents to review in detail the events around birth and the early days of the infant's hospital course. It is surprising how differently the two parents may recall the early minutes and hours, how confused they may be about what went on, and how often their concerns are completely different from those of the nurses and physicians. Because this 1-hour interview is never sufficient time to cover everything, we encourage the husband and wife to continue the discussion, in minute detail, between themselves and then to call a day later to discuss the interview with us. (See Dr. Cramer's work for further details on pp. 181-185.)

By helping the parents start to work through their difficult recent experiences, will the incidence of complications such as the vulnerable child syndrome be reduced?

The 12 interventions we have described reflect a remarkable interest in studying how to help parents become attached to their small infants, how to provide support for mothers and fathers during the difficult days of hospitalization, and how to prepare them for the stressful first weeks at home. In the next pages we will discuss clinical considerations for the parents and premature infants in more detail based on the studies we have already described.

CARE OF THE PARENTS—CLINICAL CONSIDERATIONS

We believe there should be no limit on parental visiting in nurseries. Inflexible regulations isolate mothers and fathers from their infants, drastically increasing their anxiety about the baby's condition. The nursery should be open for parental visiting 24 hours a day and open, or at least flexible about, visits from others— grandparents, supportive relatives, siblings (after discussion and preparation), and a friend of the mother if the father is unavailable or unable to visit. Studies have shown that infections will not be a problem, providing proper precautions are taken such as informing parents that they can only enter if they are feeling well, have no upper respiratory tract problems or other infectious diseases, and wash their hands thoroughly for 4 to 5 minutes. Our suggestions concerning parental visiting are presented on the opposite page.

Health professionals have six tasks in their work with parents:

1. To help the mother adapt her previous conceptualized image of an ideal normal infant to the small infant she has produced
2. To help relieve the mother's guilt about producing a small infant
3. To help the mother begin building a close affectional tie to her infant, developing a mutual interaction so that she will be attuned to her baby's special needs as he grows

4. To permit the mother to learn how to care for her infant while he is in the hospital so that after her child's discharge, she will be competent and relaxed when caring for him
5. To encourage the family to work together during the crisis of the premature birth, helping the father and mother to discuss their difficulties with one another as they attempt to arrive at satisfactory solutions
6. To help meet the special needs of individual families

NEONATAL INTENSIVE CARE UNIT GUIDELINES FOR PARENTS

1. The nursery is open 24 hours a day for you to visit with your baby. We would like to welcome and encourage all parents to come into the nursery. You may touch your baby now and help to care for him or her.
2. The safety of the baby depends on everyone's thoroughly washing their hands before picking up any baby. You must wash your hands for a period of at least 4 minutes, using the large sinks at either end of the nursery. The outline for the hand-washing technique is above the sink. After hand washing please put on a gown. It is important to tie the gown snugly at the back.
3. If you have any questions about your baby, please do not hesitate to talk to the nurse or the doctor. We find it helpful to chat with you each visit, telling you about the progress of your baby. We may be busy when you call or visit and may find it necessary to ask you to call back later. At times we might be unable to talk completely at every visit.
4. Your observations about your baby are important, so if you notice something that has changed or if you are concerned about something, please be sure to discuss it with the nurses or the doctor caring for your baby.
5. At certain times the nursery appears busy, sometimes hectic. Even at these times there is always room for you to come into the unit. Once in a while we may have to ask you to wait a few minutes.
6. If you have any concerns in the evening or during the night when you are home, please do not hesitate to call. The nurses enjoy talking with you, even at 2:00 in the morning. Someone is always here. Call directly to the floor.
7. Please do not come into the nursery if you have any disease that your baby might catch from you such as diarrhea or a cold (this includes a sore throat, cold sores or water blisters on your lips, a runny nose, cough, and fever). While they are young and in the nursery, premature babies are more susceptible to infectious disease, and so we do not permit anyone into the nursery unless they are feeling well. Please check with the doctors and nurses if you have questions about whether it is safe for you to visit, and after an illness, when it is wise to resume your visits.

COMMENT: All six points suggest that a major role of the health professional is to support efforts of the parents. I would add a seventh task, which is to assist families in the transition that occurs after the infant is discharged. This involves connecting the family with other community resources more directly involved in home-based care. Parent support groups are an extremely important resource. Many states now have a developing network of parent's groups.
K. Barnard

To accomplish these important tasks, one must begin by talking with both the mother and father immediately after birth. The choice of words will have far-reaching effects. The entire medical and nursing staff should be particularly cautious about suggesting that the infant is not normal. Early remarks, such as, "Oh, it's very blue . . . It's so small . . . Do you think it will live? . . . Look, it's grunting . . . Why won't it breathe?" are indelibly fixed in the parents' memories. Obstetricians must remember that their words will have particular weight because they have a close tie with the mother. Parents have often remarked long after the birth that they will never forget the physician's comment, "I doubt if the baby will live. It looks too small and immature." Statements such as these reflect the belief of many physicians that if a mother is prepared for a death, she will go through the experience with less emotional upheaval. This assumption has been proved incorrect in studies of parents who have lost newborn infants (Chapter 7).

The physician who shares all of his or her concerns with the parent is attempting to be helpful. Although on the surface this approach appears to be reasonable, it is contraindicated in this situation. At present most premature infants do survive. If a woman is to mother her child adequately throughout the rest of childhood, she must begin by building a firm and close tie with her infant at birth. Pessimistic remarks in the first hours of life cause a premature infant's mother to hold back, stifling the development of this essential bond at the time of inception. As a result of such remarks, the mother may embark on the process of anticipatory grief. Once this process is fully under way, it is extremely difficult to reverse its course. If by the end of the second or third day, the obstetrician and pediatrician feel optimistic about the premature infant's survival, they may have already begun to lose the mother. It may be several days before the mother will believe that her baby will live, and she may not be completely convinced for years or ever.

The physician must be frank and, if the situation warrants it, must state that in some cases it is difficult to predict how a small premature infant will do. Unfortunately, this situation often leads to a suspension of communication with the mother, adding to her concern. We have found that it helps for the physician to describe how he or she visualizes the baby, leaving out some of the negative factors. We do not give the mother any statistics about the baby's chances. However, if the child has been home for some time, has successfully elicited his parents' attachment, and then returns with meningitis or some other acute disease, physicians should share their worries with the mother from the beginning.

Parental adjustments

In the previous chapter we discussed how the mother of a normal, healthy newborn must adjust her idealized image of her infant to the actual infant before her. Naturally, this adjustment is much more difficult for the mother of a premature infant. She must realign her idealized mental picture with a thin, scrawny, feeble infant. Because the mother of a premature infant has difficulty recognizing that her tiny baby will ultimately grow into a normal, husky, vigorous, healthy youngster, her adjustment to his appearance is far from easy.

The anxieties of a parent about to enter the nursery for the first time, whether in the 1950s or today, are naturally much greater than those of the physician. The average mother who comes to visit her infant—let us say a daughter—was not prepared physically or emotionally for the early birth, and she is still shaky from it. She is extremely anxious about the health of her daughter, wonders about any abnormalities, worries about whether she will be criticized for producing an unfinished, feeble, imperfect product, and fears that she may carry germs which will harm her daughter. She enters the brightly lit, stainless steel and glass citadel, filled with unfamiliar sounds and smells, densely populated by intense young men and women who rush from incubator to incubator, manipulate complicated equipment, and spend long periods of time hovering over individual babies with serious expressions on their faces. These activities appear ominous and suggest an air of great tension—even after several visits. It is not until she has been told that her daughter is definitely progressing well or, far better, until she has touched and seen for herself, that she can begin to relax. But there are usually frightening surprises at the early visits. Complicated wires, fine tubes, large tubes, bandages on the head, arms, or legs, and bright lights and bandages on the eyes cover the baby. She is so tiny, so different from a normal baby. Her head is large, her extremities thin, her movements jerky, and her respirations irregular and labored. Fig. 5-10 pictures what a mother may see when she comes to visit her baby in the first days of life. We may gain further understanding of how the nursery and a very tiny premature baby appear to parents from Fig. 5-11, which shows how the nursery is viewed through the eyes of school-age children (7 to 8 years old). At each visit a new problem may be discovered or announced, and with every problem the mother feels a sharp visceral pain. "Do babies with jaundice live?" "How will she ever stand the strain of breathing so hard when she is already so small and fragile?" "Does such a tiny thing ever grow up to be a full-sized child or adult?" "Are they really telling me the truth?" "What have I done to my poor child?"

While we acknowledge the inappropriateness of using any set script, we would like to offer here some potentially useful comments which the physician might use. If a 1500-gram infant is grunting but pink at 30 minutes of age, we find it helpful to say, "Mr. and Mrs. Jones, you have a fine, strong baby, even though he is small. He is showing some of the adjustments to life outside of you that we commonly

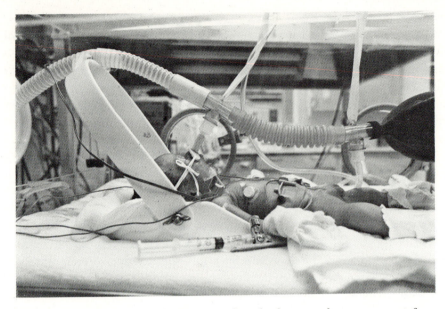

Fig. 5-10. A picture of what a mother sees when she first visits her premature infant.

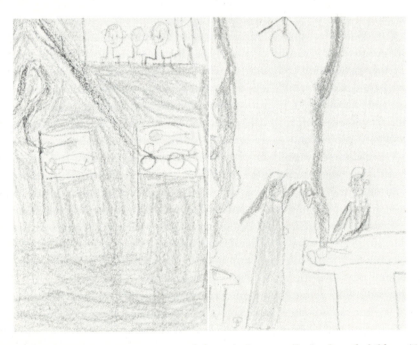

Fig. 5-11. The premature nursery as viewed through the eyes of school-aged children (7 to 8 years old).

encounter. Although there may be some setbacks along the way, we believe he is going to do well after he gets through this early period of adjustment over the next few days. He is pink, active, and beautifully formed. He looks perfect to us except for some difficulty in fully expanding his lungs, but we often see that during this period. There have been many developments recently in the care of premature infants and we have many new techniques. We will undoubtedly be using some of these to help your baby, and we'll let you know about them as they are used. For now, I am pleased by his progress and will be seeing you later in the day. You have done a great job. You should be pleased with yourself and your beautiful baby. If you are feeling well enough, I think you would enjoy coming to see your son later today."

It is also important at this point to ask the mother how she is doing and what her concerns are. If she has had a chance to see her baby, we might ask, "How did the baby look to you? What did you notice? How do you feel about the baby and what we just told you? What questions do you have?" Each woman has individual needs, and if we are not careful, we run the risk of overwhelming a mother with unwanted and unnecessary descriptions. She may well be concerned about something entirely different from what the physician imagines. During the early period of evaluation and stabilization, which may take an hour or more, parents appreciate contact with the nurse or physician every 15 to 20 minutes, even when there is nothing new to report.

To some readers a recommendation for optimism at this point may seem dishonest or misleading—not playing the game "fair and square" with the parents. A physician should never deceive a mother if the baby is expected to die, and we do not intend to imply that deception should be carried out. It is important for the physician first to determine what the chances for a baby will be, and then, on the basis of the current expectations, adjust what he or she says accordingly. Physicians who have had experience with the high infant mortality of the past may find it difficult to be optimistic and may want to have someone else talk to the parents during the period of intensive care.

The physician must be careful to involve both the father and mother. At the time of the first discussion, the physician would be wise to reassure the parents that there will be no secrets, that they will be informed about the baby's progress, and that both will be told about the developments together whenever possible.

If the mother is anesthetized (this is extremely rare in our hospital), the physician should discuss with the father how his infant is doing and allow him to see the baby at close range. Then, just as soon as the mother is awake, it is important to talk with both parents together. Many physicians believe in sparing a woman from the stress of hearing about her sick infant soon after the birth, but it is clear that a mother's and father's worries are often far worse than reality warrants. The physician may talk directly to the mother for convenience and have her in turn tell her husband, but the physician must be certain that she is confident that no developments are being kept from her by her husband.

Many small or sick infants are transported from the hospital where they are born to a hospital with an intensive care unit. At the time of transfer, even if the infant is only being moved for observation of a slightly elevated bilirubin level, most mothers are worried about their infant's survival (Benfield et al., 1976). They think the baby is dead or dying. This is important to remember, since in these cases the mother and father will require additional help (Fanaroff and Baskiewicz, 1975). Before the infant is transported, we show him to his mother and father and attempt to describe to the parents, in simple terms, the care their baby will receive. We ask the father to help us care for his infant, impressing on him that he has a very special role to play. There are really two sick individuals in his family— his wife, in one part of the hospital or in another hospital, and his baby in the neonatal center. In addition, the father sometimes has responsibility for other children at home. We have observed that, by bringing him into the situation early, he can better master his own anxieties. For these reasons we suggest that he come to the intensive care nursery and discuss the baby's condition with the physicians and nurses and familiarize himself with the routine before visiting his wife. In this way he can report current information to his wife and help to allay her fears. We also encourage him to visit and talk with his wife at least once a day.

Before the mother comes to the nursery, the physician should clearly describe the baby's appearance to her. She should know that he is in an incubator wearing only a diaper, that there is a small, fine plastic tube in his navel through which small blood samples are drawn to regulate his treatment, that there is another fine tube in his arm through which he is receiving some nourishing sugar solutions, and that there is a small plastic hood over his head to permit precise oxygen control. She may be told that the infant is pink, active, moving around, and waiting for his mother to put her hands into the incubator so he can feel her touch. At this time we also explain to the mother that a number of recent studies demonstrate that simply touching the infant will help to relax him as well as to improve his breathing, physical development, and rate of weight gain. Thus the visit is important not only to the mothers but to the baby as well.

Frequently, a mother will say that she does not want to touch her baby for fear that she will hurt or infect him. This may stem from her belief that she is an inadequate or "bad" mother because she has not been able to produce a normal baby. It also has been, and still is, common for a mother to have too much respect for the expert nurses and feel inferior to them. It is beneficial to let the mother express these feelings, but it is equally important to convey our acceptance of her concern, our encouragement and confidence in her. By telling the mother, "You can come in," we are essentially letting her know that we consider her a good person and a wholesome, important influence on her baby.

The longer the mother must wait before she can see her baby the more time she has to imagine that her worst fantasies are true. On the other hand, the sooner she sees her baby the more rapidly she can reconcile her image of him with his true physical condition. The first sight and first handling of the infant are never easy for the mother. We suggest that a chair (preferably a high stool with a back) be placed near the incubator in case she feels faint.

Each mother brings to this experience a different set of worries, problems, and past history. Some can adjust faster than others. For those who are extremely hesitant about coming in, we say, "How are things going? How have you slept? How are you managing these days? How is your husband managing? How are both of you getting along?" Encouraging her to talk about her thoughts is most helpful. She should never be forced to put her hands into the incubator nor be pressured to enter the nursery if she is not ready and willing to do so. Many people believe that the mother who denies the illness, withdraws, and is passive has a much more difficult time adjusting. The mother who is able to face the difficulties of the small baby, to talk about them, and to wrestle with her guilt feelings, copes more quickly and easily. Once these feelings are verbalized, the family is on the road to becoming attached to the newborn.

The following note is part of a letter written by a mother about her experience in the premature nursery.

> I felt angry when I would look up at a small group (doctors) standing next to me talking about my baby and not one would look at me. So I quit looking up. I quit expecting to be treated the same way one would in usual circumstances. I tried to learn the "rules." I was for the most part ignored. I was not a worker and had little in common with the work group.
>
> I think I'm mad at the world. I'm mad at all the people who work in the premature nursery. Even the ones who aren't taking care of John. They're all in it together. They stole him from me. They have control over him. They tell me whether he's OK or not. They affect my well-being with the intonation of their voices, their moods, their work load.
>
> I mean: I can't tell you in this hostile environment with all these beeps and lights and where you have work responsibilities that I know will take you away in a few minutes. I can't tell you in front of this little plastic bed where my baby is imprisoned, my baby who is such a mystery to me, who looks like a *baby* but whose insides don't seem to work right, and who may have had a serious mysterious bowel disease. I can't tell you in this *unsafe place* that I'm afraid my baby will die, because it hurts too much and I don't want to feel it right now.
>
> But I didn't have to say anything. She (a nurse) put her hand on my shoulder and said some small things like, "It must be tough," and that was all she had to do. She acknowledged my feelings and helped a great deal in doing so.

Involving parents in the care of their premature infant

The care of the mother and her baby during the period in the intensive care nursery will influence their relationship throughout the child's life. We have been impressed with the ingenuity of some nurses in developing techniques that allow a

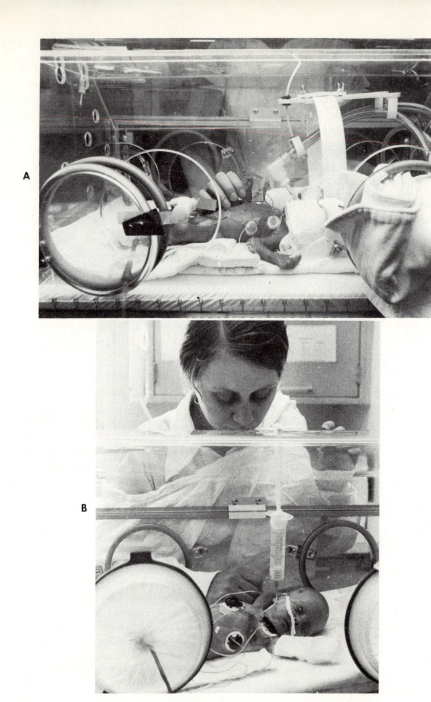

Fig. 5-12. A to **C,** A pictorial essay of a family in our nursery who were actively involved with the care of their infant for many days before the baby could be removed from the respirator and incubator. **D,** The parents and their son one year later. (From Alderman, M.M.: Patient care, Feb. 1, 1975. Copyright, 1975, Miller & Fink Corp., Darien, Conn. All rights re-served.)

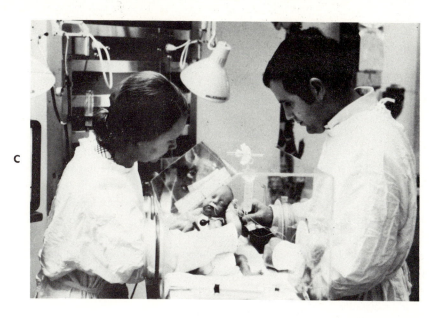

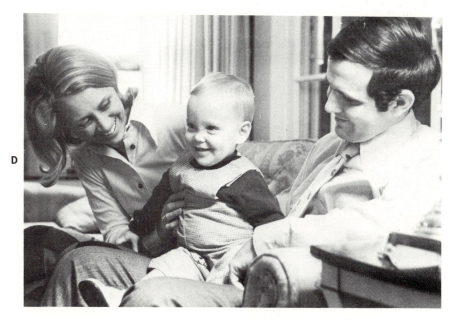

Fig. 5-12, cont'd. For legend see opposite page.

mother to hold her baby in her arms while he is being fed by nasogastric tube. They attach the burette to the mother's gown, which permits her to hold her baby until all the feeding has run into his stomach. We have found notes tacked to the baby's bed: "Please hold my 1:00 feeding for my mother. She will come to give me this feeding. Boy will I be glad to see her! Signed, Susie."

The mother must not be given a caretaking task if there is the slightest possibility that she will not succeed. She should not bottle feed unless a nurse or a physician has fed her baby several times and knows he can take the feedings easily. During the period when he is being fed or being nourished by intravenous hyperalimentation, the mother should have other tasks, such as changing the diaper and giving him sensory stimulation. Fig. 5-12 is a pictorial essay of a family with a small premature infant. In contrast, Fig. 5-13 shows a premature nursery before parental visiting was permitted.

Early studies of infant development suggest that contingent stimulation (stimulation related to cues from the infant) may aid the infant's development. Therefore we suggest that, as much as possible, mothers fondle and talk to their babies as they would normally if the baby were not in the hospital. Fig. 5-14 shows a mother in the intensive care nursery playing with her baby just after a feeding.

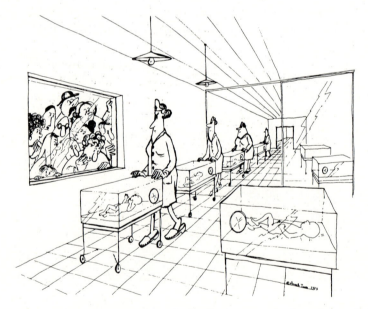

Fig. 5-13. A cartoon by Annette Tison made for her sister, Claudine Tison, showing the premature nursery before parent visiting was permitted. (Courtesy Claudine Amiel-Tison, Hospital Port Royal, Paris.)

COMMENTS: Not only is contingent stimulation important but also the temporal pattern. Recent data we have from providing a temporal pattern of rocking and heartbeat suggest that the combination of a constant factor, like regularity in the stimulation schedule coupled with opportunities for contingent stimulation, had the most positive influence on later congnitive development.
K. Barnard

The case of Benjamin G., a 900-gram infant, is an example of the importance of contingent stimulation by one person consistently. Of course, it is best if this is the mother. Benjamin was extremely immature, was fragile in appearance, and had frequent apneic episodes, of which his mother was aware. After being informed of the importance of stimulation, his mother came to the hospital early each morning and stayed until noon, returned after lunch and stayed until 6:00 P.M., when her husband finished his work. Her efforts with the baby were sensitively adjusted to him and consisted of considerable talking and stroking. Gradually she assumed more and more responsibility for his feeding and care. Her infant's significant decrease in apneic episodes, his unusually rapid weight gain, and developmental

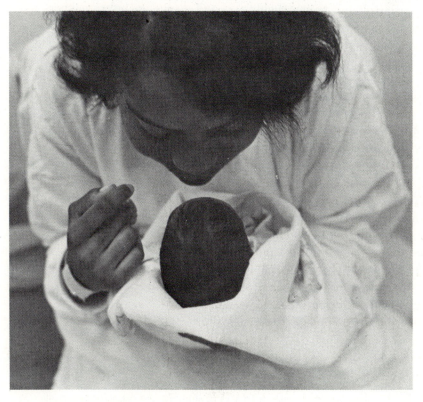

Fig. 5-14. A common sight today in the modern premature nursery.

progress in the hospital as well as in subsequent months were remarkable. The staff repeatedly told her that the baby was doing extremely well "due to her efforts." This was a sincere statement because the baby's progress was viewed as well above the normal expectations. There were several reasons for this notable progress. The mother was allowed to help care for her baby and consequently believed that she was making an important contribution. On several days the number of apneic episodes were frequent during the night and almost absent when she was present. Most importantly, this mother was able to establish a reciprocal interaction with her baby. She could send messages to him by stroking and talking and could receive messages in return, such as a change in activity level or an opening of the eyes.

Adaptation of the hospital

Each division, wing, or unit of a hospital is a social entity. The entire social environment of the nursery unit changes when parents are permitted to enter or to telephone 24 hours a day. Before shifting to a new, more flexible visiting policy, the personnel must be thoroughly prepared. In the era before mothers and fathers were allowed free access, the nursery was like a home with the head nurse as majordomo. It has been our experience that nurses in these units often develop close attachments to the babies they care for intimately day by day. As mothers and fathers entered this unit, which had been the domain of the nurses, some changes in orientation were required. There was the obvious, simple need for nurses to adjust to the fact of the parents' presence and all that it implied. Nurses must realize that it is beneficial for parents to share responsibilities for the care of their infant and his small portion of the nursery with the nursing and medical staff. It is not easy patiently to explain to anxious parents how to carry out a procedure that the nurse or physician enjoys, is in the habit of doing, and can manage more efficiently. A further complication arises from the fact that mother and nurse are often jealous of one another, and these feelings must be anticipated, discussed, and resolved before the new nursery setup can run properly. It is the long-term outcome that must be kept in mind and the fact that the parents will be responsible for providing total care for the baby after discharge.

COMMENT: In our nursery, primary care nursing is practiced. In addition, there is one nurse whose position is to coordinate care of parents. Even though our attitudes toward parents coming into the nursery have changed and we now encourage it, the fact remains that the parents get the short end of the deal when the unit is busy. Attention of the nursing and medical staff go to meet the physical and medical needs of the infants. This is as it should be. Having a person who can pull up the slack and attend to parents during these busy times helps. One task our parents' nurse helped with was to see that birth announcements got into the paper, which often does not happen with the birth of a premature infant. Nursing services need to structure staff to ensure attention to parents' needs.
K. Barnard

Meetings of the intensive care nursery staff

In our unit we have found that it is most important to have a staff meeting at least every two weeks. At this time nurses discuss the problems they have had, both with interpersonal relationships and the deaths inevitable in any unit. Some of the nurses' questions are, "Is it true you don't tell us why babies die because you don't want to hurt our feelings? We think we produce some deaths." In response to the question, "How do you feel about this baby?" one nurse volunteered that she felt as if she were his mother and that she felt terrible when he died. She had an empty feeling that lasted for several days. One nurse mentioned how quickly she became attached to an infant when she was asked to give him cutaneous stimulation and almost felt that he was her own for a moment.

In many premature nurseries specific assignments are not made. Nurses usually favor working with specific babies; often there will be one surrogate mother for each. This nurse is in a position to give the richest reports about the baby and parents.

When nurses resent implied or actual criticism, these feelings need to be discussed. As mothers come into the unit, they tend to note every little change and deficiency in care. Wet diapers or a little bit of spilled milk do not go unnoticed. They also have many questions. When the infant's condition changes, it is often the mother who is most sensitive to modifications in color, tone, or breathing. Questions and comments from the mothers can trigger resentment. When one nurse mentions that she has such feelings, other nurses with a sense of relief often admit that they feel the same way.

Anyone who has been associated with an intensive care unit for high-risk infants knows that there are acutely ill babies who demand a disproportionate amount of the physicians' and nurses' attention. Group meetings provide an opportunity to discuss these cases and also the other babies whose progress is more satisfactory, but whose parents may have shown evidence of personal problems. During this crisis period, parents may bring many of their most intimate or immediate problems to the nurses or aides. Encouraging the discussion of the nurse's intuitive observations about a mother is extremely valuable when making plans for the infant. Nurses are especially sensitive to the needs, tolerance, and ability of the mother. Heeding observations from the nursery staff permits problems to be recognized early in the course of hospitalization so that social work and psychiatric intervention may be arranged as required.

To enable the nurses and physicians to feel more at ease while discussing their difficulties with nursery policies, other staff members, and "problem" parents, some units have a person not connected with the unit to lead the group meetings.

Parents helping parents

The following letter to one of the authors best describes the effectiveness of parents helping each other.

I was having my fourth child in hospital. She was born in the late evening after a fairly rapid labor and immediately whisked away to the intensive care unit. I was transferred to a side ward off the main postnatal ward. The next day I was lying there feeling very confused. It is strange after having this constant companion during pregnancy, and the anticipation of labor, to be suddenly left with nothing. I knew with my mind that she existed and would be returned to me, but my body didn't understand.

A woman came in to see me from the main ward. She was a friend and we knew each other well. She had had her baby two days before. She asked if I had had mine and I remember saying, 'They tell me I have.' She went away and brought her baby back, full of joy and pride, and thrust him into my arms.

Holding the baby, I had a startling and intense sensation of release. It really was as if some lock had been undone, and the tension could disappear, and I could understand the events of the previous day. I cuddled the baby for a few minutes and admired him and gave him back.

After that everything seemed normal. I believed in the existence of my baby and was able to wait for her peacefully.*

I explained this to myself by thinking that some hormone had been released by the trigger of holding the baby. My body felt different afterwards, and as if something necessary had happened, without which the normal postnatal events and changes could not take place. The experience was so strong that I have wondered ever since whether it might be necessary for every mother to hold and cuddle a baby, not necessarily her own, in the first day after birth. I don't think there would be any danger of bonding to another woman's baby, there was no feeling of that, only of allowing something to happen that would enable the bonding process to take place later, as appropriate.

Discussions with parents when the health of the infant is not in doubt

The possibility of brain damage while a small premature infant is in the hospital troubles physicians and nurses. Usually these concerns are not borne out by difficulties in the future. In a follow-up study in our unit, we found that predictions made by pediatricians and neurologists with electroencephalograms and other neurological tests were accurate only 50% of the time—one half of those for whom dire predictions were made proved to be normal.

It is our strong belief that disturbances of the brain should *never* be mentioned to parents, unless the outcome can be accurately predicted, as in the case of Down's syndrome. Parents can erase questions that are raised about other organ systems in the baby, but once the possibility of brain damage has been mentioned, it cannot be easily forgotten. Many concerned parents have read about the brain and a closely related organ, the eyes. The physician should be aware of their concern and open to answer any questions. When questions are raised about the future development of a premature infant, the physician can quote the recent optimistic reports. The physician should indicate that although it is never possible at such an early age to predict conclusively the outcome for any baby, full term or premature,

---

*Her infant was well at two days, taken out of the special care unit, and given to her.

the parents have no reason for worry. The existence of eye problems such as retrolental fibroplasia should be acknowledged, but it should be pointed out that babies are monitored closely, which diminishes the chances of occurrence of these conditions. The parents should be further reassured that the baby's eyes will be checked in the hospital and after discharge to make certain that all is as it should be.

> **COMMENT:** Again, a simple demonstration of neonatal interactive behaviors, such as those on the Brazelton Neonatal Behavioral Assessment scale gives the nurse a chance to show the parents, just prior to discharge, that all systems are functioning. Demonstration of seeing and hearing may be more convincing than reassuring words.
> **T. Field**

Milestones and worrisome signs

As the days progress and the small premature infant starts to grow, the mother begins to believe that he will most likely survive. As she starts caring for him, she readjusts her previous image of the imagined baby to one which is closer to her own infant before her. It is remarkable to notice that a mother may comment on how much bigger her baby appears when there is evidence of improvement, whether it be a slight weight gain, a feeding taken by nipple, or a decrease in the use of monitors or other support equipment. Most parents consider the removal of catheters or monitors, the onset of weight gain, and the change from feeding by tube to feeding by nipple to be major milestones in the development of the infant, whereas the staff takes them as routine.

We have always found it helpful to present the positive developments to the mother. If the infant loses a few grams of weight (something seen often in the premature nursery), we do not emphasize it. If the mother expresses concern, we point out that this is normal, that weight gain is not straight line but rather a slow process containing brief plateaus or drops. If a mother is prepared for these fluctuations ahead of time, she will worry less.

Most mothers have mentioned that they do not feel close to their baby until they actually have him in their arms during a feeding and do not feel really close until they are feeding him at home. The glass-walled nursery is a barrier to their feelings of attachment. The more privacy they have the warmer they feel toward their infant. This is an important fact to remember when building new units for premature and sick infants. Small rooms should be provided for mothers so that they will have privacy while interacting with their infants.

It is important to recognize as soon as possible any mother who is not becoming attached to her infant, since she will need help. The longer she delays in attaching herself to her infant the greater will be her difficulty in finally achieving a close and warm relationship. Therefore during the hospitalization it is wise to assess the infant's physical progress and clinical care continually and to be equally alert to the progress of the other patients—the mother and father.

One of the best indicators of the parents' progress is their visiting pattern. For example, is the number of visits decreasing or increasing? Is the mother beginning to consider the baby a member of her family?

We try to keep track of the length of time the mother visits and her actions during the visits. Does she hop from one incubator to another looking at all the babies, or does she spend the time with her own? What comments does she make about her infant, and what skill does she show during her visits? There seems to be a correlation between poor outcome and a mother who travels from incubator to incubator, looks out of the window when she puts her hands into the incubator, or actually turns the baby's face away from hers. Are the parents starting to make plans at home for their infant—painting the room or buying new curtains and equipment they will need? Are they preparing the nest?

The overly optimistic mother who appears unconcerned about her baby's clinical state, who does not ask any questions, and who is passive or indifferent presents some worrisome signs. In other words, we are concerned about the mother who denies. The mother who grapples with the problem seems to get through much better. For example, throughout the hospitalization of her twins, Mrs. B. was outwardly extremely confident about her ability to care for her infants, not concerned with them, and frequently telling the nurses to change their way of managing and handling the twins. Because Mrs. B. ignored the nurses' suggestions, it was difficult for them to communicate with her and to learn how much she understood. After she took her babies home she was unusually anxious and made many frantic telephone calls to the nursery.

COMMENT: In cases such as the mother who incubator hops or appears unconcerned, care should be taken to detect the pattern of behavior the mother establishes rather than the isolated incident, since all parents' behavior shows a great deal of variability. It is the consistency of a worrisome response that is most important.
K. Barnard

Discharge requirements

There are three patients in the nursery—the mother, the father, and the infant. When discharging the infant, it is necessary to know about both the baby and the home situation. In some nurseries the infant's attainment of physical milestones (feeding ability, taking at least $1\frac{1}{2}$ ounces at a feeding, weight gain, and adequate temperature control) determines discharge dates. However, before discharge we attempt to measure the degree of maternal confidence and attachment. Previously, these assessments were made from observations of feeding and caretaking. Now several techniques allow more accurate predictions. We suggest the following guidelines.

1. Noting the nurses' observations of the mother
2. Inquiring about preparations the mother has made at home

3. A visit (with the parents' permission) if any question about the home situation arises
4. Determining whether the mother feels she is prepared for the discharge
5. Keeping a notebook in which to record every mother's telephone calls and visits so that we can assess if she is likely to be a high-risk mother

With the discharge of babies at 4 to $4^1/_2$ pounds, most parents are anxious about the care of their fragile infant. There are no available data about the long-term effects of caring for such precarious infants, but we believe that, prior to discharge, the mother should spend a period of 3 to 8 hours for several days providing full care, including the administration of medications that will be continued at home. We believe that two or three days of round-the-clock care provided by the parents, such as described under Nesting (pp. 177-178), ensures even better preparation. This might be compared with learning to fly with a copilot first prior to soloing.

Follow-up—what to watch for after discharge

After discharge we must be alert to situations in which the mother feels inadequate or disturbed. Key signs are frequent telephone calls and more than one visit to the emergency room at a strange hour with a completely normal infant. If the mother appears in the emergency room more than once, or if she appears to be signaling for help, we readmit the baby.

From our own studies we have found that the following considerations may be helpful for the pediatrician. At three to four weeks after discharge we ask the mother whether she has gone out, and if so, who stayed with the baby. We also ask how everything worked out while she was away.

We have found that the mother's answers fall into one of two categories: She is either concerned about the baby or about herself. The most successful attachments seem to be associated with replies which indicate that the mother is concerned about leaving her baby and thinks about him while she is away.

During the physical examination a physician can make important observations. Does the mother stand close to the physician, watch the handling of the baby, and soothe him when he cries, or does she appear detached and look around the office and concern herself with other matters? These latter behaviors can be important warning signals.

If possible, the physician or nurse should observe a mother feeding her baby. In general, positive features are eye-to-eye contact, close contact with the baby during the feeding, and fondling, kissing, stroking, and nuzzling. Evidence of disturbance in attachment and caretaking are a loose, distant hold on the baby, a propped bottle whether the baby is held in her arms or not, and a failure to hold the bottle so that milk can flow out of the nipple.

With these kinds of considerations in mind it is possible to make semiobjective measurements of mothering behavior with a few questions and simple observations during the physical examination and the feeding. None of these requires additional time.

In the follow-up of very small premature infants, Hack (1980) identified a group of infants who were gaining and progressing well prior to discharge but then showed a drop-off or slowing of weight gain. These were incipient cases of nonorganic failure-to-thrive syndrome occurring at a time of rapid mental development and brain growth. If weight percentile corrected for gestational age drops below the 10th percentile, investigation and intervention should not be delayed. The concern is similar, but the approach is different, when a baby has failed to progress appropriately in length, weight, and head circumference in the nursery.

We have become increasingly attentive to the mother's emotional state during the period of the infant's hospitalization and in the first weeks at home. It has been striking how many mothers report later about their extreme depression during this early period with sadness, crying, and an inability to get out of bed.

The surge of interest in perinatal and neonatal care, coupled with the desire to apply these latest ideas to benefit premature infants and their families, has unleashed a flood of innovative, humanistic changes in premature nurseries. The absence of innovation between 1945 and 1960 was almost complete. All the ideas about care were ossified in the pattern derived from Martin Couney.

AVOIDING OVERUSE OF INTENSIVE CARE NURSERIES

Richards and Roberton (1978) state "that babies are being unnecessarily separated from their mothers. Even if the evidence that separation may cause long term problems (including battering) is not conclusive for infants admitted for a comparatively short time, unnecessary maternal anxiety and unhappiness is caused by unjustified admission to the special care nursery. A newly delivered mother wants her baby: unless there's a very good reason, she should be allowed to have him."

Richards and Roberton (1978) have identified an important iatrogenic disease, which results from admitting normal infants to intensive care units because of prior high-risk conditions such as cesarean birth, fetal bradycardia, or short periods of rapid breathing for minutes or an hour after birth. They also noted a remarkable variation in the percentage of infants with these problems who were admitted to different units.

An increasing number of sick infants are being transported into our own intensive care unit. However, we have also been impressed that many more infants are brought back to the normal newborn nursery in the maternity unit of our hospital to be with their mothers at a much earlier time than in the past. As more intensive care units are built, we must be watchful that we do not admit normal infants to intensive care units simply to keep up the bed occupancy.

Our transitional care nursery has proved to be a valuable facility where an infant can receive care for an hour or two under the watchful eyes of a nurse. After care in this nursery an infant can be quickly reunited with his mother as soon as rapid breathing or increased oxygen requirements are normalized.

INTERVIEW

The following interview with the parents of a premature infant highlights some of the concepts already discussed in this chapter. The experiences of the parents and their reactions are representative of many parents with an acutely ill infant in a neonatal intensive care unit, transferred from another hospital. Kimberly Dixon* was born after 34 weeks of gestation, required assisted ventilation with continuous positive airway pressure (CPAP) provided in a negative pressure transparent box within an isolette for moderately severe respiratory distress syndrome. The pulmonary disease improved, and she appeared to be progressing well when a delay in her recovery occurred. A patent ductus arteriosus with mild congestive heart failure was diagnosed, so she was digitalized. After this setback her subsequent course was satisfactory. This interview with Mr. and Mrs. Dixon was obtained one month after discharge.

MRS. DIXON: I was really shocked. I was really tired out and I hadn't seen my baby, and all I could think of was, "My baby's very sick and they're going to take her away." I was really afraid she wasn't going to be with me very long. I was ready to run down to the nursery. You know they don't want you to get out of bed right away and you're supposed to take it easy after delivery. I got out of bed, and the nurse came in and said, "You can't get out of bed, dear," and I said, "Well, then, you'll have to get me a wheelchair because I'm going down there and I'm going to see my baby because they're taking her away." So they took me down there, and she looked terrible. I thought, "Oh, my poor little baby."

MR. DIXON: The doctors that came with the ambulance to pick her up brought her into Ann's room and said, "The baby is sick, but we've seen babies that are a lot sicker than this one." I was somewhat reassured.

MRS. DIXON: The next thing I knew they were wheeling her in, and the doctor was very nice and explained everything to me. He said, "I'm sure that you're worried about this tube and that tube, and we're going to do this to her and give her more oxygen." He was very reassuring. It was raining that night, and I said, "Please don't let her get wet—she'll get a cold." All I could think of was, "That's all she needs—to get a cold on top of all of this." He was very reassuring and told me not to worry and told me he would arrange it with the nurse so that after my husband saw her here, no matter what time it was, he could call back and tell me what they were doing.

MR. DIXON: That was good. Usually the husband feels kind of left out in a normal birth because he's not allowed in at some hospitals and is not allowed with the mother and child as much as probably a lot of fathers would like to be, but in this situation it's just reversed. I'm here all the time with the baby and trying to get back to my wife once or twice a day and relate to her what I'm seeing.

*The family's name has been changed.

COMMENT: Our experience has indicated that many fathers express the feeling that they are closer or more attached to their premature infant than their other children. They relate this to the fact that they had more involvement with the infant in the hospital during his early period of life.
K. Barnard

MRS. DIXON: I was still worried. I don't think until I got over to the premature nursery and got to hold her and make sure that she was still really a baby, that she was really OK, that everything was put together right, and that you were doing everything so she would be all right—I still had this empty feeling. I felt very bad. I called over here all the time—almost every hour.

A large percentage of mothers, separated from their premature infants, describe this empty feeling either while they are still hospitalized in the maternity unit or after they have gone home. The mother's uterus has been physically emptied, but there is no baby for her to hold. In contrast, the mother whose full-term infant remains with her in the maternity unit does not mention this type of feeling.

MR. DIXON: Probably the biggest thing that helped was when she could actually get over here. She can trust me, but she wanted to see the baby.

MRS. DIXON: I felt very empty because with all the other mothers and the other mother in my room—she'd get her baby every 4 hours and it was terrible in the hospital—at 6:00 in the morning they would come in and say, "Would you please wake up, Mrs. Dixon, your baby's coming in," and I was there for six days. Every day they'd come in and say, "Please wake up, Mrs. Dixon, your baby's here—it's time to feed her," I'd say, "My baby isn't here." The nurse said, "Honey, you're just asleep—your baby's here." I said, "I know my baby is not here—please don't wake me up." That was very hard. The girl next to me got her baby and fed her baby and she sort of felt bad. She said, "Do you want me to pull the curtain because I have my baby and you don't?" When I went home, there was another mother who had her baby all huddled in her arms—and I just left with my flowers. That was bad. I went to church a lot. I lit every vigil light you could name—I lit them all.

The large staff required for the operation of a modern hospital combined with the efforts to achieve maximum efficiency may result in impersonal care unless strong and repeated efforts are made to discuss the needs of mothers with every member of the hospital staff. Because the nursing and medical care of the baby is separated from the care of the mother, unfortunate situations of this sort do happen. However, if the mother-infant pair is cared for as a single unit, these situations do not occur. Mothers whose babies have died or have been transferred to a nursery for premature or sick infants have repeatedly told us that it would be best to transfer the mother to a separate room or another division so she would not be caught up in the routine care for the normal healthy newborn infant. Mrs. Dixon's report also makes it clear that if a woman has the mother of a sick infant as her roommate, some of the bloom is taken off her exciting postpartum period.

MR. DIXON: At that hospital I would change the hours that a father could be there. I had to wait until 7:00 at night after being here during the afternoon or morning, then I could not get into the hospital to see my wife until 7:00 at night, and then only from 7:00 until 8:30. There were so many things I was trying to relate to her—show her the pictures, trying to explain to her what was going on, what they were doing, how the baby was doing. Not that the telephone isn't convenient, but you just want to *be* there, and there isn't enough time. That's kind of a bad situation.

MRS. DIXON: If you had your baby, the father could be there from 3:00 till 8:30—*if* your baby's there.

Every hospital has a multitude of rules and procedures that are written and unwritten. Although at one time there may have been a good reason for establishing a rule, that reason may no longer exist. Often personnel have failed to consider the overall consequences of a rule that focuses just on the hospital care of the mother or the baby. It is difficult to see why a hospital would allow the majority of fathers to be present with their wives from 3:00 until 8:30 P.M. *but not allow the husband of a woman who has been separated from her baby*. Most of the restrictive regulations in maternity hospitals were originally established to protect the mother and baby. But with the infant absent, the reason is even less evident. It is imperative that we begin to reconsider many of these regulations.

MR. DIXON: But in our situation the baby wasn't there so the father is just another visitor. I was angered—they stood like a guard at the door and said you can't go up there till 7:00. They have regulations, and I guess we have to live with them, but I think in certain instances the regulations should be bent a little. I'm sure this is harder on the staff, but it's nicer for the people—and I think that's what hospitals are supposed to be for—the people.

Hospitals are built and operated for the benefit of sick people, and most have been built from funds contributed by lay people. It is easy to see why parent groups, as well as some professional groups, are working toward making hospitals less like military installations and more like home for patients and their families.

MR. DIXON: But I found the way that we operated in terms of coming and going to the premature nursery whenever we wanted was very beneficial to me, and once my wife got out of the hospital, it was very beneficial to her. Because a couple of nights we stayed here till 11:00.

MRS. DIXON: I hated to leave.

MR. DIXON: I felt like an ogre, saying, "Come on, I've got to work in the morning."

MRS. DIXON: He was so tired, one night he went into the lounge and fell asleep. I just didn't want to go home. I wanted to sit there and hold her and rock her. I read all these articles about premature babies—if they don't get enough oxygen to their brain or there can be too much oxygen . . . it can hurt her eyes or she could be mentally retarded. Or I thought, "If she has a heart murmur, then she'll never be able to run around and play with other children." I'm going to have to say, "Kimberly, sweetheart, you can't do that—you can't jump on the bed, you can't climb up on the stairs, you've got to sit down and play quietly." I wanted her to be normal, and all I could think about was, "What next?"

It is interesting to note that this is the first time either parent has mentioned the baby by name. Parents of premature infants often delay selecting a name for their baby for many days or even weeks. During the hospitalization and sometimes during the first weeks at home, they may not use the baby's name, referring to her as "it" much more than will the parents of a normal healthy infant.

> MRS. DIXON: The digitalis scared me to death. When I was in the hospital, I didn't want to think of it, but it did run through my mind—what's going to happen if this baby doesn't live? When I was over there and she was over here in the nursery, and I didn't really see her, and all I had was second-hand information from everyone, I kept thinking, "If my baby dies, they're not going to tell me and I never held her. I don't want her to die." I kept saying to her, "Now, Kimberly, you wanted to come early, you were so impatient—you're not leaving. Now remember that. I'm going to be very mad at you if you decide to leave. " I talked to her all the time—I think the nurses thought I was crazy.

No matter what the parents' level of education, intelligence, or experience, it is not unusual for them to resort to magical thinking in times of stress. Many physicians can remember occasions when parents talked to a baby in this manner when they had been told he may not live.

> PEDIATRICIAN: When you came in and she had the digitalis, what did you begin to think about?
> MRS. DIXON: Well, I didn't think she was going to die—I thought, "She's going to have a heart problem all the rest of her life." So many things can happen with heart problems . . . and digitalis—that's what they give older people when they have heart attacks.

The parents of every premature infant have different previous experiences with physicians, illnesses, and medications. Any diagnosis, symptom, or medication may bring back memories. It is not unusual that the Dixons believed that since Kimberly received digitalis, she would be on lifelong therapy. This emphasizes the importance of easy and free communication between the parents, nurses, and physicians. The physician should be sensitive to the reactions of overconcerned or underconcerned parents. Fortunately, Mr. and Mrs. Dixon were able to bring up their question so that an explanation could be given promptly. Many parents are too frightened to do this.

> MR. DIXON: The first thought when I found out about the digitalis—I don't know much about medicine—but that is what they give heart attack patients for the rest of their life. I must have been a classic example of worry. My parents had driven in from Detroit. We were waiting. Christ, it was my first baby. You know the old thing about whether you want a boy or a girl. I really didn't care, honestly, as long as it was healthy.
> MRS. DIXON: You know I never thought, and I've never known a baby that was born sick or with anything like that. It never crossed my mind. I'd read articles when I was pregnant about birth defects. It never crossed my mind that my baby would be born

and they would have to take her and she would be sick. I was just going to have my baby, and I was going to bring her home, and grandma and grandpa would come and see and say, "Oh, how cute." Everything was going to be typical, stereotyped, having a baby, if that's what you want to call it. But everything was quite different.

PEDIATRICIAN: You mentioned you had some fears the first night?

MR. DIXON: I would have done anything. There really wasn't anything that I could do at that point, but I said, "What can I do?"

MRS. DIXON: That's the thing. I felt very helpless. It was like you go and visit this baby, and they're taking care of her. They put her monitors on her, and I could talk to her through her isolette, and they did most everything for her. It was like their baby.

"It was like their baby" echoes the words of hundreds of parents of premature infants. This statement by these parents in the nursery, and after discharge, contrast vividly with the attachment of parents of normal full-term infants, and it started us searching for the factors that led parents to feel this way. Mrs. Dixon had lived with her baby in utero for 34 weeks. Now after birth she felt as if the baby belonged to someone else. This raises the question whether her attachment would be different had she played a larger role in the care of her premature infant. Even though the baby was ill and surrounded by monitors and tubes, a mother like Mrs. Dixon would benefit from contributing something that was uniquely her own to the baby's recovery.

> COMMENT: Occasionally, even parents of full-term babies express that they only felt that the baby really belonged to them a week or so after they got home from the hospital.
> **K. Barnard**

MR. DIXON: She didn't want to go home, and that was one of the reasons—"This is my baby. If she can't be at home with me, I want to be with her as much as I can."

MRS. DIXON: I guess I was very jealous. I know that they're taking care of her and I could have never done that, but yet I was very jealous because here she is, my baby, and I felt very empty because I couldn't do anything for her. There was nothing I could do for her. And so I sat and cried.

This is a criticism of the arrangements for the care of the baby. Although Mrs. Dixon had been welcomed into the nursery and had been allowed to touch and talk to her baby, she had not been given a definite role in the infant's care. Probably optimal mother-infant attachment cannot be achieved until the mother feels she is making an important contribution to the care of her baby.

PEDIATRICIAN: Were you jealous of one nurse specifically, or of all of them?

MRS. DIXON: The entire hospital.

MR. DIXON: I didn't feel that as much as I did the fear part of it. Babies are small and men are supposed to be somewhat clumsy, but I think that fear kind of carried over because even afterwards, when she was coming along much better and you said it was just a matter of time before she came home, I was still very much afraid to even hold her. I'd get cramps in my arms after holding her for just 5 minutes because my arms would be clenched so tight. Now I feed her. I change her—I'm still probably not as much at ease with her as Ann is, but that fear part of it is gone.

MRS. DIXON: Now she's a real baby.

PEDIATRICIAN: When did she become a real baby?

MRS. DIXON: When she got out of her isolette and got into that little bassinet.

MR. DIXON: Ann says she's got rid of her plastic house—now she's a real baby. When we realized that was coming up, we'd say, "Come on, Kimberly, let's get into your own little bed instead of that isolette. You can be a real baby then."

MRS. DIXON: I know it's silly, but I thought perhaps it was my fault that she was born early, and I kept thinking, "But I did everything I was supposed to do—I took my vitamins and I took the iron and I did everything the doctor said."

For the Dixons, Kimberly did not seem real until she was in a bassinet where she could be handled as a normal baby. It is a universal and normal reaction of mothers to wonder what they did that resulted in the early birth, even though they may have the education and intelligence to appreciate that it was not their fault. Later on, Mr. Dixon clarifies how perplexed he was, and Mrs. Dixon comes closer to the heart of the matter. She felt that there was something the matter with her, something bad about her, that resulted in her baby's premature birth. It is helpful to discuss the mother's fears. It is also important to demonstrate to the mother that we do not consider her responsible for the prematurity of her baby, that she must play an important role in the baby's care, and that she must touch her because it will be helpful to her progress.

MR. DIXON: She did all these exercises the doctor said, and I'm not sure the exercises didn't contribute to it in a way.

MRS. DIXON: But they tell you to do these to prepare for delivery.

MR. DIXON: We'd gone to these Stork Club classes, and I guess in a way they're good and in a way they're a waste of time.

MRS. DIXON: I don't think I'd recommend them to anyone.

MR. DIXON: They tell you the classic symptoms of labor. I went to bed one night and she said, "I have a bad backache." As I woke up, I saw that she was crying and I said, "I don't understand what's going on, so I'm going to call the doctor." So we called her obstetrician, and the doctor talked to her and got me back on the phone, and he said, "It sounds as if your wife may be in labor." But the Stork Club classes make everything seem so regimented—Ann didn't feel any of that—it seemed to come on so quickly. Of course you're not expecting it six weeks early, so maybe it happened and we didn't recognize it.

MRS. DIXON: I felt great that day until about 11:30 that night, when I got this horrible backache.

PEDIATRICIAN: You said that after the baby came you wondered what had happened or what you might have done. What sort of thoughts went through your mind?

MRS. DIXON: I didn't know. I wanted to know why she was early. Was it my fault—did I do something wrong? Was there something the matter with me?

MR. DIXON: She asked me that question one time on the phone: "What did I do that made the baby come early?" The doctor said she could still drive a car—she was still six weeks away.

MRS. DIXON: I'd go to the grocery store at the corner of the street.

MR. DIXON: That's about it, but that's what I couldn't understand. I couldn't understand why she felt maybe it was her fault. I said, "That happens sometimes."

MRS. DIXON: But I wanted to know why. For a while, and when she got so sick, I thought, "Maybe there's something the matter with me and that's why she was born so early." Everything wasn't ready for her to be born so early.

MR. DIXON: Especially with the first one. I think if it were to happen again, it would be a little easier to take. It was a very frightening experience for both of us. She kept saying, "What did I do? Is it something that I did? Aren't I right because the baby came early?" That was difficult for me to comprehend because I kept thinking to myself, "We conceived the child and carried it for almost nine months, almost full term." Six weeks early isn't 11 weeks early. You didn't have a miscarriage in the first month or something, so maybe it's a biological thing. I don't know, but I couldn't comprehend why she would tend to think it was her fault.

This lengthy discussion about Mrs. Dixon's guilt feelings illuminates the mother's intense and persistent preoccupation with her guilt about the premature birth. Also highly significant is her statement, "Everything wasn't ready for her to be born so early." Parents of a premature infant are deprived of about six weeks of psychological preparation. The changes that occur in the last six weeks are very important. The parent prepares for the birth of the baby, both physically and psychologically. The parents of a normal full-term infant experience a labor that is not associated with concern for the welfare of the baby. In contrast, the entire experience of labor, birth, and attachment for the mother of a premature infant takes place under a cloud of fear.

MRS. DIXON: I just felt that she's my baby and I'm supposed to be taking care of her while she's there and maybe I didn't do that. I don't know—I thought I did everything.

MR. DIXON: The biggest thing we felt at that time was fear. Fear for the baby, and I guess in a way, fear for ourselves. What happens? You plan for a baby and if the baby doesn't make it, what do you do? How do you pick up the pieces and keep going? But I think that biggest thing that really helped us was the staff at the hospital, yourself, and all the other doctors.

PEDIATRICIAN: How did they help?

MR. DIXON: Reassurance.

MRS. DIXON: Being so kind and answering all of my questions and talking to me at 2:00 and 3:00 in the morning and not saying, "Oh, it's Mrs. Dixon again."

MR. DIXON: It's the whole atmosphere.

PEDIATRICIAN: You mean they still kept their sense at 2:00 in the morning?

MR. DIXON: Well, of course 2:00 in the morning to them may be 2:00 in the afternoon for some people; they're more awake than we are, but we've called at 2:00 in the morning, 11:00 at night, just before they're changing shifts, and nobody ever rushes you and says, "Call back in 10 minutes." Somebody always takes the time to talk to you and explain things. That's the biggest thing. I learned more while Kimberly was in the hospital here about medicine and different things, equipment and pieces of equipment, how you use it, blood transfusions—they had to give her blood.

MRS. DIXON: That scared me too. I thought, "Oh, poor baby—she doesn't have enough blood."

MR. DIXON: But after that, the change. It was remarkable. It seemed the day after she got that blood there was such a rapid improvement. Her color and activity. She became much more active and cried.

PEDIATRICIAN: Could we go back to the first time you handled her? When was that?

MR. DIXON: She was still in the incubator. She was only in 40% oxygen—no, lower than that. I think it was 30%. So they said we could hold her for a few minutes.

MRS. DIXON: Everybody knew that I wanted to hold her. Everybody knew me when I walked in. I didn't know them, but they all knew me. "Oh, you're Kimberly's mother!"

Considering the intense pressure on the staff of an intensive care nursery, it is remarkable how warm, welcoming, and thoughtful the staff in this nursery has been. The staff nurses, nurses' aides, and secretaries have been welcoming mothers into the nursery to touch and hold their infants since the early 1950s. In any nursery it may at times be difficult to show enthusiasm about the visit of parents, particularly when the work load and pressures are heavy.

It has been helpful for us to put ourselves in the place of a mother. She comes to the incredibly strange and frightening nursery, fearful that her baby is dead or dying. There are new sounds, tubes, machines, and other sick babies. All combined, these are often enough to cause beginning nurses or medical students to feel faint, particularly if blood or unusual odors are evident.

Because she has been separated from her infant, the mother's imagination has pictured a baby who may be much sicker in many respects than her baby. The mother's anxiety is heightened by her tremendous guilt and her overpowering belief that something bad about her has injured her baby and caused the infant to come early and be sick. The best remedy in these cases is for the staff of the nursery to recognize the mother, to welcome her into the nursery, to tell her what a fine baby she has, to tell her how much the baby benefits from her visits and touch, and to impress on her the importance of the care and feeding she will provide for her baby.

MR. DIXON: That's how they knew her, as Kimberly's mother.

MRS. DIXON: But I got to hold her, and I just felt like all these thoughts I had about her dying completely were gone because there was no way. I was very determined there was no way. "You're going to fight. You wanted to come early, you're not leaving now. You're staying."

MR. DIXON: We told that to her—"You can't leave now. You've fought too long."

MRS. DIXON: "You were so impatient, you couldn't wait, you're staying here, not leaving."

PEDIATRICIAN: Do you remember when you felt the baby was yours?

MR. DIXON: I think we felt that from the beginning, but in a way the jealousy comes back up. I didn't really feel that as much as I did the fear.

MRS. DIXON: I didn't feel that she was my baby until I got to stay with her—when you said I could live with her those three days in the hospital. I took care of her, I did everything for her. I fed her. Then she was my baby.

PEDIATRICIAN: It wasn't when she came out of the incubator and you held her that first day, then?

MRS. DIXON: I was still scared then. I knew she was my baby, but I didn't know for keeps, and I didn't feel she was a real baby.

The mother's fear about the survival of her baby may inhibit the normal attachment process. The opportunity for this mother to care completely for her baby did much more than the previous visits to assure her about the value of her contributions to Kimberly's well-being.

MR. DIXON: Had anything happened after that so the baby couldn't come home, Ann would have been very upset.

PEDIATRICIAN: So something changed when you had the baby down at the end of the hall in the room.

MRS. DIXON: She was a real baby. She was mine.

MR. DIXON: And she was going home. We were going to be together as a family.

MRS. DIXON: Finally we were going to be a family. I wasn't going to have to run back here and run back home and fix dinner and run back to the hospital. I was so tired of doing that. It's not that we resented coming here at all—I wanted to be here. It was just so much, going back and forth, and I hated to leave here. I really did. I thought, "I have to leave my baby now." I always told the nurse, "Please turn her head the other way so that when I walk out she won't see me leave." One night she cried and I had to go back. I felt like, "She knows I'm leaving her, and I can't leave her." So I went back in and she stopped crying and I finally left.

MR. DIXON: I don't think Ann and I have ever really talked about that. But as soon as the baby was born, of course you know it's my first child and I was so excited. The doctor said, "There is a slight problem, but don't be concerned." I didn't really become that concerned until we went back to the hospital. But that baby was mine from that moment. I was petrified, especially when we came here and saw all these incubators and here's Kimberly. But I got to put my hand in (the isolette). I was scared. I really was. You encouraged me and said, "Put your hand in." You said, "Touch her leg." If anybody could have taken a picture—I put my hand in almost hesitantly. I was frightened. But that baby was mine—or ours—in my mind anyway. The baby was sick; there were some problems. Everything that could be done was being done. I was very reassured by you and the staff. Your people are fantastic. That was what pulled me through.

MRS. DIXON: Everyone was so kind, and no one gives you, "Oh, Mrs. Dxon—again."

PEDIATRICIAN: Could we go back to the last three days when you stayed in the room? Did you feel the baby was yours right away or was it the second day?

MRS. DIXON: When the nurse left, she was mine. I had to take care of her; I had to do everything for her, and that was great. I felt like, "She's my baby now, and I have all the responsibility for her."

PEDIATRICIAN: Did you think about her a little differently?

MRS. DIXON: There was no nurse there. Before there was always a nurse around so I could say, "Hey, come here. What's this, what's that?" Here I am, right here, she's my baby and I have all the mother responsibilities now. There's no nurse here who can pick her up and say, "Well, it's time for this now."

PEDIATRICIAN: When you lived in with your baby, you were on a division where the babies weren't just getting bigger, the babies there were sick. Did the mothers talk to you or try to include you?

MRS. DIXON: Well, at night we'd go into the lounge and sit and talk. There was a mother of a girl who was six weeks early also. She is now 2 years old and has had 12 operations on her head in two years. She doesn't think that she will live beyond 6 years old. I thought, "My baby was six weeks early too!" And they didn't know this when she brought the baby home. Her baby was in the hospital for a month also, and they told her, "Oh, your baby is fine."

PEDIATRICIAN: So all the old worries quickly came back?

MRS. DIXON: Yes, they all came back. I thought, "Why is he putting me here—to make me realize how lucky I am that my baby is well? Because I know—I feel like I'm the luckiest woman in the world."

MR. DIXON: Now that the baby is home I sometimes forget she was sick. She's so well— she screams and she hollers. And I love to hear her cry—except at 3:00 in the morning.

MRS. DIXON: I think it was good that while I was in the hospital he was here with the baby. I thought that was very good because whenever he would come and talk to me about her, he was so proud. He would say, "I was touching her and I was rubbing her leg. They told me to hold her hand, and you know, she gripped my hand—just pulled on it really tight." I thought that was very good because usually the father just sits there and watches.

MR. DIXON: Here it was just the opposite.

RECOMMENDATIONS FOR CARE

1. *First hour*. When a premature infant weighing between 4 and 5 pounds is born and appears to be doing well without grunting and retractions, we have found it safe for the mother to have the baby placed in her bed for 20 to 60 minutes in the first hour of life with a heat panel above them. We do not recommend this unless the physician feels relaxed about the health of the infant.

2. *Accommodations*. A mother and her infant should ideally be kept near each other, on the same floor, in the same hospital. When the long-term significance of early mother-infant contact is kept in mind, a modification of restrictions and territorial traditions seems appropriate and can usually be arranged. Furthermore, a mother appears to develop a closer attachment if she can have some privacy with her infant in a separate room close to, or connected to, the unit.

3. *Transport*. In our transport system, if the baby needs to be moved to a hospital with an intensive care unit, we have found it helpful to give the mother a chance to see and touch her infant, even if he has respiratory distress and is in an oxygen hood. The house officer or the attending physician stops in the mother's room with the transport incubator and encourages her to touch her baby and look at him at close range. Any comment about the baby's strength and healthy features made at this time may be long remembered and appreciated. The infant must be pink and adequately ventilating before we take him to his mother. If he is gasping

and blue, resuscitative measures are taken in the referring hospital, and our transportation team stays in the hospital until we can be sure of a safe trip. Transporting the mother and baby together to the medical center that contains the intensive care nursery is occurring more frequently in many communities. This trend should be encouraged for its immediate and long-term benefits.

4. *Father's participation.* In the event that the baby needs to be transported, we encourage the father to follow the transport team to our hospital so that he can see what is happening with his baby. By using his own transportation he can stay in the premature unit for 3 to 4 hours. We urge the father to use this period of time to get to know the nurses and physicians in the unit, to find out how the infant is being treated, and to talk with the physicians in a relaxed fashion about what they expect will happen with the baby and his treatment in the succeeding days. We allow him to come into the nursery, often offering him a cup of coffee, and we explain in detail everything that is going on with his infant. We ask him to act as a link between us, the members of his family, and the hospital by carrying information back to his wife so that he can let her know how the baby is doing. We suggest that he take a Polaroid picture, even when the baby is on a respirator, so that he can show and describe in detail to his wife how the baby is being cared for. Mothers often tell us how valuable the pictures are for keeping some contact with their infant even while being physically separated.

5. *Initial visit to the nursery.* A mother should be permitted into the premature nursery as soon as she is able to maneuver easily. In all our contacts we tell her that the staff of the nursery looks forward to her visit and that we know her baby will make better progress once she is able to visit. It is important to anticipate that she may become faint or dizzy when she takes her first look at her infant. We always have a stool nearby so that she can sit down, and a nurse stays at her side during most of the visit to describe in detail the procedures that are being carried out, such as the monitoring of respiration and heart rate, the umbilical catheter, the feeding through the various infusion lines, the functioning of the incubator, and, if appropriate, the ventilator and endotracheal tube.

6. *Cesarean birth mother.* We have found it exhausting for most mothers who have had a cesarean birth to visit more than once a day after discharge from the hospital. For these mothers the single visit a day can be extended, but it is best that it not last more than a few hours in the first week.

7. *Family visits.* We encourage grandparents, brothers, sisters, and other relatives to view the infant through the glass window of the nursery so that they will begin to feel attached to him. We let grandparents and other close relatives and friends enter and touch the infant if the parents wish. If the father is not available, we invite the mother to share the visits in the nursery with her mother or another relative or close friend.

8. *Discussions with parents.* At least once a day we discuss with the parents

how the child is doing. If the child is critically ill, we talk with them at least twice a day. It is necessary to find out what the mother believes is going to happen or what she has read about the problem. We try to be sensitive to her needs and to move at her pace during these discussions to ensure that she understands everything we say.

9. *Telephone communications*. While discussing the infant's condition by telephone with the mother who is still in the referring hospital, we ask the father to stand nearby so that we can talk to them both at the same time and they can hear the same words and intonations. This group communication reduces misunderstandings and usually is helpful in assuring the mother that we are telling her the whole story.

Parents are encouraged to call our unit 24 hours a day. This permits them to get an immediate report of their baby's status, activity, and color. This practice has occasionally led to confusion because several nurses may report the same infant's condition within several hours and use slightly different words. Ideally, only one nurse should talk with the parents. However, this is not always practical, since shifts last only 8 hours. Confusion can be avoided if the nurse will write down her message to the mother on the care record. This may be impossible in an extremely busy unit, but the development of primary care nursing in many units shows that it is feasible and beneficial. Usually the baby has one nurse with overall responsibility for primary care and then a designated primary nurse for each shift. The day secretary has the daily weights of the infants available at her desk and so can quickly report this information to the mother who calls and is waiting to speak to the nurse.

> **COMMENT:** In our nursery there is generally a nurse assigned to each baby, and the parents would know who was taking care of their baby during a particular shift. Thus when they call in, they either ask for, or are referred to, the nurse who is taking care of their baby, and the information given may be highly personal and specific to their child's progress. This has helped to develop rapport and excellent communication between the parents and the nursing staff.
> **K. Barnard**

10. *Optimistic attitude*. If there is any chance at all that the infant will survive, we maintain an optimistic tone in our talks with the parents from the beginning. If the infant is receiving 70% oxygen and assisted ventilation with continuous positive pressure airway pressure, and if he has a Po_2 of 55 mm Hg at 24 hours and a reasonable pH, we will say, "We're pleased by your infant's progress. He's active and pink. Although we're not in the clear yet, if we went to see Jimmy the Greek at Las Vegas or any other gambler, he'd certainly be betting with us and with good odds. We expect he will come through this illness in good shape unless unexpected complications develop." The next day, when the blood gas values are about the same, we might say, "The baby has had an excellent 24 hours. You have made a strong baby with good stamina. We're really pleased that everything is remaining

the same. Now, after going another day, the baby's condition is obviously improving." There is no evidence that if a favorable prediction proves to be incorrect and the baby dies, the parents will be harmed by this early optimism. There is almost always time to prepare them before a baby actually dies. If he lives and the physician has been pessimistic, it is sometimes difficult for parents to become closely attached if they have already anticipated and perhaps even begun to accept the child's possible death. We recognize that this recommendation is contrary to many old customs and places a heavy burden on the physician. It is our belief that if the infant does die, we must continue to work closely with the mother to help her with the mourning process.

11. *Possible brain damage*. Once the possibility that a baby has brain damage has been mentioned, the parents will never forget it. Therefore, unless we are 100% sure that the baby is damaged, we do not mention the possibility of any brain damage or retardation to the parents. On many occasions we have had neonates who have appeared to be brain damaged, but who later were obviously perfectly normal. Of the premature and full-term infants in our hospital suspected to have brain damage, only one half were correctly diagnosed, as normal or as brain damaged, in spite of multiple diagnostic studies and skillful neurological evaluations. If we had told the mother and father that we were concerned about damage to the brain, we might have indelibly inscribed on both parents' minds a concern which might have continued for many years. This parental concern can be transferred to the children involved and often drastically affects how they are reared. We have had these children, about whom there was a question of brain damage in early infancy, return years later and tell us how much it has affected their lives. Even after 20 years of normal progress some tell us they are still concerned that they are subnormal in mental ability and that they avoid competitive situations and worry excessively about examinations.

12. *Explaining findings*. It is important to emphasize that if we have a clear, objective finding, such as a cardiac abnormality or a specific congenital malformation, we see no reason to hide this from the parents. We would never lie to a parent. It should be remembered, however, that in overwhelming situations some parents can only assimilate a small amount of information every day. Explanations should be kept as simple as is appropriate to the situation. There is no need to add an unnecessarily wide variety of diagnostic possibilities or to speak of potential complications that may never develop.

13. *Touching*. As soon as possible we describe to both the father and the mother the great value of touching their infant. It helps them get to know him, reduces the number of apneic episodes (if this is a problem), increases weight gain, and hastens the infant's discharge from the unit.

14. *Feedback from infant*. We believe that the human mother must receive feedback from her baby in response to her caretaking for her to develop a close

attachment. If the infant looks at her eyes, moves in response to her, quiets down or shows through any behavior that he appreciates her efforts, he will encourage his mother's feeling of attachment. Practically speaking, this means that the mother must catch the baby's glance and be able to note that some maneuver on her part, such as picking him up or soothing him, acutally triggers a response or quiets him. We suggest to our mothers, therefore, that they think in terms of trying to send a message to the baby and of picking one up from him in return. Usually when we say this to the parents, they laugh; they think we are joking. We then explain that small premature infants do see, being especially interested in patterned objects, that they can hear as well as adults, and that there is evidence they will benefit greatly from receiving messages.

Because the baby often sleeps for 2 or 3 hours, waking up for only short periods of time, the parents need to stay in the nursery for long periods to be able to see one of these short periods. This usually requires special help from the nurse or some other caretaker.

It is important to remember that feelings of love for the baby are often elicited through eye-to-eye contact. Therefore, if an infant is under bilirubin lights, we turn them off at the time of a visit and remove the eye patches so that the mother and her infant can really see each other.

> **COMMENT:** We have found that premature infants sleep more hours during the 24-hour period than full-term infants all during the first four months after discharge. The amount of sleeping, particularly at 4 months of living age, shows a relationship with 24-month mental development. Infants who slept more had lower scores. Part of the nurse's guidance for a sleepy baby should be to help the parents modulate state. This would involve helping the parent keep track of sleep schedules and to try gradually to increase the times when the infant is awake. It is more difficult to get feedback from a baby who is sleeping a lot and for long periods each time.
> **K. Barnard**

15. *Breastfeeding.* It is especially helpful for the mother to make some tangible contribution to her infant, such as providing breast milk. Breast milk may be helpful in reducing the number of infections and other complications that the infant might encounter both in the nursery and after discharge. We are presently suggesting to all obstetricians referring patients to our unit that they enthusiastically recommend that the mother supply some of her own milk to meet the nutritional needs of her infant. Many mothers of premature infants had not planned to breastfeed and may not succeed. It is desirable to encourage and praise the mother for even a small amount of milk production, but at the same time we must avoid overselling its value so she will not feel a great deal of disappointment if she is unable to provide sufficient milk for her baby or wishes to stop for other reasons.

The mother-to-mother support provided informally by a friend or by a member of an organized group such as La Leche League has been extremely helpful for some mothers of premature infants with regard to breastfeeding and adaptation to their care.

Table 5-3. Visiting frequency and outcome in the intensive care nursery*

	> 3 visits/2 weeks	< 3 visits/2 weeks
Number	111	38
Follow-up	108	38
Disorders of mothering	2 (1.8%)	9 (23%) $p = <.001†$
Abandoned	1	1
Battered	0	2
Failure-to-thrive	0	5
Fostered	1	1

*From Fanaroff, A.A., Kennell, J.H., and Klaus, M.H.: Follow-up of low birth-weight infants—the predictive value of maternal visiting patterns, Pediatrics 49:288-290, 1972.
†Chi square.

16. *Recording parental performance.* We have found that keeping a book in which to record parental telephone calls and visits is useful in determining which mothers are likely to require additional help from a social worker or extra discussions about the health of their infant. Fanaroff and co-workers (1972) studied the visiting patterns of mothers in a nursery where they were allowed unlimited telephone calls or visits. They determined that 25% of those mothers who visit or phone on an average of less than three times in a two-week period will exhibit significant mothering disorders (Table 5-3).

If a mother visits fewer than three times in two weeks, the probability of occurrence of some sort of mothering disorder, such as failure to thrive, battering, or giving up the baby, increases. If we observe that the visiting pattern of a mother is less than that of most mothers, she is given extra help in adapting to the hospitalization.

17. *Staff meetings.* Nurses should feel comfortable about reporting any worries or problems that they have about a mother's and father's behavior. To accomplish this there must be a good working relationship between the physicians and nurses. Meetings with the nursery staff in the intensive care unit should be held every one or two weeks. This provides an opportunity for the expression of concerns and problems.

COMMENT: The necessity for team work is as great in the high-risk nursery as anywhere, and it is important that the staff have the opportunity to develop knowledge of each other's skills and abilities. Thereby they will gain a respect that will enhance the working relationship and the team work required in caring for the infant and the family.
K. Barnard

18. *Nurse-mother interaction.* Nurses should take mothers under their wing, teaching, supporting, and encouraging them when they first handle the child. The nurse's guidance in showing the mother how to hold, dress, and feed the infant can be extremely valuable in helping her overcome her mothering paralysis. Often

mothers need special reassurance and permission before they can develop good mothering practices. In a sense the nurse assumes the role of the mother's own mother, teaching her the basic techniques of mothering.

19. *Communication of information.* When a mother does not ask for explanations, the physician should be alert to difficulties and attempt to establish a rapport with her to help her express any feelings of low self-esteem and guilt. This does not require a highly skilled interview technique but can be done by a sensitive nurse or pediatrician who knows how to listen to a mother's concerns.

20. *Lack of maternal behavior.* If maternal behavior fails to develop, the pediatrician should suggest psychiatric consultation. Cases of frankly pathological deviations can be spotted whenever mothers show pronounced avoidance behavior (no visits), demonstrate marked denial when there are problems, evidence an absence of affective response, resort to constant accusation of the staff, or reveal consistent lack of maternal behavior.

CHAPTER 6

CARING FOR THE PARENTS OF AN INFANT WITH A CONGENITAL MALFORMATION

NANCY A. IRVIN, JOHN H. KENNELL, and MARSHALL H. KLAUS

The world breaks everyone and afterwards many are strong in the broken places.
Hemingway in *Farewell to Arms*

A newborn blighted with a malformation is a crushing blow to the parents and to everyone else who has shared in the event. The baby is the culmination of his parents' best efforts and embodies their hopes for the future. Human societies' responses to malformations are not uniform and may range from protection to exclusion.

The early recorded history of human society indicates that malformed infants have been treated in widely differing ways and have evoked a broad range of emotional reactions. The reactions parents experience today after the birth of a malformed baby are not novel. Warkany (1971) noted that when "a monstrosity was born, then man's emotions were aroused and he reacted to such misfortune with admiration, awe, or terror. His emotions toward reproductive anomalies often have led to extreme measures; he exterminated or adored the deformed of the species— and sometimes he did both."* After killing an infant with a disfiguring abnormality, he "often made an image in its likeness and set it up as an idol-god or demigod. Sculptures, carvings, and drawings of abnormal births by ancient peoples antedate the arts of reading and writing; they reflect early teratologic knowledge and interest in rare and unusual human beings. That such deviants were made gods or goddesses is understandable. During times when human deities were worshiped, it was the unusual human being who assumed divine status."*

---

*From Warkany, J.: Congenital malformations: notes and comments, Chicago, 1971, Year Book Medical Publishers, Inc.

Although United States society has elected to include most sickly or malformed infants through medical treatment, some societies have practiced euthanasia. For example, a tribe of African bushmen, the Zhun-twasi, practice infanticide with certain children. When a baby is born with a malformation such as agenesis of a limb, ear, or nose, with a malpresentation such as breech birth, or if he is one of a pair of twins, he is buried seconds after birth, even before he has breathed (Konner, 1972). This extreme, however, is rare and is often related to population or sex ratio control, not to the elimination of malformed infants.

Despite new scientific knowledge about the origins of congenital defects, ancient superstitions still plague modern parents. Because of the strong emotional reactions accompanying the birth, it is not surprising that the lore of the past surfaces to haunt parents of children with congenital malformations.

BASIC AND CLINICAL CONSIDERATIONS

The birth of an infant with a congenital malformation presents complex challenges to the physician who will care for the affected child and family. In the United States a major malformation occurs in two of every 100 births. Thus almost every nurse or physician will have a part in the care of these babies. Yet despite the relatively large number of infants with anomalies, understanding of the development of parental bonding to a malformed infant remains incomplete. A number of investigators agree that the child's birth often precipitates a major family crisis, but relatively few have described the process by which the parents and family members adapt.

The objective of this chapter is to describe methods for helping parents from widely diverse backgrounds develop ties to their malformed infants. This is difficult, since parental reactions are turbulent, and the usual pathways for the development of close parent-infant bonds are disrupted. The final absolute goal is best described by Bettelheim (1972): "Children can learn to live with a disability. But they cannot live well without the conviction that their parents find them utterably loveable. . . . If the parents, knowing about his [the child's] defect, love him now, he can believe that others will love him in the future. With this conviction, he can live well today and have faith about the years to come."

The strength and character of the original parent-infant bond will influence the quality of the child's bonds with other individuals in the future. During this early period the design and weave of future interactions and attachments, which determine the personality structure, are set.

During the course of a normal pregnancy, the mother and father develop a mental picture of their baby. Although the degree of concreteness varies, each has an idea about the sex, complexion, coloring, and so forth. One of the early tasks of parenting is to resolve the discrepancy between this idealized image of the infant and the actual appearance of the real infant (Solnit and Stark, 1961). The dreamed-

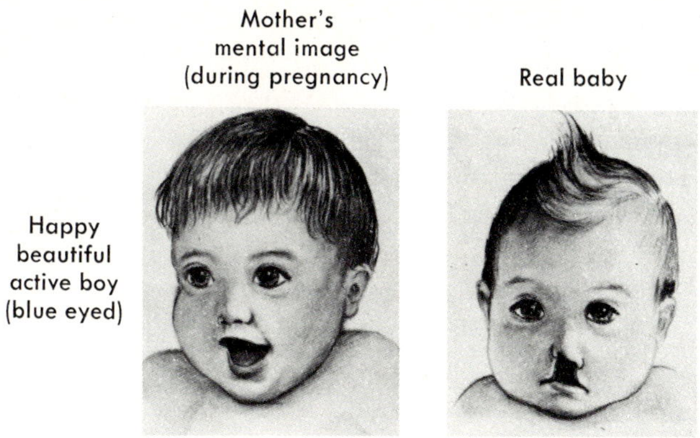

Mother's
mental image
(during pregnancy)

Real baby

Happy
beautiful
active boy
(blue eyed)

Fig. 6-1. The change in mental image that a mother of an infant with a malformation must make following childbirth.

about baby is a composite of impressions and desires derived from the parents' own experience. Therefore, if the parents have different cultural backgrounds, the tasks of reconciling the image to the reality is more complicated. However, the discrepancy is much greater if the baby is born with a malformation, and the parents must struggle to make the necessary major adjustment (Fig. 6-1).

The reactions of the parents and the degree of their future attachment difficulties depend in part on the properties of the malformation:

Is it completely correctable or is it noncorrectable?
Is it visible or nonvisible?
Does it affect the central nervous system?
Is it life threatening?
Will it have an effect on the future development of the child?
Does it affect the genitalia? The eyes?
Is it a single or multiple malformation?
Is it familial?
Are there other members of the family with a malformation?
Will there be a need for repeated hospitalizations?
Will repeated visits to physicians or agencies be needed?

COMMENT: Does the malformation have a specific meaning for the parents because of their occupation or their cultural background and expectations?
A.J. Solnit

The initial reactions of the parents largely depend on the answers to these questions, which will determine the long-term problems they will have to face.

Few studies have separated the different impacts of various malformations, but a number of investigators have noted that the more visible the defects are the more immediate will be the resulting concern and embarrassment. Even a minor abnormality of the head and neck results in greater anxiety about future development than an impairment of another part of the body (Johns, 1971). This is in agreement with the findings that disabled adults with visible impairments experience more disruption in their interpersonal relationships than do those with nonvisible impairments (Zahn, 1973).

> **COMMENT:** Recent studies have shown that even in nursery school, children tend to select as their friends their better looking peers. This trend remains through the life of the person, and everyone is naturally initially drawn to a handsome-, or strong-, or sweet-looking person and withdraws from a physically unappealing person. The homely or malformed child, and later, adult, will have to compensate for his unattractiveness by an unusual personality. Parents may react with the same initial negative feelings toward their visibly malformed child, but through increased contact the infant's own personality should facilitate the overcoming of these feelings.
> **N. Josefowitz**

In several studies parents have reported that when they saw their infants for the first time, the malformations seemed less alarming than they had imagined. Seeing the children allayed some of their anxiety. In our own studies one parent reported, "We had been conjuring up all kinds of things—that there could be something wrong with every organ. But then what I saw was a relatively normal baby" (Drotar et al., 1975). Others (Daniels and Berg, 1968; Johns, 1971) report similar parental reactions—the information that something was wrong with the baby was often far more disturbing than the sight of the child. Mothers found that the time spent waiting to see the baby after being told about a congenital amputation was the most difficult to endure (Daniels and Berg, 1968). Both the mothers and the fathers were greatly relieved when they actually saw their children.

Some parents were reluctant to see their babies at first, expressing a need to temper the intensity of the experience. When these parents did see their babies, it seemed to mark a turning point, and caretaking feelings were elicited where previously there had been none. Roskies (1972) studied the mothers of children with phocomelia due to thalidomide. She describes four mothers who were debating whether or not to institutionalize their children. The issue was settled when they saw their infants and found aspects they could "cherish." "When one mother looked into her baby's eyes he seemed to plead not to be abandoned." In our studies the parents of children with visible anomalies had a shorter period of shock and disbelief than did the parents of a child with a hidden defect. The shock of producing a baby with a visible defect is stunning and overwhelming, but attachment can be facilitated by showing parents their newborn baby as soon as possible.

> **COMMENT:** "Possible" includes when the parents feel ready, since enabling parents to be active in the decisions and care that affect their child will enhance their capacity to cope with the challenge of having a child with a congenital malformation.
> **A.J. Solnit**

When 194 mothers of babies with spina bifida were interviewed, two thirds of the mothers preferred to be told about the diagnosis as early as possible and were satisfied with the information they had received about the defects. Any delay tended to heighten their anxiety. They objected to being given an unneccessarily gloomy picture at first on the one hand, and on the other hand they objected to having the seriousness of the condition minimized at first and aggrandized later. For example, one mother of an infant with myelomeningocele was told that the baby had "just a small pimple on her back, but that was nothing for her to worry about." The parents attached great importance to the approach and general attitude of the medical and nursing staff. Most importantly, they often did not recall the words of the nurse, obstetrician, or pediatrician but did remember their general attitude. Mothers who were hurt by an apparent lack of sympathy tended to attribute the abruptness to a lack of feeling in the informant, rather than to the likely cause—the difficulty of imparting such painful information. Most mothers were impressed by the kindness and sympathy extended to them by the nursing and medical staff. Small acts of kindness were clearly remembered years after the event. D'Arcy (1968) concludes that "the initial counseling of the mothers of malformed infants makes a deep and lasting impression."

In our studies, despite the wide variations among the children's malformations and parental backgrounds, a number of surprisingly similar themes emerged from the parents' discussion of their reactions. Generally they could recall the events surrounding the birth and their reactions in great detail (Drotar et al., 1975). They went through identifiable stages of emotional reactions, as shown in Fig. 6-2 which

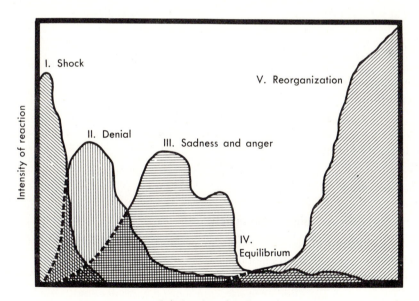

Fig. 6-2. Hypothetical model of the sequence of normal parental reactions to the birth of a child with congenital malformations.(From Drotar, D., Baskiewicz, A., Irvin, N., Kennell, J.H., and Klaus, M.H.: Pediatrics **56**:710-717, 1975.)

is a generalization of the complex reactions of individual parents. Although the amount of time that a parent needed to deal with the issues of a specific stage varied, the sequence of stages reflected the natural course of most parents' reactions to their malformed infant.

First stage: Shock

Most parents' initial response to the news of their child's anomaly was overwhelming shock. All but two of the 20 parents reported reactions and sensations indicating an abrupt disruption of their usual states of feeling. One mother said, "It was a big blow which just shattered me." One of the fathers explained, "It was as if the world had come to an end." Many parents confided that this early period was a time of irrational behavior, characterized by much crying, feelings of helplessness, and occasionally an urge to flee.

Second stage: Disbelief (denial)

Many parents tried either to avoid admitting that their child had an anomaly or to cushion the tremendous blow. Each reported that he or she wished either to be free from the situation or deny its impact. One father graphically described his disbelief: "I found myself repeating 'It's not real' over and over again." Other parents mentioned that the news of the baby's birth did not make sense. One man admitted, "I just couldn't believe it was happening to me." Although every parent reported disbelief, the intensity of the denial varied considerably.

> **COMMENT:** Between the second and third stage there is another stage that you mention later under doctor shopping. It is kind of a bartering stage. There is often a return to religion or to giving to charities as if to say on a primitive, unconscious level: I have been bad, and I am punished, now if I promise to be good, my child will be made normal. One wishes to make "a deal" with God. It is also at this stage that there is the most danger of succumbing to quackery in the form of faith healers.
>   It is also my belief that anger precedes sadness or depression. The anger can be turned against God (who did not answer) and fate, but also against hospital staff, and as you mention, friends or relatives of the spouse. Doctors, nurses, and relatives can be warned that no matter how much one does for the mother or father, it is not enough, never right, and not appreciated. Of course the only help really wanted is to have the child made whole again, and nothing short of that will do.
>   **N. Josefowitz**

Third stage: Sadness, anger, and anxiety

Intense feelings of sadness and anger accompanied and followed the stage of disbelief. The most common emotional reaction was sadness. One mother reported, "I felt terrible. I couldn't stop crying. Even after a long while I cried about it." A smaller, but significant number of parents reported angry feelings. One father said, "I just wanted to kick someone." a mother reported that she was angry and "hated him (the baby) or hated myself. I was responsible." In most instances mothers feared for their babies' lives, despite strong reassurance. One mother said that she initially perceived her child as "nonhuman." "Holding him with that tube distressed me. Initially I held him only because it was the maternal thing to do." Almost all of the mothers were hesitant about becoming attached to their babies.

Fourth stage: Equilibrium

Parents reported a gradual lessening of both their anxiety and intense emotional reactions. As their feelings of emotional upset lessened, they noted increased comfort with their situation and confidence in their ability to care for the baby. Some parents reached equilibrium within a few weeks after the birth, whereas others took many months. Even at best, this adaptation continues to be incomplete. One parent reported, "Tears come even yet, years after the baby's birth."

Fifth stage: Reorganization

During this period parents deal with responsibility for their children's problems. Some mothers reported that they had to reassure themselves that "the baby's problems were nothing I had done." Positive long-term acceptance of the child involved the parents' mutual support throughout the time after birth. Many couples have reported that they relied heavily on one another during the early period. However, in some instances the crisis of the birth separated parents. In one case the parents blamed each other for the baby's birth. Another mother wanted to be isolated from her husband. "I don't want to see anybody. I just want to be by myself."

Despite the important similarities in parental reactions to various malformations, parents progressed through the various stages of reaction differently. Some parents did not report initial reactions of shock and emotional upset but tended instead to intellectualize the baby's problem and focus on the facts related to the baby's condition. Other parents were unable to cope successfully with their strong emotional reactions to the birth and, as a result, did not achieve an adequate adaptation; they were in a state of sorrow that lasted long after the birth.

A lack of opportunity to discuss the infant's diagnosis can create a situation in which the parents feel overwhelmed and unable to gauge the reality of their child's abnormality. If the mourning process becomes fixed as a sustained atmosphere of the family, the ghost of the desired, expected, healthy child sometimes continues to interfere with the family's adaptation to the defective child. These findings confirm the original creative work of Solnit and Stark (1961), which has become the foundation of most therapeutic approaches to the parents of the malformed infant. Their brilliant analysis consists of the following elements:

1. The infant is a complete distortion of the dreamed-of or planned-for infant.
2. The parents must mourn the loss of this infant—a process that may take several months—before they can become fully attached to the living defective infant.

3. Along with this process of mourning there is a large component of guilt that takes many forms (such as the "mother's dedication of herself unremittingly and exclusively" to the welfare of the child while excluding others in the family) and requires great patience of the individual helping the family, since the parents may repeat the same questions and problems many times.

4. There is resentment and anger, which nurses, pediatricians, and obstetricians must understand, since it is sometimes directed toward them.

5. The physician, nurse, and social worker should *not* interpret to the parents that the grief they are feeling is due to the loss of the expected perfect child, nor should they attempt to compare this mourning response with any others the parents might have experienced, since it may rob the mother of the full strength and depth of her own grief by intellectualizing it.

6. The mother's attempts to withdraw her strong feelings from the lost expected baby are disrupted by the demands of the living blighted child. The task of becoming attached to the malformed child and providing for his ongoing physical care can be overwhelming to parents at the time around birth, when they are physiologically and psychologically depleted.

7. The mourning cannot be as effective when the damaged child survives. The daily impact of this child on the mother is unrelenting and makes heavy demands on her time and energy. For example, based on interviews with 96 mothers after the birth of an anencephalic infant, D'Arcy (1968) observed that the mothers' sense of loss and grief was more acute than that of mothers of a surviving infant with a severe malformation. However, these mothers recovered sooner than mothers of infants with severe congenital defects who survived.

It is remarkable that families who must cope with the intense emotional experience engendered by the birth of an infant can assimilate the child into the family and begin responding to his needs as readily as they do.

As with other crises, successful mastery often strengthens people's ability to cope in other areas. The father of a boy with a congenital amputation described his confidence and pride in his management of the especially difficult time around his son's birth, his securing of treatment facilities, and his overall management of life. "I suppose you never know until you are all finished whether you have given your family what they need, but I try and I think I do a good job" (Daniels and Berg, 1968). Voysey (1972), in her analysis of the problems which parents and their disabled child face in encounters with those outside the family, notes that they develop special interactional skills. By dealing with occurrences that other people might find embarrassing and distressing in the course of daily life with their child, parents of the disabled learn how to treat these events routinely. These special qualities, which may be characterized as "understanding" and "self-sacrifice," provide a rationale for the "deep philosophy" that persons with a stigma are said to evolve (Goffman, 1968). The parents' identity, which was so compromised by the birth, may go through changes that result in a more positive self-image (Voysey, 1972). However, this kind of psychological maturity may appear slowly.

The struggle with the complex issues involves negotiating many tasks fraught with the potential for less than adequate resolutions. Several studies note outcomes in which parents, because of unresolved guilt and anger, develop an overprotective attitude toward the child, which can thwart his development. Managing disturbed feelings by denying painful facts about the malformation can also lead to less than adequate resolutions. Other members of the family may be neglected if parents ward off the grieving process by establishing a guilty attachment to the child (Drotar et al., 1975; Miller, 1968; Solnit and Stark, 1961). If the mourning process is protracted rather than diminishing or if it develops into self-reproachful depression, the parent will not be able to actively contribute to the family.

Responding to the circumstances surrounding the birth of an abnormal child in the best way is exceedingly difficult because of the ambiguities involved. For example, what is the difference between overprotectiveness and responding to special needs? Daniels and Berg (1968) quote one mother as saying, "It is hard, sometimes, to figure out what is being motherly and what is taking over. I want to help him as much as he wants and needs, but I don't want to hold onto him." Realistically, it is true that the physical care required by such children is much greater than that required by normal children. Recurring hospitalizations for some, and uncertain developmental predictions for others, intensify parental concern and often frustrate consistent planning so that it is difficult to determine when parents cross the boundary into overprotective behavior.

Another feature to consider is the notion of just what characteristics constitute optimal adaptation. If sorrow, depression, and anger are natural responses to the birth, and if the infant evoking these feelings continues to live, what is the right balance between mourning and acceptance? Olshansky (1962) coined the term "chronic sorrow" to describe some of the enduring aspects of parental reactions in adapting to a retarded child. Chronic sorrow at some level may be constantly present in parents, especially if the child will always be dependent on them, as in some cases of retardation. To expect the disappearance of the painful impact of this child on a family, under the guise that these feelings must be "resolved," can only force parents to deny their real feelings to professionals who may want to help. A useful stance for professionals might be to consider the rewards of shepherding a child with problems to a more successful level of functioning along with the need to come to grips with the malformation in the first place.

Many parents also struggle with these issues and search for some explanation of why this happened to them. Sometimes these struggles include much concern over the exact cause of the problem, which can be frustrating if a cause cannot be determined. When there is no acceptable medical explanation for the child's birth defect, the parents' genetic competence is called into question. They may try very hard to find a specific nongenetic cause for the anomaly in order to rid themselves of guilty feelings. Parents of children who develop mental retardation due to an illness, such as meningitis subsequent to birth, for example, seem to adjust much better than parents with a baby retarded from birth.

An analysis of the anguished reactions of parents assuming the new role of parent to a defective child helps to clarify some of the obstacles that physicians, nurses, and others are likely to encounter. For example, the parents' search for causes, sometimes leading to doctor shopping, may not be due to dissatisfaction with the physician's diagnostic abilities as much as to the parents' need to alleviate their own guilt. Furthermore, the "active" search for services is often necessary because of the fragmentation of treatment facilities and can be one form of mastery in a crisis that parents are powerless to reverse.

It is disturbing for parents to encounter a discrepancy between their own intense emotional turmoil and what they believe is a lack of feeling on the part of professionals. The physician's objective professional manner may sometimes be mistaken for a lack of sympathy and may be met by generalized outrage on the part of the parents. Many physicians are able to compromise, maintaining their own standards of correct professional behavior and at the same time fulfilling some of the parents' needs for support. The baby can be presented to the parents in such a way that his attributes and normal features are highlighted. It is desirable to do this shortly after birth in the presence of both parents. This demonstrates to the parents that the hospital staff considers the baby an acceptable substitute for the wished-for baby and not a "piece of damaged goods" (Carr and Oppé, 1971).

COMMENT: This focus can be helpful provided it is not used by physicians and nurses to "turn off" the fears, questions, and resentment that many parents need to express before they can see and hear what the health personnel are presenting.
A.J. Solnit

Involving the parents in the care and planning for their infant allows them to enjoy satisfying feedback from him. It is also at this early stage that the groundwork is laid for an effective alliance of parents and professionals concerning treatment.

Nurses and physicians can facilitate the bonding of parents to their malformed infant in the neonatal period and as the child grows. Knowledge about the usual course of parental reactions helps the physician to take this into account in planning interventions. For example, a physician who knows about the disorganization which parents experience during the stages of shock and denial will realize that information about the child's condition and progress may have to be repeated many times.

COMMENT: It is important to add that to talk with angry or depressed parents is not the natural inclination of the obstetrician, pediatrician, or nurse. The gratifications of these professions lie in either the delivery and care of the healthy infant or in the use of their medical knowledge to heal

or remedy. With a congenitally malformed baby they are often helpless and therefore feel useless. This of course is not so, and although at the time it is not evident that the extra visiting is doing any good, it is important to visit repeatedly and not to abandon the parents to their grief.
N. Josefowitz

In addition to their own emotional turmoil, parents must cope with the demands and expectations of those around them. With their ability to produce a normal child called into question and their emotional reserve at a low, they must face grandparents, friends, and neighbors. In this case society has few built-in supports such as those available in other crises such as the death of a relative or a community disaster. For example, friends and relatives send gifts and cards to the hospital after the birth of a normal baby but are confused about the proper procedure when the baby is abnormal, and they may find it easiest to forget to call or send anything. The parents are often reluctant to send out announcements of the birth or even to name the baby. As a result, they are likely to experience intense loneliness during the period immediately following the birth.

> **COMMENT:** There are no flowers in the rooms of these mothers. A maternity ward is supposed to be the happiest place in the hospital. A weeping mother disconfirms this, and one does not forgive her easily for disturbing the joyful atmosphere.
> **N. Josefowitz**

The crisis of the baby's birth has the potential for bringing the parents closer as a result of the mutual support and the communication required for adaptation. On the other hand, in many of the families we have studied, the baby's birth estranged the parents. The ongoing demands of the baby's care increased the isolation between some parents, particularly if they did not share the responsibility. We have used the term "asynchronous" to describe parents who progress through the different stages of adaptation at different speeds (Fig. 6-2). These parents usually do not share their feelings with each other and seem to have particular difficulty in their relationships. Asynchrony often results in a temporary emotional separation of the parents and appears to be a significant factor in the high divorce rate after a major family crisis.

> **COMMENT:** Paradoxically, trauma such as the birth of a defective baby tends to magnify the weaknesses in a marriage more than it enhances the strengths of the relationship, and success, such as the easy birth of a normal baby will more often magnify or make more explicit the strengths of the marriage.
> **A.J. Solnit**

The availability of the pediatrician throughout the child's early years puts him or her in a position to help with the family's adaptation. The pediatrician can be sensitive to the relationship between the parents, can determine which stage of adaptation each parent has reached, can check how aware each partner is of the other's progress, and may be alert to evidence of asynchrony. Parents have told of the importance of identifying the normal features of their child, which become increasingly evident as he grows. The pediatrician has an excellent opportunity to nurture this.

As a physician, nurse, or social worker follows the progress of the parents, each will be struck by the step-by-step nature of adjustment to a stressful situation such as this. There will be a tentative and perhaps ever-changing view of the child's potential. If reality indicates a less hopeful prognosis, the professional can present the news so that the parents can adapt to it in small amounts without losing confidence in themselves. Many parents describe that the most effective way they have found to deal with the challenge is to take things day by day. They try not to worry excessively about the uncertainties in the future or to dwell on the traumatic events of the past. Sometimes this can be mistaken for defensive denial. Unless the daily care and planning for the child is affected, however, this type of reaction seems to serve to protect parents from unbearable pain.

> **COMMENT:** It presents the problems in a "dosage" that both can be taken and that does not exceed the physician's capacity to predict what will happen.
> **A.J. Solnit**

In one of our studies to assess each parent and to evaluate how he or she is managing, we have used the following interview. We have often been surprised by the unusual interpretations that parents have given about previous explanations of the defect. There are three points to consider in this interview:

Where each parent stands in her or his emotional reactions.
How the parent views the baby and the defect.
How each parent views the spouse and his or her emotional progress.

An outline of an interview that we use in our hospital is included on pp. 240-241.

INTERVIEW

Following is an interview with Mr. and Mrs. Colfax,* the parents of Laurel, their 6-week-old daughter with Down's syndrome. This is their second child.

> MRS. COLFAX: Every mother in pregnancy must think, "I want a healthy baby," and you do have thoughts of having a baby with a problem. But the thought of mental retardation never entered my mind. When I thought about a problem with my baby, it was always something physical. When she was born and I looked at her, she was all in one piece and had 10 fingers and 10 toes. I thought, she's fine. When they brought her to us and we looked at her, she looked physically fine. I will mention that there was one thing I noticed, and I said to Dick (husband) because she weighed 7 pounds, 1 ounce, when she was born, which was a nice size. Joshua (first child) was 6 pounds, 3 ounces, and very long and skinny. I guess every mother thinks her baby is pretty,

---

*The family's name has been changed.

but Joshua was really a pretty baby. I noticed her neck was very thick, and we later found out that is a characteristic. Of course, we never thought anything more than we had a girl with a fat neck. But it really gave us a chance to look her over, and we really studied her, turned her over, just looked at her, loved her, and we were already building that love. I think you already love the baby before they are even born, but having that time with her, you hold them and you really had already built that love.

To have had such a good beginning with their baby is important, perhaps critical. It allowed the parents to complete the process of pregnancy and birth. The mother had delivered a "real" baby with identifiable characteristics to whom she could direct her active "mothering" impulses. Thus when she received bad news about her baby, she was well under way with her bonding to the baby and so did not have to initiate loving responses at the same time she was struggling with rejecting responses. She had been active in mothering already, and this was useful in coping with her mixed feelings. There is considerable debate about whether it is better to tell families that their baby has Down's syndrome right away or whether to wait for several hours (unless the family suspects there is a problem). We have no firm data, but based on our own experience we believe it is desirable to take some time to be sure about our diagnosis and to allow the process of parental bonding to the infant to begin before we give the parents the bad news (hours or days).

PEDIATRICIAN: How did you find out about the baby?

MR. COLFAX: We really found out two different ways. Kitty found out first.

MRS. COLFAX: I think I had been awake almost the whole night. I was so excited, even though I was tired, I just couldn't sleep. I had requested a private room but there was none available so they put me in a semiprivate. The girl who was in the room had delivered the same night also. She and I stayed up the whole night talking. It was her first baby, and she had some problems before her baby was born. She had high blood pressure and had been in the hospital for about three months before the baby was born. So, I was telling her how sick I had been and she was saying she had been in the hospital. We were comparing notes. They had moved many more times than we had, so we were commiserating and then sharing our happiness. When I woke up about 9 o'clock the next morning, our pediatrician, whom we also had not met because we had just moved to Cleveland, happened to be on vacation and was not here. So somebody else, an associate of his, came in to tell me about the baby. I might mention that Dick had come down to the hospital in the morning at about 7:30.

MR. COLFAX: I think I ate part of your breakfast.

MRS. COLFAX: You probably did. We called some of our friends in Cincinnati and told them about the baby—said we had a girl and everything was great, fine. The night before we had only told our parents. So, anyway, Dick was there I'd say until about 8:30 and it seemed like he had just left when the doctor came in and said, "Mrs. Colfax, I would like to talk to you about your baby." I was up at the moment, and I

Outline of first counseling sessions
(for parents of children with congenital anomalies)

A. **Introduction and explanation of goals.** Early in the first session it would be useful to review with parents the purposes of the counseling with a statement such as the following:

> Based on our experience with families who have infants with significant physical difficulties, the time after the child is born can be extremely trying for the parents and family. Thus it is usual for parents to feel upset and to have some difficulty handling this situation. It's a time when we have found that a great many families need extra support and help from people. In this regard many parents have expressed an interest in talking with their physician and other people about not only their child's physical problem but also about their reactions to the baby's birth. Such discussions seem to help the family cope more effectively with what is usually a very difficult situation.
>
> As we related to you earlier, I'd like very much to meet with you both for _____ times to try to provide help to you during the baby's first year. Although we will be discussing many issues, such as your own reactions to the situation, how you might handle the situation, and issues related to the baby and your other children, it is important that you feel free to use this time to discuss issues related to the situation that are important to you. From your acceptance you must have felt that such counseling might be useful to you. Have you thought any more about how it might be useful to you? (Both parents.)

The aim of this introductory communication is to structure the intervention, clarify some of the expectations we have of the parents, and state what they might expect of us. In addition, it is important to find out their perception of how we can help them and their notions about what they need most. The parents will have already been infomed of their commitment in terms of time, and so on, and will have agreed to participate.

B. **Assessment of the parents' reactions.** One of the main objectives of the first hour, in addition to establishing rapport with the parents, is to assess how they have been coping with the situation both individually and as a family. From this assessment it would be possible to formulate goals regarding future sessions.

1. PARENTAL FEELINGS. The following questions might be useful in assessing the status of parental feelings:

   a. What was your initial reaction when you found out what was wrong with your child? How did you feel? (*This is asked of each parent. The aim here is to help them recognize what their reactions are.*)

   b. Can you recall your expectations of what the baby would be like? How you felt before the baby was born? (*This question allows a beginning focus on the discrepancy between the parents' hopes regarding the baby and their present feelings.*)

   c. What has been the most difficult thing about the situation?

2. PARENTAL PERCEPTION OF THE CHILD'S DIFFICULTY
    a. Can you describe what is wrong with your child?
    b. What have you been told about the baby's condition? By whom?
    c. What do you anticipate for the future?
    d. Is there information that would be useful to you that you don't have? (*The parents' appraisal of the baby's problem is yet another focus of the later counseling sessions.*)
3. PARENTAL REACTIONS TO THE BABY. The aim here is to obtain an assessment of the parents' attitudes about, and interactions with the baby.
    a. How do you feel about handling the baby? Do you feel close, etc.? Is the baby enjoyable?
    b. Does the baby present problems with feeding, etc.?
4. PARENTAL COPING. Given the parents' recognition of how they are feeling, it would be useful to assess how the parents are handling the situation.
    a. What do you do when you feel that way?
    b. Since the baby was born, have there been significant changes in areas such as mood, activities with freinds, or physical complaints? (*The objective here is to note the family's style of coping and eventually to have the parents relate their feelings to this, particularly if it is a maladaptive, defensive maneuver.*)
5. PARENTS' RELATIONSHIP TO ONE ANOTHER. Throughout the session it will be important to note differences in parental response to similar issues; the focus here is on how the parents are communicating regarding the child and how they are handling the situation as a family unit.
    a. Have you been aware of each other's reactions?
    b. Have you discussed your reactions with each other?
    c. How are your reactions similar? Different?
    d. Has the baby's problem been discussed with the other members of the family? How have they reacted?
6. FAMILY'S ATTITUDES TOWARD OTHERS. The family's capacity to make productive use of other people, such as friends or family, during this period may be an important mental health support that should be assessed.
    a. Have you told your family or friends about the baby's problem? What have you said?
    b. What was your family's reaction to finding out your baby's problem? Your friends?
    c. How do you feel about their reactions?
    d. Have there been changes in your relationships to friends or family since the baby's birth?

said, "Oh, O.K." I felt that this was just routine—I remember with Joshua the pediatrician came in and wanted to talk to me about the baby the first morning—so I said O.K. So, I jumped back into bed, and the first thing he said to me was, "Do you see anything different about your baby," and I said yes, I did, I noticed that she has those little white bumps all over her nose, but everyone has told me that those will go away so they are nothing to worry about. He said, "Yes. Did you see anything else?" I can't remember now what it was, but I noticed some other minor thing. He said, "Yes, but was there anything else?" Well then, I knew that he was fishing and I said, *"Is there something wrong with my baby?"* At that point, I—my heart—it was just like when you know something is wrong. I can't even think of any way to describe how I was feeling, waiting for him to say—and he said, "Yes, your baby has Down's syndrome."

The physician was trying to use any piece of reality that the mother might have wondered about as a way of "anchoring" the reality of the bad news to come. Since such a diagnosis will produce shock reaction and an unconscious protective attempt to deny the diagnosis, he knows that some observable reality will serve to reduce the period of denial. It is also desirable to explore what ideas or fantasies parents already have so that the physician or other professional can structure what he or she is about to say by confirming or correcting what the parents already think. In this case it may be that the physician kept her on the hook a bit too long, but his questions did serve to change gradually her mood from euphoric to a sharp alertness that something was wrong—an extremely difficult transition for the physician to endure also.

PEDIATRICIAN: Do you know what that is?
MRS. COLFAX: Well, I did know what it was and for a reason. We had been visiting with Dick's family about a year before. We had vacationed with Dick's cousin many years. They had a little girl 1 year old, and I said to Pam, "Is there something bothering you?" She said, "Well, nobody knows this, but they're checking Samantha for Down's syndrome." Well, I said, "What is that?" She said, "Well, it is retardation or mongolism." After that they found out she was not a Down's syndrome child. She did have some of the physical characteristics, which made them check to see. She had sort of slanty eyes. We have since found that most people don't know what Down's syndrome is. But, when he said that, I was just devastated. I don't think I have ever heard anything worse in my whole life, except maybe when I heard that my sister had died. I don't think I heard much of anything else he said after that.

We may not always be aware that this is happening because of a compelling need we feel to finish all the bad news as quickly as possible, and because parents continue to ask questions as though they are still functioning. This "not hearing anything after that" accounts for the repetitive questioning and going over old territory that we experience with parents in the early days and weeks after the diagnosis is made. It reminds us to hold back on detailed explanations early and to give information gradually and in small doses as the parents appear to be ready for it.

MRS. COLFAX: He asked me if I knew anything about it, and I really didn't. I conjured up in my mind all the—trying to think of the people that I'd seen and I always thought of adults. I don't know if I can describe the feelings at that particular moment. It was like I was numb. I guess this goes back to the fact that the children didn't live a long time because I think maybe the one question that I asked him was, "How long will she live?" and he said, "Well, that all depends on a lot of things, and I don't want to go into any of that right now."

We do know more about the life expectancy of a child with this diagnosis, barring other complications, than the physician seemed willing to share. An equally accurate but more optimistic statement could have been, "Many children with this diagnosis survive to adulthood, and we will have a more complete picture as we see how she progresses." This would also have made the mother feel that the physician was aligned with her and ready to stick with her through whatever might come. Notice in her next statement how quickly she expresses her feeling of abandonment right after his statement. Probably the most important message a physician can convey at this time is that he or she will "be there" and bit by bit will help piece together a future which will have meaning for them all. This message can be given before much is known at all about an individual infant, and the physician need not feel helpless if there is little factual information to give to the parents. What needs to be transmitted is that you, the physician (or other professional), and they, the parents, are embarking on a journey together and that the physician feels confident about the process.

MRS. COLFAX: He's a very businesslike person. I just felt like he doesn't—nobody cares. He doesn't care. I don't know how I felt, but I was terribly upset that Dick wasn't there at the moment when they told us. I know there is no easy way to tell a mother or father that their child had any problem, no matter if it is Down's syndrome or whatever. You would always like to hear that your child is perfect. But, I do think, especially in my particular case—Dick and I are very close—that I needed him there at that very minute and he wasn't there. My immediate reaction was I wish I would die. I wish I would die and this baby should die with me.

She feels abandoned and without strength to continue and wishes to blot out the struggle that at this point feels too painful to endure. (The discovery that a newborn infant has a malformation results in an almost universal wish to flee. Fathers may flee to another woman or to alcohol, but these options are usually not available to the mother.) We can feel confident that in the case of Mrs. Colfax, these feelings will probably be only temporary and of the kind which occur to most people at a devastating time, since she has already pointed out that she can use support from people when she described her intense wish that her husband be there. To be able to use support is one of the attributes that we look for in people who are going to make it through an intensely stressful time. It means that they are not feeling totally helpless with only one way out.

MRS. COLFAX: I remember when I talked to my sister that day, and I told her about the baby's problem. I said to her, "I just feel like I should die." She said, "Don't ever say that, don't ever say that, you have so much to live for." "You have Dick, you have Joshua. What would he do without you?" She said, "I've been through something myself, of course, having a mastectomy." And she said, "I can remember thinking those things myself," but she said, "I thought about them very briefly, because I have three beautiful little girls and I have so much to live for." She said, "You don't even know anything about this child yet, you don't know what her future is going to bring. Don't ever feel that you wish you would die or she would die either."

If anyone else but someone who had a long history with her and whose love felt secure, her sister, had said this, it might not have worked. At this early stage a person who did not know her as well as her sister would have a hard time not sounding harsh and insensitive to the tragedy and her feelings about it in pointing to the necessity of being strong for other people's sake. Later on, though, it is helpful to bring someone immersed in grief back to the real world, where their functioning as a mother again to other children can restore confidence and bring solace. However, this requires careful timing.

MR. COLFAX: I arrived back at the hospital and went up to talk to Kitty. The first situation that was a little bit difficult was having the girl still in the room whom Kitty had met the night before, and Kitty was naturally very upset and crying. So, it was very difficult. Afterwards, the girl stopped back in to say "hi" to Kitty, and they became friends, but it was very hard for her being in the same room. . . . I think it would have been much better to have Kitty in a room by herself because the other lady was sharing an experience which was much happier than hers at that point.

MRS. COLFAX: I'd like to say something about that. That was another thing. Dick wasn't there and I was by myself, and when he said, "I want to talk to you about your baby," he just drew that little curtain—here she was lying in her bed, where she heard the whole thing. She was just devastated also. She felt terrible. As a matter of fact, she was crying and I thought, this isn't fair because—after I was enough together—I knew she was lying over there and heard this whole thing, because she didn't say a word. I'm sure she didn't know what to say to me. She didn't say a word, and I said to Dick "I have to get a private room. You have to get me a private room." I felt sorry for her because, well, as I mentioned earlier, the doctor left and then Dick came, and they brought the babies at 10:00, and I said, "Take her away, I don't want to even look at her." This girl had her baby and she never said a word to it, and in the night she talked to it. I knew she couldn't even react to her own baby because she didn't want me to hear any of that because she knew that I was feeling terrible anyway. I felt this isn't fair, this was her first child. This was spoiling all of her happiness, and it was just unfair to her.

MR. COLFAX: As efficent as hospitals are, I think there should have been a system to make a change at that point without my creating pressure for the change. But we did ask, and they came back and said some time later that we would be able to move the girl into another room and that Kitty would then have a room to herself.

MRS. COLFAX: I just wanted to be by myself.

MR. COLFAX: I don't think that everybody reacts the same, but my reaction was I really need somebody that can talk to Kitty about Down's syndrome. So, I went to the nurses' desk and I said, "Is there anybody that is professionally trained to deal with a situation of this nature?" She said, "I don't know, but I'll look for you." I came back feeling somewhat better because I had said, "Well, here's what I would like," and they said they would do the best they could to see if they could find somebody who could help us.

This points out how an opportunity to begin to function actively as a parent can help the process of grieving and then attachment. He felt better once he was able to do something a father does, which is to search for and obtain something his family needs.

MRS. COLFAX: It was the nurse clinician. She was such a great help to us.

MR. COLFAX: When the nurse clinician came to speak to the other girl who had roomed with Kitty, this girl told the nurse about the problem that Kitty had, and then we met this nurse clinician. We found this out later on, because I had felt that because I had gone to the desk and said I needed professional help, that they had contacted her. Well, it was one of the patients who turned the nurse clinician on to our case, so to speak, and she in fact was able to get in and see us the first day that we had known about Laurel.

MRS. COLFAX: She didn't know that much about Down's syndrome either. It was just that her job was to help people who had problems in the hospital. We can't even say enough about what a big help she has been to us. I don't think we'd be where we are right now without her help.

MRS. COLFAX: Well, we had enough time after they moved my roommate out so that I was at least rational. I mean I was at least able to stop and start to think somewhat. She came in and made us realize how important it was for us to talk out all our feelings, because I was very bitter.

This is the first time she talks about how angry she was. It must have been even harder for her to struggle with this emotion and talk about it with the roommate and her healthy baby in the room. You could hear how concerned she felt about this roommate and her first experience with her baby. This quality of concern about others at this early stage is not common, but it may be a favorable indicator for the long-term resolution of the conflicts and feelings aroused by Laurel's diagnosis through assisting others.

MRS. COLFAX: I think one of your immediate reactions after the initial blow of it is, "Why me? Why did this happen to me, what have I done?" And I think you felt that way too.

MR. COLFAX: Absolutely. I think it is a feeling that you just want to shake your hand up in the sky and just say, "Why did it happen to me?" I didn't think I was able to stay in the hospital, but because it was such an unordinary situation, I tried to get permission to stay in the hospital, which I did.

MRS. COLFAX: That was the nurse clinician's idea. She said, "I think at this time you two should be together." As I mentioned before, Dick and I are close, and I don't see how I could have gone through it without having him there. She said, "I will speak to someone and see if Dick can spend the night." Well, because I was in the double room with the extra bed, she went around and said they were going to find him a cot and I am sure he is going to be able to stay and everything will be fine. I knew that I could stay not on top, but I could be fairly under control as long as Dick was there. As long as he was there and we were together. She came back and said that everything was arranged and that Dick could spend the night here. So, it was that evening, until Dick went home.

There was one particular person in the hospital who felt that this was going against the rules and that this really shouldn't be done. She came in to see me and said, "Do you really think you need him here?" I just looked at her and said, "I *know* I need him here." Dick had taken maybe an hour to go home and see Joshua at that time, so I was by myself and I really fell apart just in that hour. I cried the whole time he was gone. My mind would just run away. And she said to me, "Well, you know we can give you a sleeping pill," and I thought to myself, "Are you telling me a sleeping pill is the same as having my husband here? I mean this is the most ridiculous thing I've ever heard of."

It is easy, sometimes, in a hospital setting to forget that the supportive effect of human contact can be more powerful than medicines—the nurses and physicians in our obstetrical unit now see the presence of fathers as an essential part of care during the entire 24-hour day.

MRS. COLFAX: I said, "I don't want a sleeping pill. Anyway I am nursing the baby and that means she would get that." She was kind of sleepy, and that's all I needed was to have her even sleepier. I said, "No, I have to have him here." So nothing more was said, and Dick came back and they never did bring him a bed that night. But because I was in the double room, he slept in the other bed. So everything was fine. But the next day they did arrange for me to move into a private room—it was the next day, wasn't it?

MR. COLFAX: It was the next day.

MRS. COLFAX: A private room opened up. So they said to me, "We can move you into a private room now. Would you like that?" They said, "We really can't guarantee that this bed will stay open you know. If we get crowded, somebody else will have to come into this room." So I said, "Oh yes, I want to go into a private room. Dick really just stayed in the hospital all the time. Every time he left, I fell apart. He was really my strength at that time. Dick really was very strong. I just kept saying, "Dick, you can't go. I can't stay here if you go." Now, I had taken the baby after 10:00 A.M. I had taken her at the other feedings and fed her and, really, I don't think right at those feedings I felt anything. I don't know. I know I must have loved her, but I was still so mixed up. I didn't feel anything, and then, I am a very stubborn person anyway. The doctor told me that I wouldn't be able to breastfeed her, and I was determined, if it was to do anything but to show him that she would breastfeed. So Dick said, "Don't worry, I'm going to stay here."

It was unfortunate that the physician could not have been more optimistic. Not many mothers are spunky enough to persist and show that the physician is incorrect under circumstances such as these. It is fortunate that this was not her first baby.

The anguish may be the same whether it is a mother's first or fifth baby, but the confidence and experience gained by giving birth to, and caring for, one healthy child makes it easier for a mother to carry out normal activities such as breastfeeding, disciplining, and separating from the child.

MR. COLFAX: Yeah. And in fact, that first night, I think she got up at 3 o'clock and she just wanted to talk. The biggest need at that point and for the five days you are in the hospital is to have a sounding board.

To be able to express feelings to another person has several effects. It clarifies for parents what in fact they are feeling, and this in itself can reduce the intensity of emotional reactions and fearfulness characteristic at this stage. In addition, some feelings may be new or frightening to a parent, such as the rage he or she feels, and to say it aloud to someone may make the emotion seem less powerful or reduce guilt about feeling it.

MRS. COLFAX: I think that is important.
MR. COLFAX: I think the other thing which happened that week was that initially you are led to believe that you are dealing with a very measurable commodity (or potential). That she can go from number 1 (and even the number 80 was used in terms of how far she can grow). Fortunately, we had the opportunity to meet with a couple who had a child named Carmen. They came in and met with us one day and told us about their child. I think it left us, first, with a deeper appreciation of what Laurel was and who she was, but more importantly, that she could go as far as we could help her go. I think to leave not feeling that you have something which is a commodity which is only measurable in numbers 1 to 80. I think that you have to leave with a feeling that she can grow as high as possible.

As is true with all child rearing, the destination really is unknown, and there is no value in trying to be unnecessarily precise about what may be accomplished when parents are trying to gather resources for the journey. Sometimes we tend to use numbers because we feel comfortable with that kind of description and it gives us a sense of control, but in this situation the parents do not want to feel as though their fate is sealed by parameters which they would gradually come to grips with over time.

MRS. COLFAX: And that we want to help her do whatever she is able to do, and we will love her and accept her for that. I might say, as each day went on it got a little easier. I think a lot of that was the help we got, and each time I had her, I knew I loved her but I was afraid Dick wasn't going to love her. I really was. Even though he was there, I was afraid he wasn't going to be able to love her. Then I knew that he loved her, and I was afraid our parents weren't going to love her. And when I talked to my mother on the phone—she didn't come down the first couple of days, even though she was here, because she was with Joshua and I would talk to her even though I still couldn't talk to anybody else on the phone. My mother and Joshua were the only people I talked to on the phone. I didn't even talk to Dick's parents, because as soon as I would get on the phone, I would start to cry. But I did say to my mother, "I just love her so much, and I love her every time they bring her to me." And my mother said to me, "Are you saying that to reassure yourself? Are you afraid you're not going to love her?" And maybe at that time I was.

She is struggling with her own opposite feelings and working them out by initially feeling that it is only other people who would reject this baby, then gradually understanding that a part of herself also may have felt that way at one time, but that loving feelings, for the most part, won out. She may also be starting to deal with her fears about how society will react. She could not talk to her husband's parents perhaps because she was not sure enough of their unqualified support, which she knew she could find from her own mother. She was hinting at the guilt one feels about producing a defective child.

    MRS. COLFAX: Now, I mean there is just no question that we love her as much as Joshua or any other child we would have. And then I said to her, "Well, I know you'll love her." And she said, "Don't worry about the fact that we'll love her." She said, "You know we'll love her." And she said, "I want you to think about one thing, and this has been said to me by somebody else who has a Down's syndrome child. Don't go the other way. Don't neglect Joshua for her. Don't try to—I don't think you can ever love a child too much, but don't forget that you have another child." The other person that I am mentioning right now is not the couple who came to see us in the hospital, but my sister, when I talked to her on the phone in Florida, said, "Well, I don't know if you remember, but I have a friend who has a child with Down's syndrome. They have since moved away from Wade Park and they live in California, but I am going to write to her immediately." And so she did write to this friend of hers. I had never met the girl, but the week after I came home from the hospital, this girl called me long distance from California. There is this special bond between parents who have children with problems. We talked like we knew each other and I had never met her. We must have talked for an hour.

Sometimes this valuable source of information and support can be arranged by hospital staff between two sets of parents who live close by.

    MR. COLFAX: One of the things which is difficult at that point is you still believe that maybe the initial interpretation by the doctor is wrong. And so it is kind of difficult to have to wait three weeks. That is not to say that we didn't leave the hospital knowing that we had a Down's syndrome child, because we did. Certainly. But you always hold that hope in reserve. Because she didn't have—she had some of the characteristics, but she was missing some of the characteristics as well. So you always want to see the test done, and you have to wait for a certain period of time at home then to get the results. That's a little frustrating.

    MRS. COLFAX: I think you always have that outside hope that somebody was wrong. I think we both admitted it when the results came.

They were able to give up their magical hopes fairly soon, when the test results confirmed the diagnosis. Other parents sometimes continue magical thinking by suggesting alternative explanations, for example, that the tests were done on the wrong baby or got mixed up at the lab, and they may come more gradually to a final realization. This is done at the parents' own pace. It is important to understand that there may be a genuine need to hold off the realization until personal resources are sufficient to sustain the impact. The normal slow development of infants in the first six weeks sometimes slows the parents' adjustment to the realistic problems of an infant with Down's syndrome because he appears similar to a normal infant during this early time and it may be hard for them to stop pretending that this is not so. Unless it is impeding their care of the infant, parents should be allowed their own rate of coming to terms with this baby's problems. Occasionally professional help is desirable if denial and magical thinking persist too long and interfere with parental judgments.

> MRS. COLFAX: I was just very happy because of my future chances of having another baby. She was a trisomy 21, but when I told Dick, he said, "Well, I'm glad she is a trisomy 21, but I have to honestly say that I was hoping that they were going to say that it was a mistake," because really I guess she seems like such a normal baby right now. I mean she does everything. She is a really good baby, but she does everything that any other baby does. Maybe because she is special, we notice everything that she does a little bit more. Every time she pushes herself way up, we notice and we get all excited. One thing that the doctor did say that was sort of a ringer in her case, is she is very active. She is quite an active baby when she is awake, and she is very alert. I do think we had ups and downs, but I think every day became a little bit easier, and now we know that there are going to be a lot of hard times to come.
>
> I was having a very good day, this particular day, and Dick walked in from his office and whether he looked at me and knew I could finally handle his coming down or whether he had a bad day that day, I would say it was the first day that Dick was really way down. Then that Friday it was nice that this couple came to see us because it brought him back up, and we both felt good.

This couple has an intuitive grasp of each other's needs and strengths. For other couples it may be more difficult to be reciprocal, to understand each other's place in the grieving process.

> MRS. COLFAX: As I said before, each day got a little bit easier. We knew that we weren't going to go home and everything was just going to be roses, especially after this couple came to see us. Now for us, in our case, that was really important. She was born on Monday and they came on Friday, so we did have a period of five days to sort of adjust ourselves. But this is interesting because Dick said to me before they came (we were a little nervous about their coming), "You know that they are going to pull out pictures of their child." And he said, "I don't think I can look at them." He said, "I don't know what we are going to do." I said, "Well, Dick, you can't be rude."
>
> And he said, "Well, just hold your breath before you look at those pictures and give them a quick glimpse." And sure enough, we talked and they said, "Well, we brought some pictures of Carmen for you to see."
>
> I looked over to Dick and he was practically white, and we said, "Oh, O.K." And

they pulled these pictures out and Dick looked at them first. And the next thing I knew, he looked at me and was smiling and he said, "She is darling! She is just darling!" Each picture he went through I watched him. And then he was taking hours looking at them. I said, "Dick, I would like to see them too." So it just goes to show that you don't know what to expect. I guess you conjure up all these things in your mind, and I don't know what we thought was going to be in those pictures.

Here is another instance of the reality being much less difficult than the fantasies were.

MRS. COLFAX: That little girl was just one of the cutest little things you had ever seen.
Almost our whole outlook on life has changed. Since we had her, we found ourselves reevaluating what we thought was important. So many things that we thought were important, were really unimportant. Because we had just moved into the house, we were talking about decorating the living room and, oh, we didn't have this and that. All of a sudden that was so unimportant.

Many people find themselves with new, deepened philosophical attitudes toward their own life.

MRS. COLFAX: And, getting back to what we were talking about making plans for Joshua. As our doctor said to us, "Once you stop and think a little bit, maybe you are lucky, because you will realize this—you have to look ahead, you can't stay where you are, but you really should realize that you never know how long each child is with you. Not only if the child has a problem. But you never know how long each child is with you. You should take each one of them for every day you have them with you." And I think that has made us do that a little bit more with Joshua.
MR. COLFAX: I think you grow out of it a little bit, but initially you are very vulnerable. This is so devastating that you almost expect something initially. You guard your other child very closely. At least I find myself doing that. So, I think you lose some of that vulnerability as you go on and get more comfortable with it.

Here, and in Mrs. Colfax's discussion with her mother earlier, these parents display remarkable sensitivity to the impact of this child on the whole family. Earlier in the interview her mother suggestd that she should not become so involved with the new baby to compensate for her mixed feelings about having a baby that she neglected her other child. Here we see the father discussing how hard it is not to overprotect the other child. By recognizing these reactions and helping each other, they seem to have avoided either extreme.

COMMENT: With the birth of a malformed baby, the unusual replaces the familiar. The growing mutuality between infant and mother, nurtured in utero for many months, seems suddenly extinguished. The air is heavy with crisis. The mood is one of sadness. The future is forbidding. The parents feel apart—cheated, faulted, and deprived. It is almost as if birth becomes conception: A new image of this baby must gestate in the minds of the parents.
This interview with the parents of a baby with Down's syndrome offers an opportunity for the reader to consider how his or her professional role in the hospital, in the home, or in the office might be extended in the care of children with long-term disorders. The following six "Cs" may

serve as stimuli for further discussion: competence, clarification, coping, communication, caring, and continuity.

1. *Competency.* Although parents cannot be prepared for the unexpected birth of an infant with a malformation, the physician and nurse should be ready. Where parents are unpracticed, we must be skilled; where they seem uncertain, we must be sure; and when needs are not expressed, we must anticipate them. Although it is part of the expected education and competency of physicians and nurses to be prepared for life-threatening emergencies, there has not yet developed a similar tradition for management of life-quakes engendered by family and personal crises such as the birth of a baby with a malformation. Yet there are few times when support is more needed, when care is more appropriate, and when the reason for a professional presence is more compelling.

These days summon the best in clinical practice. They should not be left to the vagaries of chance. The relationship between the parents and the physician or nurse begins in this time of special vulnerability and receptivity. If this opportunity is not taken, subsequent interviews are unlikely to replace the chance that was lost.

2. *Clarification.* With the birth of a malformed baby, the parents' previously formed notion of what their baby would be like, the infant's anticipated identity, is either modified strikingly or lost almost completely, depending on the character of the malformation. The baby is different from what might have been. The parents, and almost everything else, seem no longer the way they were.

As part of the reconstructive phase following the birth, physicians and nurses have a unique opportunity to help parents form a realistic and positive identity for their baby rather than allowing the infant to remain a phobic object to be avoided or wished away. Putting the shattered image back together can be facilitated at birth and in continuing visits by approaches such as examination of the baby in front of the parents; emphasis on normality while delineating the deviations; conveyance of the baby's personality so as to promote the parents' acceptance of their baby as a person; referring to the baby by name; understanding and kindness by the staff in the nursery; encouraging the parents to discuss the baby's situation with nurses, siblings, friends, relatives, and perhaps, a parent whose baby has a similar disorder; using illustrations, movies, and models to make discussions as concrete as possible; and repeated characterizations of the baby over time in interviews such as the one just described.

3. *Coping.* Whether or not parents can cope depends on many factors, including their strengths, resources, problems, and vulnerabilities. These need to be identified and discussed by parents and professionals. Strengths include the husband's presence, opportunities for privacy, a supportive marital relationship, relatives to whom the parents can turn, ability of the parents to articulate their needs, a healthy older sibling, supportive hospital staff, and a chance to talk with parents who have undergone a similar experience and with whom there is a special bond. Especially vulnerable are those mothers who face this crisis alone, without the support of the father, without close relatives, with few or no friends, and in the midst of other life stresses. Assessment of these factors permits the health professional to make a reasoned projection as to the ability of a family to cope and judge its potential for growth.

4. *Communication.* The father should be present with the mother when the physician reports a birth defect. This message needs to be communicated in privacy and with a sensitivity to the parents' readiness to know. A number of visits should be made during the newborn period to discuss both the diagnosis and outlook and to serve as a sounding board for the expression of the parents' feelings.

After discharge from the hospital, communication should continue through frequent scheduled appointments, including, if possible, home visits. Communication is, of course, a shared enterprise between physician, nurse, social worker, parent educator, and parents in which the latter gain information and, equally important, talk out their feelings, for example, the mother's wish not to see her baby, her hope that she herself would die, her belief that she is being punished by God, her concern as to how others will take the news, and her uncertainty as to whether she or the father can love the baby. Although parents may have many joint feelings such as, "Why us?" they also react as individuals such as, "Why me?"

5. *Caring.* Although the extent to which kindness and compassion in the hospital facilitate acceptance of a baby is unknown, care that attends to the parents' mind and heart, through an interest in them as persons and by ready support in periods of discouragement, is gratefully appreciated by those who endure these extremely trying nights and days. Those who take care of these families must achieve a high degree of competency. Special training and experience may be required to match modern knowledge against ancient superstition.

There is much to suggest that we are on the threshold of a major reinstitutionalization of hospital, home, and office care of infants with major disabilities. This trend will bring with it more systematized ways to provide care to these children and their families including, perhaps, special teams of physicians, nurses, and social workers in the hospital. A FACT, or Family Crisis Team, should provide specialized care in the immediate newborn period rather than leaving these challenging duties to chance or to ad hoc, "pick-up" teams of persons who are untrained and unaccustomed to working together. The observations and the actions of this organized crisis team would be shared with others involved. Its performances would be critiqued in case conferences. Such a team could also provide services to families whose babies were premature, stillborn, or critically ill.

Since parents cannot be prepared for an unexpected birth, they should have access immediately after the event to parent education and preparation centers. Infants who need secondary or tertiary management would likely be transferred to regional centers with newborn intensive care units, early intervention programs, centers for handicapped infants, or parent care pavilions. In these settings a heavy emphasis will be placed on parent participation, not only as a validation of the parents' ability to take care of their baby but also because of what they can contribute. Those babies sent home directly from the lying-in newborn service should be assured continuity of care, as discussed below.

6. *Continuity.* Although obviously important, the initial phase of management in the hospital makes a limited contribution if not followed by frequent visits during the early years. If possible, the first visit should occur in the home. If not, the baby and the parents should be seen in the office within 10 to 14 days after discharge. The interpretation of a long-term handicap is never accomplished in one visit but in segments attuned to the readiness of parents. Time and regularly scheduled visits are needed to clarify the problem. When the baby seems to behave in a primarily normal fashion in the early weeks of life, the parents' recognition of reality may be postponed. The visits to the office or to the home also help the physician, nurse, and parent educator to assess the parents' adjustment to the problem in terms of the realsim of their perceptions, the appropriateness of their expectations, their concern with current rather than distant problems, their ability to meet their infant's needs, the degree of their preoccupation with what might have been, the pertinence of their questions, their ability to utilize advice, the quality of their relationship with the child and with each other, and their decreasing need to utilize denial.

In permitting the physician, nurse, and parent educator to be psychologically as well as physically available, such visits over time build an alliance in the best interests of the child and the family. Child health professionals need also to attend to the strengths, resources, vulnerabilities, and weaknesses of the physicians and nurses as they care for the infant born with a congenital malformation.

M. Green

COMMENT: There is the risk of too many authorities, each of them "right and helpful" but tending to diffuse the effort of parents to relate to one authority or expert. An awareness of this can prevent such diffusion and enable parents to "work through" their reactions, their questions, their fears, and their hopes. It is difficult for parents to work through the trauma of the birth of a defective child if the one professional who is responsible for, and authoritative in, providing assistance is replaced by several experts, who fragment their ability to provide understanding and guidance.

A.J. Solnit

RECOMMENDATIONS FOR CARE

1. *Initial contact.* We consider it of high priority to bring a baby to the mother as soon as possible so that both parents can see him and observe his normal features as well as his abnormality. Any period of delay during which the parents suspect or know that their baby may have a problem but are unable to see him heightens their anxiety tremendously and allows their imaginations to run wild. They may jump to the conclusion that the baby is dead or dying while he is actually doing well and the problem is a cleft lip. The longer the period before they see the baby the more distorted and fixed their concept of the baby's condition may become. The parents' mental images of their infant's anomaly are almost invariably much more grotesque than the actual problem. Whatever is said to the parents initially is usually indelibly imprinted on their minds. This places a sobering responsibility on the shoulders of everyone caring for the mother and baby because the words used in discussing the baby with her may affect her initial attachment process.

> **COMMENT:** I agree with the principle but not with the paramount importance given to what is initially said to the parents or to the tendency to view the first words used in discussing the baby as having a permanent effect on the attachment process. Granted that what is said and when is highly important, it may not be possible to know how to put it to the parents until they have expressed some of what they fear and feel. The process of explaining and listening is where the emphasis belongs.
> **A.J. Solnit**

2. *Positive emphasis.* When first showing the infant with a visible problem, it is important to show all the normal parts as well and to emphasize positive features such as his strength, activity, and alertness. It is sometimes surprising that malformations that appear obvious, striking, and bizarre to the physician sometimes do not seem to the parents as frightening or disfiguring.

3. *Avoiding tranquilizers.* We have strong reservations about the use of tranquilizing drugs for the parents of a baby with a congenital malformation. Tranquilizers tend to blunt their responses and slow their adaptation to the problem. However, a small dose of a short-acting barbiturate at bedtime for sleeping is often helpful.

4. *Special caretaking.* Most maternity units are designed for the care of healthy mothers and babies. Therefore, when a baby is born with a problem such as a congenital malformation, the mother's mood and needs are out of step with the routines of the floor. Usually there is no special provision to meet the needs of the small group of parents with babies with malformations, who suffer from the assembly-line routines set up to provide care for the large volume of parents with husky and fully intact neonates. Physicians and nurses may cheerfully burst into the room and ask how the baby is doing, forgetting that he has been kept in the nursery because of the problem or has been transferred to another hospital or division. We find that it is usually best to assign a specific nurse to the mother of a baby with a congenital anomaly. This nurse should have the ability to sit for long periods with

the mother and just listen to her cry and tell about the powerful reactions, which are often disturbingly critical and negative. Not everyone on a unit will find this an easy task, so it should be given to a physician or nurse who is willing to listen and who feels prepared to assist the parents of an infant with an anomaly. This task is draining and may seem unrewarding to someone who has not had follow-up experience with families.

5. *Prolonged contact.* We believe that it is best to leave an infant with his mother for the first few days so that she can become used to him rather than rushing him to another division or hospital where the special surgery will eventually be done. Obviously, if surgery is required immediately, such as for an omphalocele or diaphragmatic hernia, this must be done without delay, but even in these cases it is desirable and usually safe to bring the baby to his mother and show her how normal he is in all other respects and to let her touch and handle him if at all possible. The father should be included in all discussions and in all periods with the baby. We try to arrange for the mother and father to have extended periods with their infant to become acquainted with all his features, both positive and negative. The mother of a normal infant goes through a period of one to three days in which she gradually realigns the image in her mind of the baby she expected with the image of the actual baby she delivered. When the baby has a malformation, the task of realigning the images is more difficult, and the result is a greater need for prolonged mother-infant contact. Lampe and associates (1977) noted significantly greater visiting if an infant with an abnormality has been home for a short while before surgery was required (Fig. 6-3).

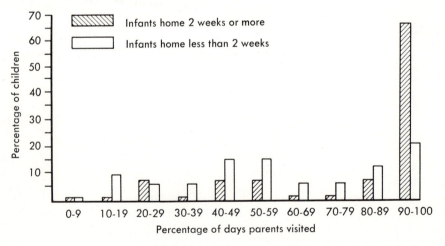

Fig. 6-3. Hospital visiting pattern of parents whose infants had been home more than 2 weeks and those whose infants had been home less than 2 weeks. (From Lampe, J., Trause, M.A., and Kennell, J.H.: Pediatrics **59**:294-296, 1977. Copyright American Academy of Pediatrics, 1977.)

COMMENT: Where the mother asks for interruptions in the closeness of the infant and herself, her tolerances, as well as those of the father, should be given appropriate weight in the arrangements.
A.J. Solnit

6. *Visiting*. It is wise to extend the visiting hours in the maternity unit to allow the father to spend prolonged periods with his wife so that they can share their feelings and start working through their sequence of reactions as synchronously as possible. Our hospital policy permits fathers to live-in with the mother and stay overnight. This emphasizes the hospital's concern for both parents, as illustrated in the interview with Mr. and Mrs. Colfax. This permits them time to work together.

7. *Questions*. It has been our clinical impression that parents who are making a reasonably good adaptation often ask many questions and at times appear over-involved in the details of clinical care. Although these parents may be bothersome at times, we are usually pleased when we see this behavior. We are more concerned about parents who ask only a few questions and who appear stunned and overwhelmed by the infant's problem.

8. *Adaptation*. The process of adaptation to a malformation requires a long period of time before the parents are able to take care of the infant easily. During the early phases, when they are mourning the loss of the perfect baby they had anticipated, they are often unable to manage rather simple procedures. For example, tube feedings that can be managed easily at two to three months sometimes cannot be handled by fairly adept parents in the first few days or weeks.

9. *Explaining findings*. Many anomalies are highly frustrating, not only to the parents but to the physicians and nurses. When things are not going well, the physicians and nurses may go through some of the same reactions—feeling defeat, sadness, anger, and anticipatory grief—as the parents. It is important for the medical staff to be aware of their own feelings and to guard against withdrawing from the parents or the infant. The many questions asked by a parent who is trying to cope with the problem and understand it often tend to be very frustrating for the physician, especially if the parent asks the same questions over and over again during the first three to four months. It is important that the physician be available during this period. It often seems as if the parent has lost his or her ability to remember and may appear quite stupid. We have been surprised how frequently parents forget that they have ever been told about a problem. The psychological reaction of denial is sometimes so strong that they may insist they have never heard about the kidney problem, or the mental retardation, or the possibility that the anomaly might be genetic, even though these may have been discussed on several occasions for periods of at least an hour.

COMMENT: For the physician or nurse these repeated questions may be experienced as an irritating reminder that they are associated with a defect, handicap, and failure in producing a healthy child.
A.J. Solnit

10. *Possible retardation*. We strongly believe that if there is a chance of the infant being retarded, we should not discuss it with the parent unless we know with almost absolute certainty that the infant is damaged. This controversial recommendation stems from the many cases in which excellent physicians expressed this suspicion, but later found that this was incorrect and then discovered that they could not convince the parents that the child was normal even years later. Many of these youngsters have subsequently experienced major developmental disturbances because their parents continued to manage them as if they were retarded. It is also extremely difficult to make predictions about such babies in the first few weeks of life. In our own high-risk nursery we found that expert neonatologists and neurologists, using all the common medical procedures, made correct predictions of normality or abnormality in complicated high-risk infants only 50% of the time (Miranda et al., 1974).

11. *Progressing at parents' pace*. It is generally difficult for parents to absorb information about several major problems in their baby all at the same time. We try to move at the parents' pace and show them one problem at a time (or wait until several can be put together in a package, such as a definite syndrome). We inquire each time how the infant seems to them and what they understand now about his health and progress. For example, "Maybe you could tell me how you see the infant today. What do you see as the baby's problems in the future that we will work on together?" If one moves too rapidly, the parents tend to flee and usually are unable to take in all the medical material.

Before speaking with a parent about a malformation, it is good to understand just what is known about the baby's problem and to be aware of the type of complications that might arise. This often requires a period of time to read about the problem so that the nurse or physician is more relaxed in talking with the parents.

12. *Discussions with parents*. The series of reactions to the birth of a baby with a malformation are such that each parent may move through the stages of shock, denial, anger, guilt, sadness, adaptation, and reorganization at a different pace. If they are unable to talk with each other about their reactions and feelings concerning the baby, a severe disruption in their own relationship may develop. Therefore we often have several private meetings with both parents, using the theory and techniques of crisis intervention. We ask the mother how she is doing, how she feels her husband is managing, and how he feels about the infant. In his presence we then reverse the questions and ask the father how he is coping and how he thinks his wife is managing. Thus they start to think not only about each other but about their own adaptation. Often communication between the parents improves after one or two of these sessions.

13. *Communication between parents*. If the parents are communicating reasonably well, we often tell them to spend some time alone together after supper and

go over how they have really felt hour by hour from the time of the baby's birth, to talk about their own feelings and impressions no matter how wild they may be. A cocktail or sherry may make it easier for them to talk. One parent is sometimes amazed by the revelations of the other, and often each one does not fully appreciate until this time that the other had some of the same thoughts but was afraid to mention them.

14. *Siblings.* The many needs of the siblings are described in detail in Chapter 3.

15. *Staff meetings.* It often appears to the physician and nurse caring for an infant with a malformation that they are impotent because they are unable to change anything important in the infant and therefore have no specific role. But this is not the case. As a matter of fact, they have an important job and in the end can look forward to greater rewards than with other patients and parents. The personnel caring for malformed infants need to discuss these issues frequently. We have found it helpful to have a meeting with the nurses in our nursery to discuss the difficult problems. We ask them to select the issues for discussion. In addition to this the physicians should also have some place to talk about their own problems and concerns and to discuss how difficult they find it to share their reactions and worries. This is especially true with young house officers. In the past we avoided these difficult topics, but it has become increasingly apparent that this was a serious oversight because of the powerful and potentially damaging reactions of both parents and caregivers. It might have been anticipated that intensive care units would put such a strain on nurses and physicians as to necessitate some means of helping them with their intense reactions.

16. *Keeping family together.* One of the major goals of the interviews is to keep the family together both during this early period and in subsequent years. This is best done by working hard to bring out the issues early and by encouraging the parents to talk about their difficult thoughts and feelings as they arise. It is best for them to share their problems with each other. Some couples who do not seem to be close previously may move closer together as they work through the process of adaptation. As with any painful experience, the parents may be much stronger after they have gone through these reactions together. We would recommend that young medical students and house officers sit in on the interviews and observe older faculty members talk to parents in a series of visits over a long period so that they may see not only the initial reaction but also the eventual adaptation achieved by the parents. Interviews with the parents of a malformed infant are usually frightening and upsetting to young physicians. The initial challenging reactions can be placed in better perspective if they follow parents over a period of time with an older experienced physician. We have included an interview to give the reader an idea of how we talk to parents.

17. *Adaptation to stress*. Each parent's adaptation depends on his or her background and adaptations in the past. For many young people this is the most difficult problem that they have ever had to deal with in their own lives. However, their own past behavior and family experiences often give us a clue as to how they will react and what their individual process of adaptation will be. Some parents have had turbulent earlier periods in their lives with their own mother and father. Under stress they may return to the behavior and problems of that period. In others, if the malformation resembles a malformation in a relative or in himself or herself, one parent may believe he or she is the cause of the malformation and so feel tremendously guilty. In most cases this can be discussed and clarified. It may be helpful to ask parents how they have reacted under stress in the past.

CHAPTER 7

CARING FOR THE PARENTS OF A STILLBORN OR AN INFANT WHO DIES

JOHN H. KENNELL and MARSHALL H. KLAUS

When a newborn infant dies, the end follows too closely the beginning. There is not enough time to comprehend what is happening. As the new life is relentlessly stalked by death, elation and sadness, hope and despair, rushing and waiting, anticipation and disappointment, the past and the future, are all intertwined in a Kafkaesque experience.

Morris Green

Over the past 50 years in the Western world, death has moved from the home to the hospital. At the same time, in modern industrial society, the death of an infant has become an uncommon event in the life history of any individual family, although there are still 45,000 perinatal deaths per year in the United States. In the past (and even today in many religions and cultures) there was a ritualized pattern of mourning behavior to be followed after the death of a close family member. For many families these grieving practices have been abandoned or forgotten. This is particularly true for a stillborn or young infant who has never gone home from the hospital. As a result, traditions that have developed over hundreds of years to ensure that the mourning reaction of survivors follows its biological course have been partly lost.

In addition, in the last decade the care of sick, severely ill, and dying infants has been concentrated in the high-risk neonatal centers, where the responsibility for a large number of deaths has been placed on the shoulders of relatively few caretakers. Since long-term studies have shown that some parents suffer a tragic outcome after the birth of a stillborn or the death of a live-born infant, it is necessary to examine in detail how to care for the family after a neonatal death.

This chapter will review the normal behavioral changes following the loss of a neonate, explore the physicians' and nurses' reactions, and offer suggestions for the management of the family, including the siblings.

BASIC CONSIDERATIONS
Normal grief

Adults experience intense mourning and grieving (usually lasting around six months or longer) only when there is an intimate affectional tie with the dead person, as with close relatives or friends. Investigators have suggested that the length and intensity of mourning are proportionate to the closeness of the relationship prior to death.

The classical studies of Lindemann (1944), on the survivors of the Coconut Grove fire in Boston and Parkes (1972), with English widows, noted that the clinical signs of acute grief in adults are remarkably uniform. Common are early sensations of somatic distress occurring in waves and lasting from 20 to 60 minutes, a feeling of tightness of the throat, choking, and shortness of breath; the need for sighing; complaints about lack of strength and exhaustion; an empty or lonely feeling; a slight sense of unreality; and a feeling of increased emotional distance from people. A feeling of guilt often torments close family members, even though their care of the deceased was completely appropriate. In addition, there is often a disconcerting loss of warmth in relationships with other people because of a tendency to respond with irritability and anger, even though friends and relatives make a special effort to maintain a thoughtful relationship. At the same time the capacity to initiate and maintain organized patterns of activity is lost. The bereaved parent clings to the daily routines, but these do not proceed in an automatic, self-sustaining fashion: "I just don't care—let me put it that way—it's just too much effort. If my husband forces me or pushes me to do something, I do it." Parkes (1965*a*) reports that "At first the full reaction may be delayed or there may be a period of numbness or blunting in which the bereaved person behaves as if nothing had happened for a few hours or days up to two weeks." Thereafter attacks of yearning or distress with autonomic disturbances begin. These occur in waves and are aggravated by reminders of the dead person. Between attacks the bereaved person is depressed and apathetic with a sense of futility. Associated symptoms are insomnia, anorexia, restlessness, irritability with an occasional outburst of anger directed against others or the self, and preoccupation with thoughts of the deceased. The dead person is commonly thought to be present, and there is a tendency to think of him as if he were still alive and to idealize his memory. The intensity of these features begins to decline after one to six weeks and is minimal by six to nine months.

Lindemann (1944) has concluded that normal grief is a definite syndrome and includes (1) somatic distress with tightness of the throat, choking, shortness of breath, need for sighing, an empty feeling in the abdomen, lack of muscular power, and an intense subjective distress described as tension or mental strain; (2) preoccupation with the image of the deceased; (3) feelings of guilt and preoccupation with one's negligence or minor omissions; (4) feelings of hostility toward others; and (5) breakdown of normal patterns of conduct.

As noted in the original work of Freud (1957), *Mourning and Melancholia,* grief is a normal and self-limited reaction to a severe loss. He described the grief process as a painful, reluctant withdrawal of attachment from a lost object, by which each memory and hope that binds the individual to the object is remembered; the deep emotional times are relived in memory and freed for new attachments. Lindemann, Parkes, and others who have studied mourning extensively have strongly emphasized that the full expression of emotional reactions in a grieving person is necessary for the optimal resolution of the mourning reaction.

Pathological grief

Lindemann (1944) observed that the grief reaction was distorted in some family members. He noted the following nine such distorted reactions: (1) overactivity without a sense of loss; (2) acquisition of symptoms belonging to the last illness of the deceased; (3) somatic reactions such as ulcerative colitis, asthma, or rheumatoid arthritis; (4) alteration in relations to friends and relatives; (5) furious hostility against specific persons; (6) repression of hostility, leading to a wooden manner resembling that in schizophrenic reactions; (7) lasting loss of patterns of social interaction; (8) actions detrimental to one's own social and economic existence; and (9) agitated depression. Patients and parents with these reactions require immediate and skilled intervention.

REACTION OF PARENTS TO THE LOSS OF AN INFANT DURING THE PERINATAL PERIOD

What, then, are the normal parental responses following a stillbirth or an early neonatal death? Although Deutsch (1945) suggests that grief after a stillbirth or neonatal death is not the same as that after the loss of a beloved adult relative but is, rather, the nonfulfillment of a wish fantasy, most observers have suggested that it is either the same as the loss of a beloved adult or that it represents a much more difficult process—the loss of a part of the self.

Although originally we believed it was similar to the loss of a close relative, we believe now that clinical studies and observations fit far more closely with the concepts proposed by Furman (1978) and Lewis (1979). Furman eloquently notes these reactions.

> Internally, the mourning process consists of two roughly opposing mechanisms. One is the generally known process of detachment, by which each memory that ties the family to the person who is deceased has to become painfully revived and painfully loosened. This is the part of the process that involves anger, guilt, pain, and sadness. The second process is commonly called "identification." It is the means by which the deceased or parts of him are taken into the self and preserved as part of the self, thereby soothing the pain of loss. In many instances, a surviving marriage partner takes over hobbies and interests of the deceased spouse. These identifications soothe the way and make the pain of detachment balanced and bearable.

For the surviving parents, the death of a newborn is special in several ways. Because mourning is mourning of a separate person, the process can apply only to that small part of the relationship to the newborn that was characterized by the love of a separate person, but there has not been time to build up strong ties and memories of mutual living. It is also not possible for parents—adults functioning in the grown-up world—to take into themselves any part of a helpless newborn and make it adaptively a part of themselves; the mechanism of identification does not work. But what about the part of the newborn which was still part of the self and that cannot be mourned? To understand this part, one has to look at the different process by which individuals cope with a loss of a part of the self, for example amputation or loss of function. Insofar as the newborn remains a part of the parent's self, the death has to be dealt with as would the amputation of a limb or the loss of function of the parent's body. Detachment is the mechanism with which the victim deals with such tragedies, but it is detachment of a different kind. Acceptance that one will never ever again have that part of oneself is very different from the detachment that deals with the memories of living together with a loved one. The feelings that accompany this detachment are similar in kind and intensity; anger, guilt, fury, helplessness, and horror. In the case of the loss of a part of the self, however, they are quite unrelieved by identification.

Next, with such a tragedy there must be a readjustment in one's self image. It is, however, altogether different to have to readjust to thinking of oneself as an imperfect human being, a human being that cannot walk or cannot see. That is a pain of a different kind and the feelings that accompany it are emptiness, loss of self-esteem, and feeling low. When a newborn dies, the parents, especially the mother, often describe these sensations. Because the internal self never materialized in those arms and has not had a chance to be detached, it is very different from the process of mourning.

These feelings are made particularly difficult because people around the parents are not there to help. At a conscious level, people say they simply do not understand about losing part of the self, and indeed they do not. Unconsciously they understand it all too well. It fills them with the fear the way an amputee fills many people with fear and anxiety and makes them shun him. This is the treatment that parents of dead newborns get. They are shunned, and they cannot rely upon the sympathy that is usually accorded the bereaved.*

This would explain the apparent anomalous behavior of women whose young sick infants are transported to another hospital for care. Even though the infant is in no danger and is doing well, they often begin to mourn the loss of the infant. If a portion of the mother's mind still considers the infant a part of herself, the infant obviously could not survive unless she is close and is caring for him. This can be compared with our own inability to conceive that one of our legs could be separated from us and could be walking and functioning several miles away.

Observers have noted intense mourning reactions after a neonatal death similar in quality to those seen after the loss of an older close family member, but lasting for periods longer than four to six months. Observers have suggested that the intensity of the mourning and grieving after the early loss of an infant is strong evi-

---

*From Furman, E.P.: The death of a newborn: care of the parents, Birth Fam. J. **5:**214-218, 1978.

dence for the presence of a close affectional tie. It is important to realize that in some women affectional relationships to their infants will begin or accelerate with the development of fetal movement or quickening. By the end of the second trimester, women who initially rejected the pregnancy have often accepted it. After she feels quickening, a woman usually begins to have dreams about what her baby will be like and may attribute some human personality characteristics to him or her. One mother commented, "If anything was to happen to her, I would have preferred it in the first three months. After that, well, after you feel life then it becomes more personal—more of a personal feeling. After that time you start feeling better physically, mentally, and everything else. When you feel life come, it is a person in your mind, you start picturing in your mind what it's going to look like when it's born. After that fourth month you'd like to have a chance to take almost anything regardless of what it is."

In a detailed study of 24 mothers who lost infants in the first 22 days after birth, common symptoms were sadness, loss of appetite, insomnia, preoccupation with thoughts of the infant, irritability, and loss of normal behavior patterns (Kennell et al., 1970). After the death the bereaved mother often reviews the period before the death for evidence of her failure (guilt) to do right by the dead infant. Mrs. G. said, "It's still so hard to believe. I can't think of anything I might have done. I've searched and searched to see if I had done anything during my pregnancy which might have harmed the baby." She accused herself of negligence: "I felt if I had put on weight, he could have been a full-grown baby, full-term. Maybe if I had eaten more, the baby could have weighed more." Cullberg (1972) found that 19 of 56 mothers studied one to two years after the death of their neonates had developed psychiatric disorders (psychosis, anxiety attacks, phobias, obsessive thoughts, and deep depressions).

STILLBIRTH

Lewis (1976*b*) and Morris (1976) have noted similar painful reactions for the mothers of a stillborn infant. Lewis (1979), noted "After a stillborn there is a double sense of loss for the bereaved mother who now has a void where there was so evidently a fullness. Even with the live birth the mother feels a sense of loss, but the consolation of a surviving 'outside baby' helps the mother to overcome her puzzling and bewildering sadness at losing her 'inside baby.'" With a stillbirth the mother has to cope with an outer as well as an inner void. Peppers and Knapp (1980) found no difference in the extent of grief between mothers having a stillbirth or neonatal death. At variance with these observations is that of Wolff and colleagues (1970), who studied 50 mothers from the age of 14 to 38 years who had a stillbirth, 40 of whom were observed for one to three years. They noted that 50% of the mothers resolved their grief with a new baby. However, a large number of mothers were adamant about not having another infant and were sterilized. The mothers talked about why the baby died. Seventeen mothers blamed themselves,

9 blamed their husbands or physicians, and 10 blamed fate or God. The investigators did not find significant psychiatric difficulties. However, the depth of their observations was not noted in the report.

> **COMMENT:** Indeed! My experience is different. Rather than resolving grief, a quick pregnancy interrupts the normal process of mourning. Frequently there is considerable difficulty with the mothering of the replacement baby, who may later have a confused sense of identity or suffer abuse. Sterilization after a stillbirth, except perhaps with severe hereditary defects, should be avoided. Sterilization, a "final solution," is rather too similar to the "black hole in the mind" that I have described as a psychic experience of stillbirth. These sterilized women would feel their lives at best to be profoundly empty, at worst they are severely depressed. The bereaved women who blame their husbands or God are unlikely to have adequately resolved their grief; rather, their failed mourning can lead to marital or family troubles, depressive symptoms, or difficulty coping with subsequent bereavement.
> **E. Lewis**

When a physician determines that a baby is dead or probably dead prior to birth, he faces the painful task of informing the mother and father and then supporting them through the macabre experience of laboring and giving birth to a dead baby. A child born dead is an overturning of the natural order of events that makes it exceedingly difficult for the physicians and nurses to cope. It is not part of their function in the delivery room to ease death into the world. As one mother said, "When a child is born dead, there is nothing. The world remembers nothing, and the gap in the womb is replaced by an emptiness in your arms." She continued, "You are not recording a birth or a death, but both at once. It is the ultimate contradiction—I felt I had created death."

After the delivery of a stillborn infant, it has often been the custom for the mother to be heavily sedated and for hospital discharge to be arranged earlier than usual. On returning home the mother may avoid contact with people because of her feelings of shame and guilt. She may not be able to communicate with her husband, who may proceed to occupy himself with activities outside the home. She may have fantasies that her thoughts or actions caused the death. One woman said, "I felt that I had failed as a woman; I hated my body as a defective machine."

Lewis (1979) urges physicians and midwives to help families re-create their memories and lost hopes, which can then be mourned. The baby can be "brought back to death." Parents are often spared seeing and touching their baby. Although this is well meant, it may deprive them of the prime chance of rooting healthful mourning in reality.

CLINICAL OBSERVATIONS

When a newborn dies in the hospital, all evidence of his existence is sometimes removed with amazing rapidity, and nothing is left to confirm the reality of his death. "Everything just happened so fast . . . my mind kept going around in circles. I didn't really understand," said one mother. "Just last Sunday I was thinking about her, thinking that my husband and I were the only ones who saw her—it's like there is no proof there ever was a baby. We were the only ones who ever saw her, and it was just for a couple of days. When a baby dies that small, there's no funeral, no masses. It seems like sort of a shame that there isn't something more. . . . I felt I was on an island by myself . . . lost. . . ."

Often no special arrangements are made for the parents. They may not have any privacy or a comforting individual who allows them to express their grief freely. There are sometimes no planned follow-up contacts with the family to see how the mourning process is proceeding, and information about the results of the postmortem examination is sometimes delivered in a letter.

Many hospital practices and efforts by hospital personnel and relatives tend to discourage or "bottle up" the mourning. One mother complained, "When I started to cry in the hospital, they wanted to give me a tranquilizer. I would say, 'Gee, if I could just cry, maybe I would get it out of my system.' " If mourning is impeded and not allowed to run its course, pathological grief can result.

Kennell and associates (1970) focused on the emotional well-being of a mother after touching her baby before his death. There were no pathological reactions in mothers who had touched their infants prior to death, except for one mother who also had a pathological reaction after the death of a previous infant whom she had not touched. The mothers described how painful it was to be located on the maternity division, in the same room as a mother who had a healthy baby, and where the cries of healthy babies could be heard. Most of the mothers stressed the desirability of being in a room on a different division, away from the maternity staff, who often caused distress. Also, as one mother mentioned, "They would keep my mother downstairs about half an hour, telling her I was feeding the baby and I didn't have a baby to feed. . . ."

> COMMENT: Although it is painful for bereaved mothers to be with women who have live babies, it can help keep the elusive memory of their stillborn baby alive in their minds, thus facilitating the normal mourning process. Furthermore, many bereaved women, as a result of their guilt, feel that they cannot be trusted with live babies. To be allowed to help a bit about the ward with the babies can reassure them that others do not blame them for what happened. Staying in the situation also prevents the all-too-common occurrence of bereaved women, who are nursed in a private room or quickly discharged from the hospital, being left alone with their grief and becoming victims of the conspiracy of silence that frequently surrounds stillbirth.
> E. Lewis

These mothers complained about hospital practices that dampened mourning responses, and they commented on the desirability of allowing a mother to decide for herself whether she wished to see and touch her baby, living or dead. Many mothers had comments about touching their babies. "I didn't get a chance to really touch him, to hold him like a mother. This is something a mother wants to do so much, to touch the baby. Even though she knows she can't pick it up. But the dreams go that I'm picking him up and holding him, and I know I didn't do it. So I wake up because I wanted to so bad."

COMMENT: This is a nice example of the healing work of dreams. In her dream this mother was able to hold the baby she had not held. In her imagination she "brought her baby back to death"; in her dream her stillborn baby became real in her arms, and this helped her to mourn. To touch a stillborn baby is so important in helping to make the event real and to facilitate mourning that I believe this mother should have been encouraged to hold her baby. It is *natural* for a bereaved mother to hold her baby herself.
E. Lewis

Another mother said, "They told me I could touch my baby, but I didn't want to. She was so small and she looked so fragile I was afraid that just the fact that I touched her would give me a little more hope and would make it harder for me if she didn't. . . . I didn't want to make anything more difficult." Mrs. G. concluded, "We had a lot of anticipation. In fact, right now, since I never held the baby or anything, it's all more or less anticipation and not reality."

In interviews many months after the death of an infant, several observers have noted that parents had been greatly comforted by the nurse or physician who expressed sadness or empathy with the parents' plight. The parents expressed at the same time great anger toward health personnel who had been abrupt or who dealt rapidly with the process of explaining the loss so that they could proceed with obtaining autopsy permission.

Many parents were surprised by the intensity of their feelings of grief and believed that they were psychiatrically disturbed or had developed a severe illness and needed help. This is important for the physician to remember.

Parents commonly reported that their close friends and their relatives were not always supportive, failing to realize that the loss of a newborn infant is a tragedy and normally results in a strong mourning response. Mrs. M. said, "After you've lost a baby, you always think about it most of the time because people want to know how it was to have a baby and lose, and you have to keep going over it for them." Traditional supportive behavior patterns that existed over centuries are usually no longer available or acceptable in situations such as the death of an infant. In addition, new cultural patterns tend to deny the reality of death. It appears that in the modern world, new behavior patterns are not seasoned to the needs of the parents. Their mourning reactions may actually be affected in adverse ways.

PARENT GROUPS

There is a need for careful studies to determine the most effective methods for helping parents after the loss of a baby. Carol Fowler's diary (a mother's account of experiences after the death of her infant) has been appreciated by a number of families. She also first began a parent group.

Several years ago we were pleased when two couples who had lost their babies, Nancy and Larry Bartels and Kathy and Bob Vincl, expressed an interest in starting a parent group, Parents Experiencing Neonatal Death (PEND). They requested that one of us (MHK or JHK) be present at each meeting, and this practice has continued. Subsequently, we have been able to bring one or two other professional persons to hear the parents' discussion of their experiences. The parent group leader initially telephones each set of parents, since in the early period after the death they have difficulty communicating. At the outset we said nothing, but this was disturbing to the group so we now make a limited number of comments during the meeting, usually in response to direct questions. When one of the caretakers attending the meeting has felt compelled to defend what a physician or nurse has done, the quality of the group discussion has deteriorated significantly.

In these meetings parents frequently state that hearing about the experience of other parents gives them the courage to carry on when parents have mentioned distressing thoughts such as concern about going crazy or an urge to commit suicide, and others have commented that they had these same thoughts. We assume, but do not know for sure, that these in-depth discussions are supportive to the others who attend. In the PEND group meetings there has usually been a mixture of parents for whom the loss occurred in the last one to two months and others whose baby died several months ago. Most of the parents who come after six months state that they are coming "to help others." We suspect that this is a positive step in the resolution of the parents' mourning.

We have been fortunate to be able to listen to the open discussion of extremely painful poignant reactions of families after the loss of an infant. Almost invariably there is a criticism of physicians, nurses, and other health personnel. It has seemed important to listen and not to defend the care or caretakers, even when the criticism is directed at our own actions.

In the early weeks it seems as if there is criticism of almost everyone who has talked or not talked to them, but at the same time there is usually appreciation of the efforts people are making to be helpful. Probably the strongest reactions arise when there are comments suggesting that the family should forget about the loss and get on with life or get on with another pregnancy, or that the baby was small and therefore they should not feel as great a loss as they would if the baby had lived longer. When their reactions to the death of a spouse or an older child have been considered, parents have consistently agreed that the loss of the stillborn or live-born infant was more distressing. They point out that there are many individuals who knew an older child or adult who has died and there are many reminders of the dead person.

In almost every group meeting parents express their great concern that others will forget about the baby, and they make strong efforts to help others remember. One father said, "You want to shout to the world that Jimmy lived. You don't want the world to forget. Even if the baby is all goofed up, he has many strengths and positive features." One mother said she was terribly concerned in the first weeks after the death that she might forget about her baby, and she told how she forced herself to keep thinking about the baby so she would not forget. The other parents quickly reassured her that the pain would decrease but she would never ever forget her baby.

Another painful issue is what parents say when asked by strangers about how many children they have. One mother said, "None" two weeks after she had a stillborn infant. She then described how depressed she was for the next several days. Parents who had progressed beyond the first one or two months usually had resolved to give an answer that included the baby so they would then answer, "I did have a daughter, but she died."

There has been general agreement about the "terrible pain" following the loss of the baby and the great feeling of emptiness. Many parents have stated that absolutely no one can appreciate the pain and misery associated with the death of a baby unless they have experienced this themselves. One mother said, "With each death a big part is taken from you and an empty spot is left." Parents described their attempts to avoid reminders that bring on a surge of this pain. However, later on there is general agreement that this pain is inevitable and that attempts to avoid it merely prolong the misery. Many parents have said that the pain was worse in the first two months, that things were somewhat better after that time, but even at six months and a year all parents were still having sad times. Some parents have described how they could really laugh for the first time about nine months after the baby's death; others described how guilty they felt if they laughed earlier. Between the monthly meetings some mothers are greatly helped by long discussions on the telephone with the parent group leader.

The group meetings are not for all parents. In our individual interviews we have considered a small number of parents to be so disturbed that we thought their reactions might be disruptive to the group, and for them we have recommended psychiatric assistance. (This is not to indicate that we have a narrow view of the reactions of parents after the loss of an infant. As a matter of fact, our concept of the normal range of reactions to the death of a baby has tended to expand progressively over the five years that we have been attending the monthly meetings of this group.) Some parents have declined the invitation to attend the group meetings and prefer a one-to-one conversation with the parent group leader. Others indicated that they knew another family with a similar loss or they had close friends or family members with whom they could discuss their mourning reactions more easily than they could in a group meeting. We are currently attempting to study the advantages and disadvantages of these group meetings. We have noted that some parents come for one or two meetings, whereas others attend for several months.

At almost every meeting one remedy for the great pain of mourning is discussed; start a pregnancy immediately. Almost all the parents in the group have been counseled individually prior to coming to the group meeting, and we have generally recommended holding off on another pregnancy until they have worked through the loss. This often means waiting six to 12 months. In spite of this, in the early weeks after the loss most mothers tell of their intense, almost fanatical desire to start another pregnancy and replace the lost baby. Often the efforts to achieve this are so determined and mechanical and intense that one wonders whether this produced a contraceptive effect. Many parents describe how they originally planned to have only two or three children, but after the loss they wanted to have four or five just in case. Six months after their baby died many parents have commented that they felt it had been wise and fortunate that they had not started a pregnancy earlier. On the other hand, those in the group who did become pregnant early have argued that they are able to mourn the first child as the pregnancy progressed so they could become attached to the new baby. In contrast, Lewis (1979) has reported that mothers usually cannot mourn a loss during pregnancy. This obviously requires further study.

> **COMMENT:** A pregnant woman becomes increasingly preoccupied with thoughts and feelings about her fetus. Mourning entails a comparable intense concern with the dead in order eventually to become free from the loss. A bereaved pregnant woman has conflicting and paradoxical needs to think and feel intensely, both about the new life and the dead baby. In my experience she usually opts for her live baby and mourning is interrupted—it is too difficult while she nurtures her new baby, and it is often impossible to resume later. This leaves her at risk.
> **E. Lewis**

The parents describe and demonstrate an insistent need to talk about the loss over and over and over again. But with whom? In the group meetings it has become clear that it is beneficial for as many family members as possible to see the stillborn or dying infant so that several close friends or relatives will have common grounds for discussing and sharing their feelings about the features of the baby, the problems of the baby, and the tragedy of the death. This has strengthened our conviction that the parents' parents, brothers, sisters, and friends should be welcomed into the nursery and encouraged to come to see the baby after death and at the funeral home so that there will be others with whom the mother and father can discuss all aspects of the baby's appearance and behavior as well as the sadness and anger associated with the baby's course.

When the meetings first started, it was more common for a number of parents to report that both parents or the mother had been given no opportunity to see and touch their stillborn infant or their baby who died shortly after birth. When a parent has not seen or touched the baby, we have been impressed that this has often been associated with a prolongation of intense mourning. One woman never saw her baby dead or alive. She told how she kept her husband awake night after night, asking him to describe the appearance of the baby in fine detail. She said that through this process she got a little clearer view of the baby each time. It was only after she finally saw two pictures of the baby taken after death that she was more contented about the baby's appearance. The baby looked very different from the way she expected. The parents' poignant comments have emphasized to us how important it is for parents to be encouraged to see and touch their baby, to participate in a simple funeral, and to arrange for a burial place that is accessible to them. When the baby is buried in another city, parents sorely miss the opportunity to go to the grave site. A large majority of parents report how helpful it has been for them to make visits to the cemetery, sometimes infrequently, but sometimes daily.

It would be unusual for a parent not to tell about the irritability and anger with the actions and words of some of their relatives and friends. Many of them did, however, recognize the efforts of others to try to be helpful in this difficult and unfamiliar situation. After several weeks a number of parents have commented that even if everyone said everything perfectly, they still could not say it in a way that would be really helpful to a parent who has lost an infant. However, there has been group agreement that it was appreciated when anyone commented that the baby could never be replaced. Mothers, in particular, tell about their almost overwhelming and unwarranted feelings of guilt in spite of the explanations of relatives, nurses, and physicians that they had no part in causing the death. Both mothers and fathers report going through a period when they kept questioning why this happened to them. Many of the parents who have attended the group for several visits have said that the experience of losing their baby had given more meaning to their lives and that simple events now meant much more to them.

Individual counseling and groups have been provided in a variety of other ways and led by psychiatrists, psychologists, neonatologists, or nurses. We will describe our plan of three visits to the neonatologist. At Downstate Medical Center in New York City, three midwives started a Perinatal Bereavement Clinic. When the client load became too heavy for them they discovered more nurses in the hospital than they needed were willing to participate in the individual counseling of parents. This clinic continues to provide care for a large number of families. In St. Louis and Denver two other groups, Association of Mothers Experiencing Neonatal Death (AMEND), serving similar purposes, have also been in existence for several years.

THE AMISH WAY

There is much about support systems for families that has been swept away with the management of birth and death in the hospital. We may be able to gain insight into helpful systems by looking at practices that have existed relatively unchanged over many centuries. In a report on the "Amish way of death," Bryer (1979) describes the customs and support systems that have been successful in coping with death for the past 400 years. Based on interviews with 24 Amish families, she reported that at the time of death, close neighbors assume the responsibility for notifying other individuals about the death. The bereaved family has only two tasks. First, they are asked to choose two or three families to take full charge of the funeral arrangements and, second, to draw up a list of the families who are to be invited to the funeral. The embalmed body is returned to the home within a day of death. As one Amish man reported, "The funeral is not for the one who died, you know; it is for the family." There are traditions about the dressing of the dead person, and he or she is placed in a plain wooden coffin in a room that has been emptied of all furnishings to accommodate the several hundred relatives, friends, and neighbors who will begin arriving as soon as the body is prepared for viewing. The Amish people see death as a part of the natural rhythm of life.

The presence of the body in the home, the repeated viewing, the continuing community support, and the family participation in the actual disposition of the body all serve as constant reminders of the fact of death. Bryer stresses the valuable effects of this approach for the children in the Amish community. She quotes Lifton and Olson (1974) that "A child's concept of death is likely to be charged with fear when earlier death imagery has overwhelmed imagery of life and continuity. Experiences that reinforce imagery of life's connection, movement, and integrity will encourage an attitude of trust and hope. . . . This is very different from having the reality of death kept from him." The high level of support shown the bereaved family is maintained for at least a year following the death.

PHYSICIANS' REACTIONS

Giles (1970) in Australia noted that physicians managed bereaved mothers by treating physical symptoms only and by prescribing sedatives liberally. They avoided discussing the baby's death in about one half of the cases. In the same study many mothers complained that junior physicians had not answered their questions but left them to be answered by senior physicians, who in fact never visited them. Of 40 mothers, 12 believed that they were mainly helped by visitors, 10 by talking to a physician, and another 10 by talking to members of the nursing staff. Bourne (1968) noted the significant tendency of general practitioners to forget details about the mother of a stillborn when compared with a live-born infant.

In Sweden, Cullberg (1972) observed that stillbirth and neonatal death evoke a sense of guilt in the staff on a maternity ward. He observed three different ways that staff members handled the anxiety associated with a death: (1) avoidance of the situation, (2) projection of personal feelings onto the patient in the form of aggressive or accusing behavior, and (3) denial and "magical repair" (". . . forget it . . . get a new child . . . give heavy doses of sedatives").

These reactions on the part of the physicians can be easily understood if one analyzes what is happening to them.

A number of strong emotional responses well up in the physician at the time of an infant's death. From past training the physician knows that the patient's total care will be reviewed for the autopsy and the perinatal pathology conference. With the myriad treatments and combinations now available, the physician wonders whether other combinations would have been successful. Young house officers and older physicians alike often raise this question: "What would the results have been if we had moved in another way—if we had raised the oxygen or given a transfusion earlier?" Thus, like the parents, the physician, who often is partly attached to the infant, is plagued by a feeling of guilt when an infant dies. On top of this the physician also has several difficult tasks, one of which is to face the family with the terrible news, realizing that this will result in tears and great sadness as well as hostile feelings. To add to the problem the intensive struggle for life now practiced in some neonatal units has some of the spirit of the sports arena, where a "loss" is almost unacceptable. In some units house officers have mentioned, with a hint of irritation, that one does not expect a baby to die these days, especially if the right things are done. We have called this the "Lombardi syndrome," after the coach who did not believe in losing a football game. Young physicians often believe they are a failure at their job and that there is little they can do now: they have no tools, no instruments, no medications. The high turnover of nurses in the intensive care units and the syndrome of "burnout" (Marshall and Kosmar, 1980) may be the result of the staff (nurses and physicians) incompletely working through these difficult emotions. Morris Green has thoughtfully commented in a slightly different vein, questioning, "How much living and dying can be experienced and normally managed by healthy young adults?"

In addition, during discussion with the parents, the physician is held back by a sensitivity to their reactions—both by tears and by the nonverbal messages of anger that are present and normally accompany true mourning and grief. However, in contrast to feelings of uselessness, the caretaker has a singular opportunity to make an important contribution to the health of the parents and to the integrity of the whole family. To do this the caretaker must assist the parents in getting under way with the expression of their grief reactions, must encourage the mother and father to communicate their feelings to each other, and then must help them to help the children at home. Obviously, future children will be affected by this loss if the parents are unable to get through their grief reactions.

It is important for the physician to realize that these beliefs are also held by all the personnel in the unit, from the secretary to the staff nurse. The physician will often pick up feelings of anger and disappointment from a nurse, since his or her directions led to failure. This is especially true when the nurses are as intimately involved as they are in the present intensive care units. For example, the nursing or bagging* of a tiny infant puts that life into their hands and leads to a strong attachment. We have found that it is difficult for the nurses to function easily unless

---

*Method of assisted ventilation.

they discuss these feelings, and we have a meeting every two weeks at which these and other problems are aired.

TASKS FOR THE PHYSICIAN AND NURSE

The caretaker has three major tasks: (1) to help the parents work through the loss and make it real; (2) to ensure that normal grief reactions will begin and that both parents will go through the process, if possible without pathological grief; and (3) to meet the individual needs of specific parents.

The work of Cullberg, Kennell, and others has shown that there are several factors which help to make the death real. First, it is important to permit the parents to visit a sick infant, even if the infant is on a respirator and appears seriously ill. (It should also be noted here that the parents should only visit when they want to and should never be forced.) Second, we have found it beneficial for the parents to be permitted, if they desire, to view or touch their dead infant (often a harrowing experience for some physicians and nurses). The infant usually does not look as he did when he was alive, but this experience helps to make the death a reality. Third, we suggest that simple or private funerals be arranged, if possible by the parents—traditional rituals promote grieving—here again the death is made real. In many hospitals it has been the custom for the hospital to dispose of small infants as a service to the parents. However, this practice removes all evidence of the infant extremely rapidly so that the infant may become like a dream to the parents, which may retard their grieving. As Mrs. D. said, "I think that all mothers this happens to should go to the burial. My doctor was against it. Some of the family was against it. Some of the family was against having anything at all. I don't believe in that. I couldn't see lying in a hospital bed or going home while my son was being buried. I had to be there."

We have found several steps to be helpful when assisting parents through the normal mourning process. We meet with the parents three times. The *first* time is right after the death. At this moment they are so overwhelmed by the news of the infant's death that they are unable to hear anything else. However, we do describe the details of the mourning process in simple terms. We explain that they may have pains in their chest and have waves of sadness come upon them intensely for the first two weeks and then gradually diminish, tapering off until they cease at about six months. At times they may imagine that they see the baby alive. Parents will often find themselves angry with each other and their friends and feel guilty about the death of the infant, believing that actions they could have taken would have saved the infant or prevented his illness in the first place. They may believe that they are going crazy.

We meet with the parents for the *second* time in the next two or three days. At this time it is much easier to review the grieving process. It is important that they understand what the usual reactions are so that they will not think that they are ill. The most important action is to listen, listen, and listen some more. Bowlby (1979), in writing about this, gives us some guidelines.

> Those counselling the bereaved have found empirically that if they are able to help it is necessary to encourage a client to recall and recount, in great detail, all the events that led up to the loss, the circumstances surrounding it and her experiences since; for it seems only in this way that a widow or any bereaved person can sort out her hopes, regrets, and despairs, her anxiety, anger, and perhaps guilt, and just as important review all the actions and reactions that she had in mind to perform and may still have in mind to perform, inappropriate or self-defeating though many of them might always have been and certainly would be now. Not only is it desirable for a bereaved person to review everything surrounding the loss but to review also the whole history of the relationship with all its satisfactions and deficiencies, the things that were done and those that were left undone.*

We stress that the parents move together and keep up their rapport and communication. If the father has been sad during the day, he should come home and tell his wife about his sadness rather than hiding it. "He felt terrible. He'd go upstairs and cry alone. If you can cry with somebody, you're better, but he cried alone." "He doesn't think about it as much as I do. And when I do, he tells me, 'Maybe it was for the best.' He just mopes around. . . ." "All we did was talk. Stayed up until 2:00, 3:00, 4:00 in the morning just talking about anything and everything. We would always fall back on the baby. It seemed to start out with the baby and end up with the baby. I think it does good to talk." Often we have seen parents move further and further apart—the father not wanting to share his sadness with his wife. "I kept busy working. . . . We picked on each other. . . . About Christmas time we had a big argument, and I realized I had to face the baby's death. After that we seemed to get closer." "We couldn't discuss the baby with each other. Maybe that's where I got the feeling of guilt. She would start talking about the baby, and I would say, 'Forget it, the baby's dead.' I guess I was at fault. She wanted to talk it out, but I would say, 'Drop it.' " "Whenever it would come up, I would usually kind of change the subject. You know, you don't want to dwell on it too much. . . ." We suggest that is important for the husband to tell his wife about his sadness and to let her tell about her own so that they may cry together. "I tried to comfort him and he tried to comfort me, and we both ended up crying." It has been particularly striking for us to see how American fathers act after a loss. They often become extremely active, frequently taking on extra jobs or duties outside the home. As well as providing an outlet for their own feelings, these extra jobs may interfere with the husband's support of, and communication with, his

---

*From Bowlby, J.:. The making and breaking of affectional bonds, London, 1979, Tavistock Publications, Ltd.

wife. At this second interview it is important to keep lines of communication open and to make plans for another conference in three to six months. It is essential that the physician does not just talk but spends a great deal of time simply listening. Obviously, every patient's needs will be individualized. One must not be afraid of tears—there will often be a great deal of crying, and physicians should not be afraid of this, for themselves or for the parents. Many parents have mentioned that they appreciated the physician's empathy.

The *third* meeting with the parents occurs three to six months after the death. We meet with them to ensure that their grieving is progressing normally and that there is not a persistently high level of mourning or any other sign of pathological grief. As described by Lindemann (1944), these abnormal reactions often involve the same mechanisms as those seen in normal mourning but are manifested in a distorted fashion. They include the following: overactivity without a sense of loss; acquisition of symptoms associated with the baby's illness; psychosomatic symptoms such as colitis, asthma, or rheumatoid arthritis; alterations in relationships with friends and relatives; furious hostility toward specific persons; repression of hostility, leading to a wooden manner resembling that in schizophrenic reactions; and lasting loss of patterns of social interaction and activities detrimental to one's own social and economic existence. If these symptoms are noted during this interview, a referral should be made to a psychiatrist.

Helping parents through these experiences is an extremely difficult assignment, but we have been rewarded by the thanks and expressions of appreciation parents have relayed to us later.

INTERVIEW

The following interview with Mr. and Mrs. Day* took place three weeks after their infant's death. Only portions are included, since this was a long interview.

PEDIATRICIAN: It is now three weeks since your baby died. Can you tell me how things have gone since the baby passed away? The feelings you both have had?

MRS. DAY: I can't sleep. I toss and turn. I wasn't thinking about it, but as soon as I saw an article in the paper with a baby in an incubator, it all came back to me. I usually see her in the incubator with them pumping oxygen into her lungs, and she's kicking. I close my eyes and I see her. My husband . . . it doesn't bother him too much . . . it's me.

MR. DAY: It's something you have to go through. These things are bound to happen. It's one of those things you have to learn to live with. It's hard to explain what happens to you. It's very, very hard to explain. I would rather not say to anybody . . .

PEDIATRICIAN: You just hold it in?

MR. DAY: Yes, hold it in . . . this is something you cannot describe. I try to live as best as I possibly can. My wife is doing a great job. It's been a tremendous strain upon

---

*The family's name has been changed.

her, and she has come through victorious. I want to commend the doctors and the staff of people who worked so hard on the child. They did a wonderful job.

This is an unusual interview because the father has told about holding back his reactions very early. It would probably have been appropriate at this point to indicate to the father and the mother that it is natural for parents to feel distressed as they recall this sad experience and that it is all right to cry. Such favorable comments about the doctors and staff at this stage tend to make us a bit wary that criticisms will be forthcoming. Let us see how this interview progresses.

PEDIATRICIAN: Tell me about your sleeping.

MRS. DAY: I don't get to sleep until 3:00 or 4:00 in the morning. I just toss and turn in the bed all night. And then either my daughter calls me or my son calls me and I get up with them. So the only time I can sleep is about 9:00 in the morning, when I fall asleep.

PEDIATRICIAN: What can you tell me about your mood?

MRS. DAY: It's low, terribly low. My daughter noticed something was wrong. She looked at me and said, "Mommy, your stomach hurt?" But now she just looks at me. My husband told her we were bringing a new baby home, and she's been looking for this new baby. She won't say anything, but she'll look at me strange and she'll look at her father strange. You know, she was looking for a new little baby. She just looks at me now—she doesn't say any more, "Mommy, does your tummy hurt?" She'll just sit there and look at me.

Children's reaction to death

The mourning reactions of parents are extremely difficult for children to interpret and understand unless the parents communicate their own feelings and give explanations. A helpful explanation might be, "Mommy is sad about the baby dying. That is why I am crying and look so unhappy. I don't feel like talking or doing the things I usually do right now, but I still love you." The ideas that arise from a sibling's death may be devastating. This girl may well be imagining that her mother's thoughts and reactions are entirely different from what they really are. She may feel guilty because of her angry thoughts about the baby. She may have wished that the baby would die and may believe that the mother's quietness is because of this. Obviously there is a problem of communication between this mother and father and their children. It sounds as if the children are also having a sleep disturbance. It would be appropriate and probably helpful for the mother to point out the similarity of the children's reactions of sadness to her own. Both the children are sufficiently old that it would be appropriate to help them put their feelings into words.

PEDIATRICIAN: What did you tell her about this baby?

MRS. DAY: Well, my husband didn't want to tell her anything. He only said the baby didn't come home, so I just told her the baby died. And she just sat there and looked at me kind of strange—she didn't know what I was talking about. She's almost 3 years old. But my son, he doesn't understand. He just runs around the house. He knows that I look different, that's all. He'll be 2 years old in five months.

PEDIATRICIAN: Do you find yourself crying sometimes?

MRS. DAY: Yes.

PEDIATRICIAN: What does this mean to the children?

MRS. DAY: At first when I came home, I was crying and my daughter didn't understand. She wouldn't come to me. She wanted to go upstairs to my mother, and she didn't want to be bothered with me, so my husband said, "You should have spoken to her before you went in the house and hugged her," but I just looked at her so strange because she reminded me of the new baby, and I just stared at her. And my husband said, "You shouldn't do that with a baby like that because she's not used to it." I don't know, I was completely numb, and my son was completely numb with me. I couldn't say anything to my two kids. I just looked at them. For two days they rejected me. All she wanted to do was to go upstairs.

As is often the case, the young children are going through severe reactions to the separation from their mother for the birth and postpartum period. This probably accounts for the daughter's unwillingness to approach her mother.

> **COMMENT:** There is more to this. A child imagines attacking the rival inside his mother. When the baby dies, this seems to confirm the child's fear that his thoughts could harm the baby. His guilt and fear of retribution from his mother may make him avoid her. These bereaved mothers often feel themselves to be unsafe with babies. Their child may sense this, which is an added reason not to approach the mother.
> **E. Lewis**

The children have found that their mother is not only different in appearance because of the birth but radically changed in behavior and responsiveness. What comes to mind are the striking observations of Brazelton and co-workers (1974) that even 2- to 4-month-old infants are drastically disturbed and depressed when their mothers sit in front of them mute and without facial response for 2 or 3 minutes. One of the features of mourning behavior is that it is self-centered. In spite of this, with some encouragement, a mother can usually find the extra ounce of strength to embrace her children and give them some explanation. The husband's criticism does not help the situation, but by holding back his own mourning reaction, he has been able to think of the needs of the children.

> MR. DAY: The children were in a kind of trance. Their mother comes home and has lost a child. She's so cruel all at once that she doesn't see anything around her, like she's closed in a tube or something, rejecting everything else on the outside, so that when she came in the house the first thing she did was reject the children, which she shouldn't have done. She should have extended more love and affection and kindness to the children, which is hard to do in some situations.

Because he has repressed his own mourning reactions, the father does not realize how stunned, shocked, and self-centered a mourner becomes. He vividly describes the mother's inability to see and respond to things around her.

PEDIATRICIAN: You were all prepared for the baby and there was no baby?

MRS. DAY: Yes. That brings it back to me. I think about her a whole lot. I told my husband that I didn't even *name* her. The nurses were calling her Pinkie. And my mother's upset too because she never did see the baby. She wanted to see the baby, but she didn't want to see her like that. She got all excited Friday and called my father at work and told him about it. She wanted to know if I would have a funeral, and one of my relatives called and wanted to know what I was going to do. I told him there was nothing I could do about it. So he called up his mother and told her and his Aunt Rosie. His cousin wrote him a letter, a sympathy card. She put on it that her daughter had a baby and it was the same way and that he came out of it and now is 15 months old and acts like he is 6 months. He doesn't do anything; he doesn't move around, just flops around. I didn't want my baby to be like this—just flop around. Now I sit around and just wonder about it. All the baby's things I have, from my other baby. I never threw them away, and she never used them up; there are no holes in them or anything like that. We still have all that stuff at home, and you look at it, and the more you look at it the more you think about it. I'm going to give all that stuff away so that I can't look at it anymore.

The cousin who writes about the 15-month-old who acts like a 6-month-old is characteristic of many relatives and friends who believe it will relieve the pain if they indicate that it is fortunate that the baby died because he or she would probably have been damaged. This matter is considered later on by the interviewer. This episode indicates the importance of good communication so that a physician can counteract this by explaining that the baby would have been perfectly normal if she had not died of respiratory symptoms. The baby clothes remind the mother about her baby and cause her great emotional pain. It is important to appreciate that the pain of mourning cannot and should not be suppressed or eliminated. We would not interfere with the mother's plans to put away the baby's clothes, but we might indicate that there would be many other reminders of the baby and that there is nothing one can do to eliminate the pain associated with mourning.

PEDIATRICIAN: How did you feel day after day when you saw the baby?

MR. DAY: Gradually, as the baby was getting worse, I began to feel different, but I still held high hopes. The doctor told me that there had been a great change in the baby in a matter of 3 or 4 hours, that the baby was getting worse.

The father had the advantage of seeing the baby during this period. In spite of the baby's poor clinical condition, the opportunity to see that the baby was breathing and that her heart was beating gave him a much more optimistic impression than the mother, who probably did not know about this bad turn of events but, because of the separation, was imagining that the baby was in poor condition.

MRS. DAY: That's right. Thursday night, I took a sleeping pill. I don't usually take sleeping pills but I asked for one, and I tossed and turned all that Friday morning until 5:00 A.M. I figured that something was wrong. I couldn't eat breakfast. I knew my baby was dead, but I didn't want to say anything, but I had a feeling that she was—my whole insides felt like they were falling out. I couldn't eat and I was sick, so the nurse said, "What's the matter?" I said, "I don't feel right." So she says, "Why don't you call and see how the baby's doing?" I did, and the doctor told me there was nothing else they could do for her. Well, then I knew she was dead. But they wouldn't tell me—but I just had a feeling she was dead. Then they called and told me she was dead.

At this point some comment about the mother's feelings would be appropriate. We might make a comment such as, "What terrible news! You know it is perfectly natural to feel like crying as we go back over these sad events." In retrospect we can see that the jump to the next item was much too rapid. It would have been wise to wait longer to obtain her reaction to the news about the baby's death, and perhaps the reaction to this information being given by telephone.

PEDIATRICIAN: Could you tell me about the first time you saw the baby? Do you remember how you felt then? Were you optimistic?

MRS. DAY: Yes, when I looked at her . . . but she was so tiny. She was breathing hard; I knew she wasn't going to make it.

PEDIATRICIAN: You were not as optimistic as your husband.

MRS. DAY: I told him I wasn't. But he said, "Have hopes." He said she was going to be all right, but I knew she wasn't. I said she was going to die, but he said, "She's going to be all right, have hopes." She moved for me. She kicked for me, but she didn't have any life in her hands—she would only move her little fingers. I would have liked to see her when she died, though, I mean . . . to say goodbye to her, you know. She was still mine, but in a way she wasn't mine.

This mother expresses a desire to say goodbye to her baby, a request that many other parents have made. As a result, we have been offering parents an opportunity to be with their babies as they die or after they die. It is desirable to provide as much privacy as possible.

PEDIATRICIAN: You felt badly that you didn't see her. . .

MRS. DAY: Yes, afterwards. I would still have liked to see her. She was still my baby. But my husband said no, and I listened to him. I didn't see her (very softly).

Based on Mrs. Day's comments and those of other parents, we started several years ago to offer parents an opportunity to see their dead baby and to touch and hold him or her. We believe that when a baby dies, a caretaker can make a major contribution to the long-term well-being of the parents and their family by doing his or her best to help them be aware that the baby really was born, did live, and is now dead. Confirmation of the baby's death will usually help to initiate and facilitate their mourning response.

PEDIATRICIAN: How have you felt since? Have you ever felt irritable in the last few weeks? Do you find yourself getting upset more easily?

MRS. DAY (laughing): It doesn't take much for me to get upset. Sometimes when my husband says something, I get mad at him, you know—but it doesn't last long.

PEDIATRICIAN: Is this different than usual? Do you jump on him often?

MRS. DAY: I snap at him, see (laughing), and he'll say, "You're so evil." My mother says, "You'd better cut that out." But we don't get into many arguments. He'll say, "You know it's for the best. Don't think about it. Think about something else." He's been taking me out to make my mind go somewhere else, but as soon as I get back home and get into bed, I lie there and just think—I don't know (sighs), I don't think I'll ever get over this (louder), and I don't think I'll ever have another baby. I couldn't take it.

The mother's irritability and anger are part of the mourning reaction. The father's tendency to label her reactions as cruel or evil is understandable because he does not appreciate the intensity of her mourning. His attempts to keep his wife from thinking about the baby are not very successful, but we would usually try to help a husband appreciate that his efforts to take his wife out and divert her mind were going against her natural inclinations and were suppressing her mourning response. In Cullberg's (1972) study in Sweden, efforts to delay or suppress the mourning reaction resulted in a prolongation of the mourning response and a longer period of time before mothers were able to get back to normal.

PEDIATRICIAN: Do you think about the baby more when you have time to yourself?

MRS. DAY: Well, I go upstairs to keep from thinking about it. I go upstairs with my mother, and we'll talk about something else different, see, and I kind of forget about it until I go back downstairs. My daughter keeps me busy.

These parents demonstrate the support that comes from an extended family. The outcome might have been much less satisfactory if Mrs. Day had not had her own mother nearby to listen understandingly to her tell about her sadness or whatever else she wanted to discuss.

PEDIATRICIAN: Your daughter helps a lot?

MRS. DAY (laughs): She talks a lot, so she helps.

MR. DAY: I think that's the only approach to get over a thing like this. Keep busy as much as possible.

This father describes an approach that is characteristic of many men in the United States, British Commonwealth, and Sweden. As a boy grows up, he is trained to act "like a man" and not to cry or show feelings such as sadness. Following the model of his own father, he develops a pattern of keeping busy to keep his mind on other matters when a death or serious illness occurs. Many fathers take on additional employment and assume extra community responsibilities so that they are constantly occupied, often traveling great distances each day to meet these obligations and avoid facing their feelings. This often has the effect of interfering with their communication with their wives.

Based on our initial series of interviews with parents after the death of a newborn, at the first two interviews we have made a point of discussing with the parents the problems of a male in the United States. We encourage the wives to help their spouses expess their feelings and tell their husband that it is perfectly all right to cry and to talk about how sad or mad or disappointed or guilty they feel.

PEDIATRICIAN: That's one approach.

MR. DAY: That's the one I know of. And like she mentioned before, I thought it would be nice if I took her out to dinner and to socialize and to make various little suggestions to her as to her liking . . . where she would like to go out.

Again the common reaction is seen of the father that he has to fight against his mourning reaction not only by keeping himself busy but also by keeping his spouse busy. It is our practice to anticipate this possibility at our first contact with the parents by saying that it is desirable to arrange to lighten up on commitments and responsibilities.

PEDIATRICIAN: Have you ever had any feelings or thoughts that there was something that you had done, or that we had done or hadn't done that would have made a difference for the baby?

MR. DAY: I understand now. What could we have done? Medically speaking, we couldn't have done anything because we're not doctors. At the time that the baby was in such distress, we had suggested to the nurse who was taking care of her—since they had to spend round-the-clock hours with her—we had suggested, both of us, that if possible, we would like to do the things that they were doing, *if possible*.

This comment was surprising to the interviewer. Since that interview with Mr. and Mrs. Day, several parents have expressed an interest in becoming involved in the care of their babies in the last minutes or hours of their lives. When we consider that the average parents have spent 20 years plus seven to eight months preparing for a baby, we realize that they believe they have done an incomplete job in producing such a small baby. Because their baby has been taken away from them for care by the experts, it is understandable that many parents may have a strong desire to have a part in their baby's care—and in the process to have a chance to touch and really get to know their baby, who will probably live for only a few more hours. When faced with a baby whose outcome is clearly going to be fatal, Dr. Raymond Duff at Yale–New Haven Hospital, Connecticut, asks parents if they would like to have all of the tubes and apparatus removed so that they can hold their baby while he or she dies.

PEDIATRICIAN: Do you feel that you are getting back in the swing of things? Or do you feel there is still something different about life from day to day in the way you feel?

MRS. DAY: Well, I miss my baby, I know that, and as I say, I'm not going to get over it. I have a certain feeling for her, you know. I carried her for seven months, and I came to the hospital to have her, but then I had to leave without her. You know, when you see other people leaving the hospital with their babies, well, it makes you wonder why your baby isn't there, and why you aren't taking your baby home. And the lady who was leaving at the same time I was leaving had her baby all wrapped up in a bundle in her arms—and our baby was down in the basement.

Several mothers who have lost their own infants have told us about an almost overpowering urge to grab another newborn baby and run away with him or her. These mothers tell us how they have seen a baby of about the same size as their own in front of a supermarket or some other public building and have found themselves touching or almost ready to seize the baby and run off.

MR. DAY: There's a kind of mysterious missing link in an individual when suddenly he loses a part. This is something that's very, very hard to explain. I'm trying to do my best to explain. My feeling is that there is something missing from day-to-day living.

PEDIATRICIAN: Something isn't right.

MR. DAY: Something isn't right. Now I can enjoy myself. I can go out. I sleep well. I eat well. I have other children that I enjoy. I have a wonderful wife, a wonderful home, but there's still that missing piece. This is the way I feel, and I think it will always be there. I don't think that you can eliminate it.

Many parents have described a feeling of great emptiness, reporting how their arms or body ache because of the emptiness left by the loss of their infant.

PEDIATRICIAN: I wanted to go into two or three points. Your feelings are normal for someone who's just lost a baby. Your difficulty in sleeping, in taking up the care of your children, and in getting back into the swing of things is really very normal.

MRS. DAY (quietly): Last night I couldn't sleep, and every time I think about her, I always say I didn't get to name her. And my husband says, "Why didn't you? Forget about naming her, she's gone now." But I will say, "I didn't name her." And my husband looks at me and he says, "Well honey, you didn't name her, so don't think about it so much. Think about the other two kids and raising them." But that's always in my mind.

PEDIATRICIAN: Do you worry about your other two children more than before the baby died?

MRS. DAY: Yes. Is she going to get into anything, is she going to take anything, is she going to wander off, or is somebody going to pick her up?

PEDIATRICIAN: What do you mean?

MRS. DAY: Well, that she'd go outside into the street, and you know, how young fellows sometimes pick babies up. I just sit down and sometimes the craziest things come to me all of a sudden.

PEDIATRICIAN: But you have more of these worries now than before the baby died?

MRS. DAY: Yes. My husband is worried too.

MR. DAY (laughs): I've always worried about them. Of course, I'm health conscious. I want to know how they're feeling all the time. When I'm away, I call to see how they're doing, whether they're eating or not eating—this is the sort of thing I'm worried about, I worry about their health.

At this point the autopsy findings were presented and discussed. The baby's lungs showed many hyaline membranes, and there was an intraventricular hemorrhage. The interviewer emphasized that the baby was physically perfect in all other respects.

MRS. DAY: Do you know why she came early?

PEDIATRICIAN: This is a very important question. Along with our obstetricians we are trying to figure out how to predict which mothers are going to deliver prematures. But at the present I can tell you that we don't know. We have no answers but many questions.

MR. DAY: I was telling my wife about premature babies. I was telling her that when something happens to a baby, I don't know, I am assuming that this is Mother Nature's way of letting you know that something's wrong—a premature child.

It is a common practice to attempt to comfort the mother whose newborn infant has died by explaining that there was really something wrong with her baby, that she never would have been normal and healthy. This type of statement just reinforces the belief of mothers that they have really been very inadequate and have produced very unsatisfactory babies.

PEDIATRICIAN: You mean that something might be wrong with the baby?

MR. DAY: Yes.

PEDIATRICIAN: In the first month or two a large number of babies are lost. When these babies are examined, many have abnormalities. But this isn't true if they are born after the sixth month.

MRS. DAY (to husband who is mumbling): Are you nervous or something?

MR. DAY: Yes, I am.

There is a question whether this nonverbal behavior indicated that the interviewer has challenged one of the beliefs that supported Mr. Day's confidence that the outcome had been reasonably satisfactory. There is always the risk that a physician will say too much and remove one of the props supporting a parent during this difficult period.

MRS. DAY: My mother always tells me about . . . I was fooling with my husband, you know, we always wrestle, and I always pull on him and I used to pick up things—strain—I don't know about straining myself. I think I'm the hard-head type, when you say don't do things.

MR. DAY: Lots of mothers do the same things.

MRS. DAY: I carry my son—you know, he's quite heavy, I was carrying him on my hip to take him up to the barbershop to get a haircut, and the baby kicked me all the way back home.

MR. DAY: I don't think this has anything to do with what he's talking about . . . this brain damage and . . .

MRS. DAY (interrupts): No, no, but he's talking about the baby coming early. . . . This is my mother's old-fashioned talk, and she says that if you play, you must pay. My husband and I play a lot, and I run up and down the steps a lot. I run up and down the street a lot.

MR. DAY (voice rising): People have been pregnant and been in the Olympics and swimming, and running. I don't think this has anything to do with it.

Mr. Day tries and tries to eliminate his wife's guilt and sadness when it would be desirable for her to continue to express her concerns.

(Mr. and Mrs. Day talk together.)

MRS. DAY: Their babies weren't down at the bottom of their stomachs. My baby was.

PEDIATRICIAN: This is one of the things that is under question. One group says that exercise is better. Other people say that rest is better, and I can tell you that neither group knows the right answer.

MRS. DAY: That's right, that's right (laughs loudly).

PEDIATRICIAN: So the doctors are just like you and your wife. Do you have any other questions that we can help you with right now?

MR. DAY (softly): No, no other questions. Jean, is there anything you would like to say? What about the physical and mental condition of the mother at the time of carrying the child with this respiratory disease?

In retrospect we wish we had asked Mr. Day further about what he had in mind. It may well have been that he was relating certain aspects of the physical or the mental state of the mother to the baby's problem.

Although this interview was long and became repetitious, new information continues to emerge. It was difficult to understand the father's early optimism, but it can be appreciated much more easily when we realize that he was a premature infant himself.

PEDIATRICIAN: Were you really?

MR. DAY: Yes, $2^{1}/_{4}$ pounds.

MRS. DAY (laughs): Thanks a lot.

MR. DAY: Yes, I was proud to say that. Yes, $2^{1}/_{4}$ pounds. I weighed $2^{1}/_{4}$ pounds. I didn't have the medical advisors' service that they have today, either.

PEDIATRICIAN: Isn't that interesting. $2^{1}/_{4}$ pounds! I would like to have you come back to see me in about two months, mainly to see how you're doing.

MRS. DAY: It's been very helpful when the doctor is interested like this. It keeps your mind clear. As I was coming up here now, I looked in where the babies are—I can't think of the name right now—and there were little babies in there, and I was thinking, once my baby was in there. That's why I hate to go past that room.

PEDIATRICIAN: It was hard for you to come up here?

MRS. DAY: No, it's not hard for me to come up here, but it's hard for me when I go past. . . . See, I can look in and see the babies in there, and I think, well, my baby was once in there (sighs heavily).

MR. DAY: Well, as I said before, if these discussions can help you in the future with other patients, to improve the individual, I'll be glad to help as much as possible . . . as much as we can.

We have been repeatedly impressed by the cooperativeness of parents and particularly by their appreciation for an opportunity to improve care for other patients and the education for physicians. This may give the parents a greater meaning for the life of their baby.

MRS. DAY: It helps me to talk about it. . . . My husband says, "Don't talk about it so much." It kind of eased my nerves a little bit.

PEDIATRICIAN: We have the impression that if you talk about something which worries you, it's better. There have been some studies about grieving after death, and they indicate that if you tend to hold everything back, it tends to make the resolution more difficult years later.

MR. DAY (interrupting): What about the individual that *never* talks about it?

PEDIATRICIAN: We don't know.

MR. DAY: This would be a finding also. You would have to study into this. This is something now that I have . . . (long pause) . . . I think, as I said before . . . it's part of life. These things are bound to happen. And we have to learn to cope with them. And I just go on living day to day, and I have other things and other duties to perform. If I break down now, somebody will have to pick these people up . . . somebody's going to have to pull them together and help them if I break down. So I just keep going and try to keep busy (louder) and keep from thinking and keep from worrying about these things. So I just don't talk about it. With some people it's just the opposite. I can see how talking may help you, but it keeps you from doing a lot of other things.

PEDIATRICIAN: What you say is very true, but maybe in life there has to be a period where you recover . . . we don't know. In general, we have known that it takes a lot of emotional and physical work to bottle things up. Sometimes things just have to get out.

MR. DAY: It takes a long time.

PEDIATRICIAN: Oh, yes.

MR. DAY: Maybe I'm doing this under a tremendous strain, but I'm the only one to determine this.

PEDIATRICIAN: Yes.

MR. DAY: By closing this door upon something that has happened, as if it didn't happen, maybe it's wrong. Maybe it's wrong for me 4 or 5, 10, 15, 20 years from now . . .

MR. DAY (loudly): I'm doing what I think is right because I have other responsibilities.

MRS. DAY: Put that ruler down—you're making me nervous (laughs).

MR. DAY (continues loudly): Because I have other responsibilities.

MRS. DAY (laughs again): You make me nervous . . . you know, this is what I was thinking about. When . . . I suffered with her so long . . . and then to lose her . . . from 7:00 that Monday morning until 6:35 that Tuesday to have her. It's a wonder I don't lose my mind . . .

MR. DAY: What do they call it when they . . .

PEDIATRICIAN: A cesarean section.

MRS. DAY: Yes, that's what he was going to do when she hadn't moved.

This was a long interview. If the physician's time is limited, it is likely that the information will come out at a subsequent interview if the physician is ready to sit and listen.

COMMENT: The Days show how useful it is to talk to parents together. We then enable each spouse to take responsibility for their own feelings and fantasies rather than lose them in their partner. When Mr. Day denies his sense of guilt by giving it to his wife to look after, he deprives

himself of help with the understanding of his own feelings while at the same time overburdening his wife, who then feels like an evil witch. Mr. Day eventually owns up to a source of his anxiety, his fantasies about his own premature birth. This case underlines the importance of taking a detailed obstetrical history, not only of the bereaved mother but also of both grandmothers. Mr. Day's feelings could then have been more quickly brought into the discussion.
E. Lewis

COMMENT: Although it may be helpful to mention possible manifestations of distress, it needs to be emphasized that each individual copes with it differently. When individuals understand and respect each other's ways of grieving, they will be able to find the necessary and mutually helpful opportunities for sharing painful thoughts and feelings. The parents' need for activity and restoration of self-esteem is best channeled into the task of supporting each other and especially into assisting their children in mastering the stress. Hard though it may be to help youngsters to understand the tragedy and to meet their needs, ultimately a parent's self-esteem is augmented most by being an effective parent. He could never forgive himself if, in his concern over one lost child, he were to lose the continuity of his relationship with the other children. Even very young children prove to be caring companions in grief, if given the chance. In working it through with his child, the parent often gains mastery himself. It would seem wise in the second interview, if there are children at home, actively to direct the mourning parents to this task for the children's sake but also their own. Clinically, one of the best indications of the parents' healthy progress in mourning is their ability to discuss and feel the loss with their children.
E. Furman

RECOMMENDATIONS FOR CARE

1. *Parental contact with infant.* If a mother loses an infant any time after she has felt fetal movement, she will usually go through a long period of intense mourning. To help with the mourning process, we encourage mothers to see and handle their infant after he has died. Some of our mothers have cleaned and diapered the baby after his death. Others have gone to the mortuary, looked at the baby closely in private surroundings, and picked him up. In the situation where the mother is still confined in another hospital, parents have requested a picture of the infant after he has died. Each of these arrangements is upsetting to some of the nurses and physicians, but it has been our experience that each helps make the death real. At first one might think that it is only good to remember the baby as a normal active infant, but it is our present belief that it is important for some parents to see the infant after he has died so that they have a clear, visual proof that the baby really died, and they should be offered this opportunity. Many mothers have told us about having lost a baby in the past and wishing for years that they could have seen, touched, handled, or even seen a picture of him before he was taken away. Many had none of these opportunities.

2. *When the baby is stillborn.* When the diagnosis of stillbirth is established in utero, both parents should be fully informed and the events surrounding labor and delivery explained throughly. The father and mother should be together during labor and delivery. As much as possible, an atmosphere of understanding and mutual support should be established between the bereaved parents and the medical staff.

Lewis (1978, 1979) emphasizes the importance of establishing the stillborn infant's identity and reminds us that a death without a body which has been seen by a family member seems unreal. Grief following stillbirth is susceptible to distortion, since there are no postpartum experiences with the baby to remember, and the infant is often perceived as someone who did not exist, a person without a name. This sense of nonexistence is exaggerated in women who are heavily sedated or anesthetized during delivery and thereby deprived of the memories necessary for normal grief. The infant's identity can best be established if the bereaved parents are encouraged to look at, touch, and hold their child.

Sometimes the parents may find the idea of holding a dead baby abhorrent at first. But after the baby is dead, there is no need to rush. We have found that parents will frequently change their minds and want to see and hold the baby an hour or a few hours later, even though they refused the first time this was offered. To facilitate this we may keep the baby on the delivery floor for a few hours. We can explain that almost all parents have been pleased that they saw and held their stillborn infant. We have been impressed that the mourning process is particularly prolonged and difficult to resolve when the stillborn infant has not been seen or held by the parents. On the other hand, parents who have held their stillborn infant or dead neonate report that this was a positive and meaningful experience they "never would have wanted to miss."

We were hesitant at first about suggesting that parents see and hold macerated or severely deformed stillborn infants. However, we have gradually come to appreciate that almost no baby is so deformed that the parents will not benefit from viewing the infant—if they wish. It is often possible to present such babies, for example, a baby with anencephaly, to parents using receiving blankets in a way that minimizes any shock which might arise from seeing the malformation. Even with extensive malformations most of the baby is "normal" and well formed.

The experience of seeing and holding a stillborn infant may temporarily deepen the sadness of both parents, but it provides concrete memories which will facilitate normal mourning. If they have any inclination to do so, it is helpful if the parents name their baby. This is another way of acknowledging the child's reality and will help the parents later when they think and talk about the child. Some parents have expressed anger that stillborn babies are not given birth certificates.

It is highly desirable to obtain a photograph of every stillborn or live-born infant who dies, even if the parents do not wish to see it at that time.

3. *Hospitalizing the family.* Thanks to the cooperation of the nursing staff in our maternity hospital, we have now had experience with several fathers living in the maternity hospital in the same room with mothers after the death of their infant. It is our impression that this opportunity for the parents to be together and to hold each other and support each other and to discuss their intense reaction has been helpful in starting a process of communication between the parents. It appears to

enhance their willingness to discuss disappointments, anger, sadness, and pain openly and freely. The experience in the hospital provides an isolation for the parents from the pressures of the outside world. Arrangements can be made for telephone calls to be held during the days and nights that the father lives in with the mother.

4. *Funeral arrangements.* We have found it valuable, if the parents choose, to have a funeral. This facilitates the grieving process. Our own suggestion is a simple funeral with only the immediate family present. We do have arrangements for our hospital to dispose of the infant with cremation and burial in the hospital's plot, without charge, if the family so desires. When parents decide to have their baby cremated, we encourage them to go ahead with a small private service in their own place of worship.

5. *Second interview.* After the death of an infant we meet with both parents together, and sometimes with their own parents, usually within the first three days but at least within the first week (first interview immediately after the death, p. 273). This meeting generally lasts for about an hour. We discuss the importance of accepting one's feelings instead of pulling oneself out of the depression or trying to get back to normal activities. We especially advise husbands to be honest with their wives, to tell them if they have a sad or a rough day. They will often be afraid of expressing their emotions for fear that they will hurt their wives and cause them to cry. This openness permits the wife to express the difficult feelings she has had, and the couple can communicate and work out their grief together.

Bowlby (1979) has noted other important facets of this care:

> If we are to give the kind of help to a bereaved person that we should all like to give, it is essential we see things from his point of view and respect his or her feelings—unrealistic though we may regard some of them to be. For only if a bereaved person feels that we can at least understand and sympathize with him in the task he sets himself is there much likelihood that he will be able to express the feelings that are bursting within him—his yearning for the return of the lost figure, his hope against hope that miraculously all may yet be well, his rage at being deserted, his angry, unfair reproaches against those "incompetent doctors," those unhelpful nurses, and against his own guilty self; if only he'd done so and so, or not done so and so, disaster might perhaps have been averted.*

It is valuable to have the couple's parents present at this early discussion so that they can appreciate the needs of their children and can provide a major support and listening post for them. If a grandparent is not available, we encourage the mother to share her thoughts with another close friend. It is necessary to explain to the parents that many of their friends will not know how to react to the death of

---

*From Bowlby, J.: The making and breaking of affectional bonds, London, 1979, Tavistock Publications, Ltd., p. 69.

their baby. They will often say something to the effect that if the baby was damaged, he is better off dead. And in the United States they may believe that since the mother and father never took the baby home, there will be little grief and mourning. In other words, there will have been little attachment and therefore little feeling of loss.

Since most young people have had minimal or no experience with neonatal death, the parents appear to benefit from hearing how other people react to the loss of an infant. We explain that normal healthy people generally feel angry after they have lost someone close to them—angry at themselves, at the doctors, and at the nurses. Guilt is also experienced for things that were or were not done. We explain that the most valuable thing they can do is to let their feelings out and not rush to pull themselves back to any of their usual daily tasks, such as work, cleaning the house, visiting friends, going out to dinner, parties, and shows, or watching television unless they really feel like it.

It is important that this long discussion take place at least a day after the death of the infant. The parents are usually too overwhelmed on the day of the death to think about their own future and their own needs. Generally they only hear that the infant has died. In our discussions we encourage them to telephone and talk with us, to continue the relationship. We make an appointment for the parents to come back in three months.

6. *Benefits of a telephone call.* If parents for any reason do not come for an appointment, Schreiner and co-workers (1979) have documented that a telephone call nine days after the death, ranging in length from 15 to 40 minutes (mean 26 minutes) significantly decreased the number of major emotional problems assessed at an interview eight to 26 weeks later. They stress the importance of calling at night to involve the father.

7. *Avoiding tranquilizers.* We strongly encourage that parents take no tranquilizers. This tends to dull the mourning reaction in such a way that it may never fully develop, and the parents are left without having fully worked through the experience. On a few occasions we recommend a sedative to be taken solely at bedtime.

8. *Planning for another baby.* During the initial discussions we strongly encourage the parents to refrain from having a replacement infant until they have completed their mourning reaction. We explain that it is difficult to take on a new baby at the same time one is giving up the baby who has died. These two processes are moving in the opposite directions and are extremely difficult to accomplish simultaneously. Therefore we ask the parents to wait six months to a year before planning for another baby. We encourage them to plan for a new baby in its own right, not to replace the baby who has just died. This has been noted by Engel (1964).

9. *Group discussions.* Recently we have found that many mothers who have just

lost babies find it helpful to read the diaries of other mothers who have experienced the same loss. We organized a discussion group for mothers whose infants have died. Many of these mothers have mentioned that only a mother who has lost a baby can really appreciate the pain involved. A similar group has been helpful for mothers in several large cities whose babies have died from the sudden infant death syndrome (SIDS). Up to the present time it has been difficult for parents who have lost a newborn to find any other parents who have had a similar experience. The parents' experience in these groups has appeared to be especially helpful in dealing with many issues.

10. *Third interview*. At this time we discuss any questions the parents may have. On the surface it appears that the parents are coming back to ask questions or to learn something more about the autopsy data, if there has been an autopsy. However, the major reason that they should come back is for us to determine whether the mourning process is progressing normally or whether there is evidence of pathological grief as defined by Lindemann (1944). This may show itself by no grief at all or by continuing, unremitting grief. (A more complete definition can be seen on p. 261.) During this session we chat with the parents to see how they are doing and ask some of the following questions:

> Have you gone out at all?
> How are your other children doing?
> Have you been able to talk about the death with each other and with the children?
> How is your eating?
> How are you sleeping?
> Are you watching television yet?
> Have you had friends over?

In other words, we are trying to learn about their daily patterns of living, focusing on whether grieving at this time is still going on, is slightly lessened, is felt in dips of sad periods each day with some crying, or whether there is a change in daily habit patterns, such as sleeping, eating, interest in television, movies, visiting, hobbies, and eating out. It is often helpful to ask each parent to comment about changes in the behavior of his or her spouse and ask how the spouse's mourning process is progressing. In our experience grief usually continues for a period of seven to nine months. Generally by this interview it has lessened, since the parents have had the opportunity to release their strong feelings about the infant and hence are able to resume their normal way of life. Often we have noticed that the marriage appears to be stronger after this period of mourning, the parents appear to be better prepared to face the ups and downs of life. We usually discuss the autopsy results near the end of the meeting.

We make the appointment for the three-month visit, and if the parents do not keep it, we call them, since we believe the visit is important. About one half of the parents find the thought of returning to the unit very difficult, although they usually seem relieved once they do come.

11. *Pathological grief.* Each year a small number of mothers, even those with special interventions, experience pathological grief. As soon as we are aware of this, we believe that it is extremely important that they be referred to a psychiatrist.

12. *Distorted mourning.* The loss of a close relative (father, husband, or one of twins) during or shortly after pregnancy may inhibit or severly distort the mourning process. Lewis (1979) has reported that when a woman loses her husband or a very close friend or relative during her pregnancy, she has to choose between mourning that loss or proceeding with the positive aspects of her pregnancy. He points out that mothers almost invariably choose the latter course, which postpones the mourning. This may have harmful effects for the mother and baby later on. The optimal management of this is not clear. If the event occurs early in the pregnancy, can the mother be encouraged to proceed with her mourning? If not, it is important to discuss what is going on and to help the mother plan to let down and experience her mourning reactions after her attachment to the baby has been firmly established and the baby is doing well. This situation is similar to the dilemma when parents lose one of a pair of twins.

13. *Other children.* If there is another child in the family, it is important to explain to the child what is happening. The surviving children sometimes feel overwhelmed and somehow guilty or responsible for the infant's death. It is important to help these children discuss their feelings. It is also wise to remind the parents to explain that they themselves are crying because of the sadness of the loss of the baby, not because they are angry at the other children, and how good it is to have them nearby.

It is not unusual for some of the siblings to need special guidance. When this is the case, it has been most useful to have the parents discuss the problems with a child guidance worker.

14. *Value of listening.* The specific suggestions just presented are misleading because there is so much emphasis on what the physician says. During visits with the parents much of the time is spent listening, often with long periods of silence or crying. On a busy day this sitting and listening is particularly difficult for a physician, but it is time well spent.

15. *Training house officers.* Interns and residents have an extremely difficult time discussing these issues with parents in their early months and years of training. They usually believe that their job is the treatment of the infant and have severe guilt feelings, wondering if they failed to do something that could have saved the infant's life. This feeling is perpetuated by the procedures in the hospital, such as the perinatal mortality committee meetings each week. Therefore, at the suggestion of Barbero (1973), we have made a strong effort to join house officers the first four or five times they talk with parents who have lost an infant. They observe how we handle the interviews, and then we observe their next three or four encounters. After the interview we discuss it for about half an hour. We ask them what they might have done differently, how we might have talked differently to the

parents, what the strong points were, and what the difficult points were in this encounter. In a sense it can be compared with the procedure in showing them how to insert a catheter. We show them once or twice, then we watch them, and finally they do it on their own. We believe that this is an essential part of the training in perinatal care for any physician planning to specialize in pediatrics.

16. *Staff meetings*. When the nurses, physicians, and other staff members of the unit are working well, they often experience mourning reactions after the death of one of the infants for whom they have cared. We have found it extremely valuable for the nurses and physicians to have a time to talk about their feelings. Our own unit works best when we have group meetings every other week and openly discuss our own feelings about the problem. Strong reactions relating to the death of some infants are often voiced. In one case a nurse asked, "You don't tell us why the baby died, Dr. _____. We wonder if we caused the death by our bagging. Did we produce the intraventricular hemorrhage? Would you please explain why each of the infants died? It would help us." We have had some house officers who experienced considerable difficulty with the newborn service because they expected themselves to be almost perfect in preventing the death of every infant under their care. In any active neonatal intensive care unit there are a number of deaths each week. This is difficult for certain house officers and nurses, and they need special personal help in coping with this high mortality. Surprisingly, it has usually been those house officers who demand perfection in themselves and expect to give an extremely high quality of care who have been most distraught in the nursery. Some have developed diarrhea, weight loss, and other worrisome symptoms. In a true sense the nursery is like an extended family, with the director and head nurse playing an important role in maintaining high morale.

REFERENCES

Adamsons, K., Mueller-Heubach, E., and Meyers, R.E.: Production of fetal asphyxia in the rhesus monkey by administration of catecholamines to the mother, Am. J. Obstet. Gynecol. **109**:248-262, 1971.

Ahrens, R.: Beitrag zur Entwicklung des Physiognomie und Mimikerkehnens, Z. Exp. Angew. Psychol. **2**:412-454, 1964.

Ainsworth, M.D.S., and Bell, S.M.: Attachment, exploration and separation: illustrated by the behavior of one-year-olds in a strange situation, Child Dev. **41**:49-67, 1970.

Ainsworth, M.D.S., Bell, S.M., and Slayton, D.J.: In Richards, M.P.M., editor: The integration of a child into a social world, New York, 1974, Cambridge University Press.

Ali, Z., and Lowry, M.: Early maternal-child contact: effects on later behaviour. Accepted for publication in Dev. Med. Child Neurol.

Als, H.: The newborn communicates, J. Communication **27**:66-73, 1977.

Als, H., Lester, B.M., and Brazelton, T.B.: Dynamics of the behavioral organization of the premature infant, In Field, T., editor: The high risk newborn, Jamaica, N.Y., 1978, Spectrum Publications, Inc.

Als, H., Lester, B.M., and Brazelton, T.B.: Dynamics of the behavioral organization of the premature infant: a theoretical perspective, In Field, T., et al., editors: Infants born at risk, Jamaica, N.Y., 1979, Spectrum Publications, Inc.

Altmann, M.: In Rheingold, H. R., editor: Maternal behavior in mammals, New York, 1963, John Wiley & Sons, Inc.

Ambuel, J., and Harris, B.: Failure to thrive: a study of failure to grow in height or weight, Ohio Med. J. **59**:997-1001, 1963.

Anderson, S.V.D. Siblings at birth: a survey and study, Birth Fam. J. **6**:80-87, 1979.

Anisfeld, E., and Lipper, E.: Effects of perinatal events on mother-infant bonding, presented at Society for Research in Child Development Biennial Meeting, April 3, 1981.

Anthony, E.J., and Benedek, T.: Parenthood, its psychology and psychopathology, Boston, 1970, Little, Brown & Co., Inc.

Apley, J., Barbour, R.F., and Westmacott, I.: Impact of congenital heart disease on the family: preliminary report, Br. Med. J. **1**:103-105, 1967.

Arms, S.: Immaculate deception, New York, 1975, Bantam Books.

Avery, J.: Personal communication, 1973.

Bakeman, R., and Brown, J.V. : Early interaction: consequences for social and mental development at three years, Child Dev. **51**:437-447, 1980.

Ballard, R.A., Ferris, C.B., Read, F., et al.: The hospital alternative birth center (ABC): is it safe? (abstract), Pediatr. Res. **14**:590, 1980.

Ballou, J.W.: The psychology of pregnancy, Lexington, Mass., 1978*a*, Lexington Books, D.C. Heath and Co.

Ballou, J.W.: The significance of reconciliative themes in the psychology of pregnancy, Bull. Menninger Clin. **42**(5): 383-413, 1978*b*.

Barbero, G.: Personal communication, 1973.

Barnard, K.: A program of stimulation for infants born prematurely, Seattle, 1975, University of Washington Press.

Barnett, C.R., Grobstein, R., and Seashore, M.: Personal communication, 1972.

Barnett, C.R., Leiderman, P.H., Grobstein, R., and Klaus, M.H.: Neonatal separation: the maternal side of interactional deprivation, Pediatrics **45**:197-205, 1970.

Barton, M.D., Killam, A.P., and Meschia, G.: Response of ovine uterine blood flow to epinephrine and norepinephrine, Proc. Soc. Exp. Biol. Med. **145**:996-1003, 1974.

Bateson, P.: How do sensitive periods arise and what are they for? Animal Behav. **27**:470-486, 1979.

Beckwith, L., and Cohen, S.E.: Preterm birth: hazardous obstetrical and postnatal events as related to caregiver-infant behavior, Infant Behav. Dev. **1**, 1978.

Bell, J.E.: The family in the hospital, Bethesda, Md., 1960, National Institute of Mental Health.

Benedek, T.: Studies in psychosomatic medicine: the psycho-sexual function in women, New York, 1952, Ronald Press Co.

Benfield, D.G., Leib, S.A., and Reutor, J.: Grief response of parents following referral of the critically ill newborn, N. Engl. J. Med. **294:**975-978, 1976.

Benfield, D.G. et al.: Grief response of parents to neonatal death and parent participation in deciding care, Pediatrics **62:**171-177, 1978.

Ben Shaul, D.M.: Notes on hand-rearing various species of mammals, Int. Zoo Yearbook **4:**300, 1962.

Berg, R.B., and Salisbury, A.: Discharging infants of low birth weight: reconsiderations of current practice, Am. J. Dis. Child. **122:**414-417, 1971.

Berkson, G.: In Lewis, M., and Rosenblum, L.A., editors: The effect of the infant on its caregiver, New York, 1974, John Wiley & Sons, Inc.

Bernal, J.F., and Richards, M.P.: In Barnett, A., editor: Ethology and development, London, 1972, Little Club Clinics in Developmental Medicine, Vol. II.

Bess, F.H., Peek, B.F., and Chapman, J.J.: Further observations on noise levels in infant incubators, Pediatrics **63:**100-106, 1979.

Bettelheim, B.: How do you help a child who has a physical handicap? Ladies Home J. **89:**34-35, 1972.

Bibring, G.L.: Some considerations of the psychological processes in pregnancy, Psychoanal. Study Child **14:**113-121, 1959.

Bibring, G.L., Dwyer, T.F., Huntington, D.S., and Valenstein, A.F.: A study of the psychological processes in pregnancy and of the earliest mother-child relationship. I. Some propositions and comments, Psychoanal. Study Child **16:**9-27, 1961.

Bibring, G.L., and Valenstein, A.F.: Psychological aspects of pregnancy, Clin. Obstet. Gynecol. **19:**357-371, 1976.

Bittman, S., and Rosenberg, S.: Expectant fathers, New York, 1978, Ballantine Books, Inc.

Blake, A., Stewart, A., and Turcan, D.: In Parent-infant interaction, Ciba Foundation Symposium 33, Amsterdam, 1975, Elsevier Publishing Co.

Blau, A., Slaff, B., Easton, R., Welkowitz, J., Springain, J., and Cohen, J.: The psychogenic etiology of premature births, a preliminary report, Psychosom. Med. **25:**201-211, 1963.

Blurton Jones, N.: Comparative aspects of mother-child contact. In Blurton Jones, N., editor: Ethological studies of child behavior, New York, 1972, Cambridge University Press.

Boston Women's Health Book Collective: Our bodies, ourselves, New York, 1976, Simon & Schuster, Inc.

Bourne, S.G.: The psychological effects of stillbirths on women and their doctors J. R. Coll. Gen. Pract. **16:**103-112, 1968.

Bowlby J.: Nature of a child's tie to his mother, Int. J. Psychoanal. **39:**350-373, 1958.

Bowlby, J.: Attachment and loss, New York, 1969, Basic Books, Inc., Publishers, Vol. 1.

Bowlby, J.: The making and breaking of affectional bonds, Br. J. Psychiatry **130:**201-210, 1977.

Bowlby, J.: The making and breaking of affectional bonds, London, 1979, Tavistock Publications, Ltd.

Boyle, M., Griffin, A., and Fitzhardinge, P.: The very low birthweight infant: impact on parents during the pre-school years, Early Hum. Dev. **1**(2):191-201, 1977.

Boyd, S.: Parental involvement in the interactive behavioral assessment process. Unpublished doctoral dissertation, Denton, Tex., 1980, Texas Woman's University College of Nursing.

Brandt, E.M., and Mitchell, G.: In Rosenblum, L.A., editor: Primate behavior: developments in field and laboratory research, New York, 1971, Academic Press, Inc., Vol. II.

Brazelton, T.B.: Psychophysiologic reaction in the neonate. II. Effects of maternal medication on the neonate and his behavior. J. Pediatr. **58:**513-518, 1961.

Brazelton, T.B.: The early mother-infant adjustment, Pediatrics **32:**931-938, 1963.

Brazelton, T.B.: Implications of infant development among the Mayan Indians of Mexico, Hum. Dev. **15:**90-111, 1972.

Brazelton, T.B.: Effect of maternal expectations on early infant behavior, Early Child Dev. Care **2:**259-273, 1973.

Brazelton, T.B., Koslowski, B., and Main, M.: In Lewis, M., and Rosenblum, L.A., editors: The effect of the infant on its caregiver, New York, 1974, John Wiley & Sons, Inc.

Brazelton, T.B., School, M.L., and Robey, J.S.: Visual responses in the newborn, Pediatrics **37:**284-290, 1966.

Brazelton, T.B., Tronick, E., Adamson, L., Als, H., and Wise, S.: In Parent infant interaction, Ciba Foundation Symposium 33, Amsterdam, 1975, Elsevier Publishing Co.

Bridges, R.S.: Long-term effects of pregnancy and parturition upon maternal responsiveness in the rat, Physiol. Behav. **14:**245-249, 1975.

Bridges, R.S.: Parturition: its role in the long-term retention of maternal behavior in the rat, Physiol. Behav. **18:**487-490, 1977.

Brimblecombe, F.S.W., Richards, M.P.M., and Roberton, N.R.C., editors: Separation and special-care baby units, London, 1978, Heinemann Medical Books.

Brimblecombe, F.S.W., Robinson, J., Edelsten, A.D., and Jones, J.: A review of infant handicap and neonatal mortality in relation to the use of a special-care unit. In Brimblecombe, F.S.W., et al., editors: Separation and special-care baby units, London, 1978, Heinemann Medical Books.

Brody, E.B., and Klein, H.: The intensive care nursery as a small society, its contribution to the socialization and learning of the pediatric intern, Paediatrician **9:**169-181, 1980.

Bronfenbrenner, U.: Early deprivation in mammals: a cross-species analysis. In Newton, G. and Levine, S., editors: Early experience and behavior, Springfield, Ill., 1968, Charles C Thomas, Publisher.

Broussard, E., and Hartner, M.: Maternal perception of the neonate as related to development, Child Psychol. Hum. Dev. **1**(1):16-25, 1970.

Brown, G.W., and Harris, T.: Social origins of depression (a study of psychiatric disorder in women), London, 1978, Tavistock Publications, Ltd.

Brown, J.V., and Bakeman, R.: Relationships of human mothers with their infants during the first year of life: effects of prematurity. In Bell, R.W., and Smotherman, W.P. editors: Maternal influence and early behavior, Jamaica, N.Y., 1980, Spectrum Publications, Inc.

Brown, J.V., LaRossa, M.M., Aylward, G.P., Davis, D.J., Rutherford, P.K., and Bakeman, R.: Nursery-based intervention with prematurely born babies and their mothers: are there effects? J. Pediatr. **97:**487-491, 1980.

Bryer, K.B.: The Amish way of death, Am. Psychol. **34:**255-261, 1979.

Budin, P.: The nursling, London, 1907, Caxton Publishing Co.

Caldeyro-Barcia, R.: The influence of maternal bearing-down efforts during second stage on fetal well-being, Birth Fam. J. **6:**17-21, 1979*a*.

Caldeyro-Barcia, R.: The influence of maternal position on time of spontaneous rupture of the membranes, progress of labor, and fetal head compression, Birth Fam. J. **6:**7-13, 1979*b*.

Campbell, S.B.G., and Taylor, P.M.: Bonding and attachment: theoretical issues, Semin. Perinatol. **3:**3-13, 1979.

Caplan, G.: Patterns of parental response to the crisis of premature birth, Psychiatry **23:**365-374, 1960.

Caplan, G.: Principles of preventive psychiatry, New York, 1964, Grune & Stratton, Inc.

Caplan, G., Mason, E., and Kaplan, D.M.: Four studies of crisis in parents of prematures, Community Ment. Health J. **1:**149-161, 1965.

Carlsson, S.G., Fagerberg, H., Horneman, G., Hwang, P., Larsson, K., Rödholm, M., Schaller, J., Danielsson, B., and Gundewall, C.: Effects of various amounts of contact between mother and child on the mother's nursing behavior, Dev. Psychobiol. **11:**143, 1978.

Carlsson, S.G., Fagerburg, H., Horneman, G., Hwang, G.P., Larsson, K., Rödholm, M., Schaller, J., Danielsson, B., and Gundewall, C.: Effects of various amounts of contact between mother and child on the mother's nursing behavior: a follow-up study. Infant Behav. Dev. **2:**209-214, 1979.

Carr, E.F., Oppé, J.E.: The birth of an abnormal child: telling the parents, Lancet **2:**1075-1077, 1971.

Carter, C.O.: Major mental handicap: methods and costs of prevention, Ciba Foundation Symposium 59, Amsterdam, 1978, Elsevier Publishing Co.

Cassel, Z.K., and Sander, L.W.: Neonatal recognition processes and attachment: the masking experiment. Presented at the Society for Research in Child Development, Denver, 1975.

Chalmers, I.: Randomized controlled trials of intrapartum fetal monitoring. In Thalhammer, I., et al., editors: Perinatal medicine, Sixth European Congress, Stuttgart, 1979, Georg Thieme.

Chard, T., and Richards, M., editors: Benefits and hazards of the new obstetrics, Philadelphia, 1977, J.B. Lippincott Co.

Cohen, R.L.: Some maladaptive syndromes of pregnancy and the puerperium, Obstet. Gynecol. **27:**562-570, 1966.

Collias, N.E.: The analysis of socialization in sheep and goats, Ecology **37:**228-239, 1956.

Collingwood, J., and Alberman, E.: Separation at birth and the mother-child relationship, Dev. Med. Child Neurol. **21**:608-618, 1979.

Condon, W.S., and Sander, L.W.: Neonate movement is synchronized with adult speech: interactional participation and language acquisition, Science **183**:99-101, 1974.

Cook, P.S.: Childrearing culture and mental health: exploring an ethological-evolutionary perspective in child psychiatry and preventive mental health with particular reference to two contrasting approaches to early childrearing, Med. J. Aust. **2**(supp.):3-14, 1978.

Corbin, J.: Protective governing: strategies for managing a pregnancy-illness. Doctoral dissertation, San Francisco, 1981, University of California.

Cornell, E.H., and Gottfried, A.W.: Intervention with premature human infants, Child Dev. **47**:32-39, 1976.

Cosnier, J.: Quelques problémes posés par le "comportement maternel provoqué" chez la Ratte, Comptes Rendus Soc. Biol. **157**:1611-1613, 1963.

Cosnier, J., and Couturier, C.: Comportement maternel provaqué chez les Rattes adultes castrées, Comptes Rendus Soc. Biol. **160**:789-791, 1966.

Crook, J.H., editor: Social behaviour in birds and mammals, New York, 1970, Academic Press, Inc.

Crosse, V.M.: The premature baby, ed. 4, Boston, 1957, Little, Brown & Co., Inc.

Cullberg, J.: In Psychosomatic medicine in obstetrics and gynaecology, 3rd International Congress, Basel, 1972, S. Karger.

Curry, M.A.: Contact during the first hour with the wrapped or naked newborn: effect on maternal attachment behaviors at 36 hours and 3 months, Birth Fam. J. **6**:227-235, 1979.

Curry, M.A.: The effect of skin-to-skin contact between mother and infant during the first hour following delivery on the mother's maternal attachment behavior and self concept, unpublished doctoral dissertation, San Francisco, 1979, University of California.

Daniels, L.L., and Berg, G.M.: The crisis of birth and adaptive patterns of amputee children, Clin. Proc. Child. Hosp. D.C. **24**:108-117, 1968.

D'Arcy, E.: Congenital defects: mothers' reactions to first information, Br. Med. J. **3**:796-798, 1968.

Darwin, C.: The descent of man and selection in relation to sex, New York, 1871, D. Appleton & Co.

Davies, D.P., Herbert, S., Haxby, V., and McNeish, A.S.: When should pre-term babies be sent home from neonatal units? Lancet **1**:914-915, 1979.

DeCarvalho, M., Klaus, M.H., and Merkatz, R.: The effects of frequency and duration of breast feeding on serum bilirubin, weight gain and milk output, Pediatr. Res. **15**:530, 1981.

DeCasper, A.J., and Fifer, W.P.: The fetal sound environment of sheep, Science **208**:1173-1176, 1980.

De Chateau, P.: Neonatal care routines: influences on maternal and infant behavior and on breast feeding (thesis), Umea, Sweden, 1976, Umea University Medical Dissertations, N.S., no. 20.

De Chateau, P.: Personal communication, 1974.

De Chateau, P., and Wiberg, B.: Long-term effect on mother-infant behaviour of extra contact during the first hour post partum. I. First observations at 36 hours, Acta Paediatr. Scand. **66**:137, 1977*a*.

De Chateau, P., and Wiberg, B.: Long-term effect on mother-infant behaviour of extra contact during the first hour post partum. II. Follow-up at three months, Acta Paediatr. Scand. **66**:145, 1977*b*.

Desmond, M.M., Rudolph, A.J., and Phitaksphraiwan, P.: The transitional care nursery: a mechanism of a preventive medicine, Pediatr. Clin. North Am. **13**:651-668, 1966.

Deutsch, H.: The psychology of women: a psychoanalytic interpretation, New York, 1945, Grune & Stratton, Inc., Vol. II.

Dillard, R.G., and Korones, S.B.: Lower discharge weight and shortened nursery stay for low birth-weight infants, N. Engl. J. Med. **288**:131-133, 1973.

DiVitto, B., and Goldberg, S.: The development of early parent-infant interaction as a function of newborn medical status. In Field, T., Sostek, A., Goldberg, S., and Shuman, H.H., editors: Infants born at risk, Jamaica, N.Y., 1979, Spectrum Publications, Inc.

Dolhinow, P., editor: Primate patterns, New York, 1972, Holt, Rinehart & Winston, Inc.

Douglas, J.W.B.: Early hospital admissions and later disturbances of behaviour and learning, Dev. Med. Child Neurol. **17**:456-480, 1975.

Douglas, J.W.B., and Gear, T.: Children of low

birthweight in the 1946 national cohort, Arch. Dis. Child 51:820-827, 1976.

Drillien, C.M.: The long-term prospects of handicap in babies of low birth weight, Hosp. Med. 1:937-944, 1967.

Drillien, C.M., Jameson, S., and Wilkinson, E.M.: Studies in mental handicap. I. Prevalence and distribution by clinical type and severity of defect, Arch. Dis. Child. 41:528-538, 1966.

Drotar, D., and Irvin, N.: Disturbed maternal bereavement following infant death, Child Care Health Dev. 5:239-247, 1979.

Drotar, D., Baskiewicz, A., Irvin, N., Kennell, J.H., and Klaus, M.H.: The adaptation of parents to the birth of an infant with a congenital malformation: a hypothetical model, Pediatrics 56:710-717, 1975.

Dubois, D.R.: Indications of an unhealthy relationship between parents and premature infant, J.O.G.N. Nurs. 4:21-24, 1975.

Dunn, J.: Distress and comfort, Cambridge, 1977, Harvard University Press.

Dunn, J.B., and Richards, M.P.M.: Observations on the developing relationship between mother and baby in the neonatal period. In Shaffer, H.R., editor: Studies in mother-infant interaction, London, 1977, Academic Press, Ltd.

Dunn, P.M.: Obstetric delivery today: for better or for worse? Lancet 1:790-793, 1976.

Eisenberg, R. B.: Auditory competence in early life: the roots of communicative behavior, Baltimore, Md., 1976, University Park Press.

Elliott, B., and Hein, H.: Neonatal death: reflections for physicians, Pediatrics 62:96-102, 1978.

Elmer, E., and Gregg, G.S.: Developmental characteristics of abused children, Pediatrics 40:596-602, 1967.

Emde, R.N., and Robinson, J.: The first two months: recent research in developmental psychobiology and the changing view of the newborn. In Noshpitz, J., and Call, J., editors: Basic handbook of child psychiatry, New York, Basic Books, Inc., Publishers, in press.

Engel, F.: Grief and grieving, Am. J. Nurs. 64:93-98, 1964.

Enkin, M.W., Smith, S.L., Dermer, S.W., and Emmett, J.O.: An adequately controlled study of the effectiveness of PPM training, Psychosomatic Medicine in Obstetrics and Gynaecology 3rd International Congress, Basel, 1972, S. Karger.

Erdman, D.: Neonatal intensive care. Parent-to-parent support: the best for those with sick newborns, Am. J. Mat. Child Nurs. 2:291-292, Sept./Oct., 1977.

Evans, S., Reinhart, J., and Succop, P.: A study of 45 children and their families, J. Am. Acad. Child Psychiatry 11:440-454, 1972.

Ewer, R.F.: Ethology of mammals, New York, 1968, Plenum Press, Inc.

Faber, H.K., and McIntosh, R.: History of the American Pediatric Society, New York, 1966, McGraw-Hill Book Co.

Fanaroff, A.A., and Baskiewicz, A.: Unpublished data, 1975.

Fanaroff, A.A., Kennell, J.H., and Klaus, M.H.: Follow-up of low birth-weight infants—the predictive value of maternal visiting patterns, Pediatrics 49:288-290, 1972.

Fantz, R.L.: The origin of form perception, Sci. Am. 204:66-72, 1961.

Ferholt, J., and Provence, S.: Diagnosis and treatment of an infant with psychophysiological vomiting, Psychoanal. Study Child 31:439, 1976.

Field, T.M.: Effects of early separation, interactive deficits and experimental manipulations on infant-mother face-to-face interaction, Child Dev. 48:763-771, 1977.

Field, T.M.: In Bond, L., and Joffe, J., editors: Facilitating infant and early childhood development, Burlington, Vt., University of Vermont Press.

Field, T.M.: Interactions of high risk infants: quantitative and qualitative differences. In Sawin, D.B., et al., editors: Current perspectives on psycho-social risks during pregnancy and early infancy, New York, 1980, Brunner/Mazel, Inc.

Field, T.M., Sostek, A.M., Goldberg, S., and Shuman, H.H., editors: Infants born at risk, Jamaica, N.Y., 1979, Spectrum Publications, Inc.

Field, T.M., Widmayer, S.M., Stringer, S., and Ignatoff, E.: Teenage, lower-class black mothers and their preterm infants: an intervention and developmental follow-up, Child Dev. 51:426-436, 1980.

Flynn, A.M., Kelly, J., Hollings, G., and Lynch, P.F.: Ambulation in labour, Br. Med. J. 2:591-593, 1978.

Fomufod, A., Sinkford, S.M., and Louy, V.E.: Mother-child separation at birth: a contributing factor in child abuse, Lancet 2:549-550, 1975.

Forfar, J.O., and MacCabe, A.F.: Masking and gowning in nurseries for the newborn infant: effect on staphylococcal carriage and infection, Br. Med. J. **1**:76-79, 1958.

Fraiberg, S.: In Lewis, M., and Rosenblum, L.A., editors: The effect of the infant on its caregiver, New York, 1974, John Wiley & Sons, Inc.

Freud, S.: Mourning and melancholia. In Standard edition of [his] complete psychological works, London, 1957, Hogarth Press, Ltd., Vol. 14.

Frommer, E.A., and O'Shea, G.: Antenatal identification of women liable to have problems in managing their infants, Br. J. Psychiatry **123**:149-156, 1973.

Furman, E.P.: The death of a newborn: care of the parents, Birth Fam. J. **5**:214-218, 1978.

Furman, E.: Some thoughts on the role of the father-child relationship. Paper presented at Birth, Interaction, Attachment Conference, Cleveland, Ohio, 1980.

Garrow, D.: Personal communication, 1979.

Gath, A.: The impact of an abnormal child upon the parents, Br. J. Psychiatry **130**:405-410, 1977.

Giles, P.F.H.: Reactions of women to perinatal death, Aust. N.Z. J. Obstet. Gynaecol. **10**:207-210, 1970.

Gillett, J.: Childbirth in Pithiviers, France, Lancet **2**:894-896, 1979.

Gintzler, A.R.: Endorphin-mediated increases in pain threshold during pregnancy. Science **210**:193-195, 1980.

Gleich, M.: The premature infant. III. Arch. Pediatr. **59**:172-173, 1942.

Goffman, E.: Stigma: notes on the management of spoiled identity, London, 1968, Penguin Books, Ltd.

Goldberg, S.: Infant care and growth in urban Zambia, Hum. Dev. **15**:77-89, 1972.

Goldberg, S.: Premature birth: consequences for the parent-infant relationship, Am. Sci. **67**:214-219, 1979.

Goldblum, R., Ahlstedt, S., Carlsson, B., and Hanson, L.: Antibody production by human colostrum cells, Pediatr. Res. **9**:330, 1975.

Goodall, J.: In the shadow of man, Boston, 1971, Houghton-Mifflin Co.

Goodell, R.: Bringing up the children by taking them to a birth, N.Y. Times, p. E9, Feb. 24, 1980.

Goren, C., Sarty, M., and Wu, P.: Visual following and pattern discrimination of facelike stimuli by newborn infants, Pediatrics **56**:544-549, 1975.

Green, M.: Parent care in the intensive care unit, Am. J. Dis. Child **133**:1119-1120, 1979.

Greenberg, M., and Morris, N.: Engrossment: the newborn's impact upon the father, Am. J. Orthopsychiatry **44**:520-531, 1974.

Greenberg, M., Rosenberg, I., and Lind, J.: First mothers rooming-in with their newborns: its impact on the mother, Am. J. Orthopsychiatry **43**:783-788, 1973.

Grossman, F.K., et al.: Pregnancy, birth and parenthood, San Francisco, 1980, Jossey-Bass, Inc., Publications.

Grota, L.J.: Factors influencing the acceptance of caesarean delivered offspring by foster mothers, Physiol. Behav. **3**:265-269, 1968.

Gubernick, D.J., Jones, K.C., and Klopfer, P.H.: Maternal "imprinting" in goats, Animal Behav. **27**:314-315, 1979.

Hack, M., Gordon, D., Merkatz, I, et al.: The prognostic significance of postnatal growth in VLBW infants, Pediatric Research **14**:434, 1980.

Haire, D.: The cultural warping of childbirth, I.C.E.A. News, 1972.

Haith, M.M., Kessen, W., and Collins, D.: Response of the human infant to level of complexity of intermittent visual movement, J. Exp. Child. Psychol. **7**:52, 1969.

Hales, D.J., Lozoff, B., Sosa, R., and Kennell, J.H.: Defining the limits of the maternal sensitive period, Dev. Med. Child Neurol. **19**:454, 1977.

Hales, D.J., Trause, M.A., and Kennell, J.H.: How early is early contact? Defining the limits of the sensitive period, Pediatr. Res. **10**:448, 1976.

Hall, E.T.: The hidden dimension, Garden City, N.Y., 1966, Doubleday & Co., Inc.

Hall, F., Pawlby, S.J., and Wolkind, S.: Early life experiences and later mothering behaviour: a study of mothers and their 20-week old babies. In Shaffer, D., and Dunn, J., editors: The first year of life, New York, 1980, John Wiley & Sons, Inc.

Harlow, H.F., Harlow, M.K., and Hansen, E.W.: In Rheingold, H.R., editor: Maternal behavior in mammals, New York, 1963, John Wiley & Sons, Inc.

Harper, R.G., Concepcion, S., and Sokal, S.: Is parental contact with infants in the neonatal intensive care unit really a good idea? Pediatr. Res. **9**:259, 1975.

Harper, R.G., Sia, C., Sokal, S., and Sokal, M.: Observations on unrestricted parental contact with infants in the neonatal intensive care unit, J. Pediatr. **89**:441-445, 1976.

Hasselmeyer, E.: Handling and premature infant behavior: an experimental study of the relationship between handling and selected physiological, pathological, and behavioral indices related to body functioning among a group of prematurely born infants who weighed between 1501 and 2000 grams at birth and were between the ages of seven and twenty-eight days of life, Dissert. Abstr. **24**:7, 1964.

Haverkamp, A.D., Thompson, H.E., McFee, J.G., and Cetrulo, C.: The evaluation of continuous fetal heart rate monitoring in high-risk pregnancy, Am. J. Obstet. Gynecol. **125**:310-7, 1976.

Hawthorne, J., Richards, M.P.M., and Callon, M.: A study of parental visiting of babies in a special-care unit. In Brimblecombe, F.S.W., et al., editors: Separation and special-care baby units, London, 1978, Heinemann Medical Books.

Helfer, R.E., and Kempe, C.H., editors: The battered child, Chicago, 1968, University of Chicago Press.

Helfer, R.E., and Kempe, C.H.: Child abuse and neglect: the family and the community, Cambridge, Mass., 1976, Ballinger Publishing Co.

Helmrath, T.A., and Steinitz, E.M.: Death of an infant: parental grieving and the failure of social support, J. Fam. Pract. **6**:785-790, 1978.

Henchie, V.: Children's reactions to the birth of a new baby. Unpublished Child Development Report, London, 1963, University of London Institute of Education.

Hersher, L., Richmond, J., and Moore, A.: In Rheingold, H.R., editor: Maternal behavior in mammals, New York, 1963*a*, John Wiley & Sons, Inc.

Hersher, L., Richmond, J., and Moore, A.: Modifiability of the critical period for the development of maternal behavior in sheep and goats, Behaviour **20**:311-320, 1963*b*.

Hinde, R.A., and Spencer-Booth, Y.: The study of mother-infant interaction in captive group-living rhesus monkeys, Proc. R. Soc. [Biol.] **169**:177-201, 1968.

Hunter, R.S., Kilstrom, N., Kraybill, E.N., and Luda, F.: Antecedents of child abuse and neglect in premature infants: a prospective study

in a newborn intensive care unit, Pediatrics **161**:629-635, 1978.

Hwang, P., Guyda, H., and Friesen, H.: A radioimmunoassay for human prolactin, Proc. Natl. Acad. Sci. U.S.A. **68**:1902-1906, 1971.

Iyengar, L., and Selvaraj, R.J.: Intestinal absorption of immunoglobulins by newborn infants, Arch. Dis. Child. **42**:411-414, 1972.

Jackson, E., Olmstead, R., Foord, A., Thomas, H., and Hyder, K.: Hospital rooming-in unit for four newborn infants and their mothers: descriptive account of background, development, and procedures with a few preliminary observations, Pediatrics **1**:28-43, 1948.

James, V.L., Jr., and Wheeler, W.E.: The care-by-parent unit, Pediatrics **43**:488-494, 1969.

Jeffcoate, J.A., Humphrey, M.E., and Lloyd, J.K.: Disturbance in parent-child relationship following preterm delivery, Develop. Med. Child Neurol. **21**:344-352, 1979.

Johns, N.: Family reactions to the birth of a child with a congenital abnormality, Med. J. Aust. **1**:277-282, 1971.

Johnson, N.W.: Breast-feeding at one hour of age, Am. J. Matern. Child Nurs. **1**:12, 1976.

Jordan, B.: Birth in four cultures, St. Albans, Vt., 1980 Eden Press Women's Publications.

Jordan, D.: Evaluation of a family-centered maternity care hospital program, J.O.G.N. Nurs. **2**:13-34, 1973.

Kahn, E., Wayburne, S., and Fouche, M.: The Baragwanath premature baby unit—an analysis of the case records of 1000 consecutive admissions, S. Afr. Med. J. **28**:453-456, 1954.

Kaila, E.: Die Reaktionen des Sauglings auf des menschliche Gesicht, Z. Psychol. **135**:156-163, 1935.

Kaplan, D.N., and Mason, E.A.: Maternal reactions to premature birth viewed as an acute emotional disorder, Am. J. Orthopsychiatry **30**:539-552, 1960.

Kattwinkel, J., Hearman, H., Fanaroff, A.A., Katona, P., and Klaus, M.H.: Apnea of prematurity, J. Pediatr. **86**:588-592, 1975.

Katz, S., Als, H., and Barker, W.: Physical anthropology and the biobehavioral approach to child growth and development (abstract), Am. J. Phys. Anthropol. **38**:105-118, 1973.

Katz, V.: Auditory stimulation and developmental behavior of the premature infant, Nurs. Res. **20**:196-201, 1971.

Kaufman, C.: In Anthony, E., and Benedek, T.,

editors: Parenthood: its psychology and psychopathology, Boston, 1970, Little, Brown & Co., Inc.

Keller, W.D., Hildebrandt, K.A., and Richards, M.: Effects of extended father-infant contact, presented at Society for Research in Child Development Biennial Meeting, April 3, 1981.

Kelso, I.M., Parsons, R.J., Lawrence, G.F., Arora, S.S., Edmonds, D.K., and Cooke, I.D.: An assessment of continuous fetal heart rate monitoring labor: a randomized trial, Am. J. Obstet. Gynecol. **131:**526-532, 1978.

Kempe, C.H., and Helfer, R.E.: Helping the battered child and his family, Philadelphia, 1972, J.B. Lippincott Co.

Kennell, J.H.: Are we in the midst of a revolution? Am. J. Dis. Child. **134:**303-310, 1980.

Kennell, J.H., and Rolnick, A.: Discussing problems in newborn babies with their parents, Pediatrics **26:**832-838, 1960.

Kennell, J.H., Chesler, D., Wolfe, H., and Klaus, M.H.: Nesting in the human mother after mother-infant separation, Pediatr. Res. **7:**269, 1973.

Kennell, J.H., Jerauld, R., Wolfe, H., Chesler, D., Kreger, N.C., McAlpine, W., Steffa, M., and Klaus, M.H.: Maternal behavior one year after early and extended post-partum contact, Dev. Med. Child Neurol. **16:**172-179, 1974.

Kennell, J.H., Klaus, M.H., and Wolfe, H.: Nesting behavior in the human mother after prolonged mother-infant separation. In Swyer, P., and Stetson, J., editors: Current concepts of neonatal intensive care, St. Louis, 1975, Warren H. Green, Inc.

Kennell, J.H., Slyter, H., and Klaus, M.H.: The mourning response of parents to the death of a newborn infant, N. Engl. J. Med. **283:**344-349, 1970.

Kennell, J.H., Trause, M.A., and Klaus, M.H.: In Parent-infant interaction, Ciba Foundation Symposium 33, Amsterdam, 1975, Elsevier Publishing Co.

Kilbride, H.W., Johnson, D.L., and Streissguth, A.P.: Social class, birth order and newborn experience, Child Dev. **48:**1686-1688, 1977.

Kitzinger, S.: Birth at home, New York 1979, Oxford University Press.

Kitzinger, S., and Davis, J., editors: The place of birth, New York, 1978, Oxford University Press.

Klaus, M.H., and Diaz-Rossello, J.: Breastfeeding 1980, Pediatr. Rev. **1:**289-290, 1980.

Klaus, M.H., and Kennell, J.H.: Human maternal and paternal behavior. In Klaus, M.H., and Kennell, J.H., editors: Maternal-infant bonding, St. Louis, 1976, The C.V. Mosby Co.

Klaus, M.H., and Kennell, J.H.: An early maternal sensitive period? A theoretical analysis. In Stern, L., et al., editors: Intensive care in the newborn, II, New York, 1978, Masson Publishing, U.S.A., Inc.

Klaus, M.H., and Kennell, J.H.: Mothers separated from their newborn infants, Pediatr. Clin. North Am. **17:**1015-1037, 1970.

Klaus, M.H., Jerauld, R., Kreger, N., McAlpine, W., Steffa, M., and Kennell, J.H.: Maternal attachment: importance of the first post-partum days, N. Engl. J. Med. **286:**460-463, 1972.

Klaus, M.H., Kennell, J.H., Plumb, N., and Zuehlke, S.: Human maternal behavior at first contact with her young, Pediatrics **46:**187-192, 1970.

Klaus, M.H., and Kennell, J.H., and Sosa, R.: Child health and breast feeding: the effect of a supportive woman (doula) during labor and the effect of early suckling (abstract), Pediatr. Res. **15:**450, 1981.

Klaus, M.H., Trause, M.A., and Kennell, J.H.: In Parent-infant interaction, Ciba Foundation Symposium 33, Amsterdam, 1975, Elsevier Publishing Co.

Klein, M., and Stern, L.: Low birth weight and the battered child syndrome, Am. J. Dis. Child. **122:**15-18, 1971.

Klopfer, P.: Mother love: what turns it on? Am. Sci. **49:**404-407, 1971.

Konner, M.J.: Aspects of the developmental ethology of a foraging people. In Jones, N.B., editor: Ethological studies of child behavior, London, 1972, Cambridge University Press.

Kontos, D.: A study of the effects of extended mother-infant contact on maternal behavior at one and three months, Birth Fam. J. **5:**133-140, 1978.

Korner, A., Kraemer, H., Haffner, M., and Cosper, L.: Effects of waterbed flotation on premature infants: a pilot study, Pediatrics **56:**361-367, 1975.

Kramer, L., and Pierpont, M.: Rocking waterbeds and auditory stimuli to enhance growth of preterm infants, J. Pediatr. **88:**297-299, 1976.

Kuhn, T.S.: The structure of scientific revolutions, Chicago, 1962, University of Chicago Press.

Kumar, R., and Robson, K.: Neurotic disturbance during pregnancy and the puerperium: preliminary report of a prospective survey of 119 primiparae. In Sandler, M., editor: Mental illness in pregnancy and the puerperium, Oxford, 1978*a*, Oxford University Press.

Kumar, R., and Robson, K.: Previous induced abortion and ante-natal depression in primiparae: preliminary report of a survey of mental health in pregnancy, Psychol. Med. **8:**711-715, 1978*b*.

Lampe, J., Trause, M.A., and Kennell, J.H.: Parental visiting of sick infants: the effect of living at home prior to hospitalization, Pediatrics **59:**294-296, 1977.

Lang, R.: Birth book, Ben Lomond, Calif., 1972, Genesis Press.

Lang, R.: Personal communication, 1976.

Lanier, B.O., Goldman, A.S., and Harris, N.S.: Plasma cell antigen-bearing lymphocytes in primary immunodeficiencies, Pediatr. Res. **9:**331, 1975.

Larson, C.: Efficacy of prenatal and postpartum home visits on child health and development, Pediatrics **66:**191-197, 1980.

Lawrence, R.A.: Breastfeeding: a guide for the medical profession, St. Louis, 1980, The C.V. Mosby Co.

Lawson, K., Daum, C., and Turkewitz, G.: Environmental characteristics of a neonatal intensive care unit, Child Dev. **48:**1633-1639, 1977.

Lederman, R.P., Lederman, E., Work, B.A., Jr., and McCann, D.S.: The relationship of maternal anxiety, plasma catecholamines, and plasma cortisol to progress in labor, Am. J. Obstet. Gynecol. **132:**495-500, 1978.

Lee, R.B., and DeVore, I.: Kalahari hunter-gatherers: studies of the Kung San and their neighbors, Cambridge, Mass., 1976, Harvard University Press.

Legg, C., Sherick, I., and Wadland, W.: Reaction of preschool children to the birth of a sibling, Child Psychiatry Hum. Dev. **5:**3-39, 1974.

Leib, S.A., Benfield, D.G., and Guidubaldi, J.: Effects of early intervention and stimulation on the preterm infant, Pediatrics **66:**83-90, 1980.

Leiderman, P.H., Leifer, A.D., Seashore, M.J., Barnett, C.R., and Grobstein, R.: Mother-infant interaction: effects of early deprivation, prior experience and sex of infant, Early Dev. **51:**154-175, 1973.

Leifer, A.D., Leiderman, P.H., Barnett, C.R., and Williams, J.A.: Effects of mother-infant separation on maternal attachment behavior, Child Dev. **43:**1203-1218, 1972.

Leonard, C.H., Irvin, N., Ballard, R.A., et al.: Preliminary observations on the behavior of children present at the birth of a sibling, Pediatrics **64:**949-951, 1979.

Levinson, G., and Shnider, S.M.: Catecholamines: the effects of maternal fear and its treatment, Birth Fam. J. **6:**167-174, 1979.

Levy, B.S., Wilkinson, F.S., and Marine, W.M.: Reducing neonatal mortality rate with nurse-midwives, Am. J. Obstet. Gynec. **109:**50-58, 1971.

Levy, D.: Observations of attitudes and behavior in the child health center, Chicago, 1951, Year Book Medical Publishers, Inc.

Lewis, E.: Inhibition of mourning by pregnancy: psychopathology and management, Br. Med. J. **2:**27-28, 1979.

Lewis, E.: The atmosphere in the labour ward, J. Child Psychother. **4:**89-92, 1976*a*.

Lewis, E.: The management of stillbirth: coping with an unreality, Lancet **2:**619-620, 1976*b*.

Lewis, E.: Mourning by the family after a stillbirth or neonatal death, Arch. Dis. Child. **54:**303-306, 1979.

Lewis, E., and Page, A.: Failure to mourn a stillbirth: an overlooked catastrophe, Br. J. Med. Psychol. **51:**237-241, 1978.

Liebling, A.: Profiles: patron of the preemies, New Yorker Mag. pp. 20-24, June 3, 1939.

Lifton, R.J., and Olson, E.: Living and dying, New York, 1974, Praeger Publishers, Inc.

Lind, J.: Personal communication, 1973.

Lind, J., Vuorenkoski, V., and Wasz-Hackert, O.: In Morris, N., editor: Psychosomatic medicine in obstetrics and gynaecology, Basel, Switzerland, 1973, S. Karger.

Lindemann, E.: Symptomatology and management of acute grief, Am. J. Psychiatry **101:**141-148, 1944.

Lott, D., and Rosenblatt, J.: In Foss, B.M., editor: Determinants of infant behavior, 4, London, 1969, Methuen & Co., Ltd.

Lozoff, B., and Misra, R.: Medical control over labour, Lancet **1:**1242-1243, 1975.

Lozoff, B., Brittenham, G.M., Trause, M.A., Kennell, J.H., and Klaus, M.H.: The mother-newborn relationship: limits of adaptability, J. Pediatr. **91:**1, 1977.

Lumley, J.: The development of maternal-foetal bonding in first pregnancy. In Zichellen, L., editor: Proceedings of the 5th International Congress in Psychosomatic Medicine in Obstetrics and Gynaecology, New York, 1980*a*, Academic Press, Inc.

Lumley, J.: The image of the fetus in the first trimester, Birth Fam. J. **7:**5-14, 1980*b*.

Lynch, M.A.: Ill-health and child abuse, Lancet **2:**317-319, 1975.

Macfarlane, J.A., Smith, D.M., and Garrow, D.H.: The relationship between mother and neonate. In Kitzinger, S., and Davis, J.A., editors: The place of birth, New York, 1978, Oxford University Press.

MacFarlane, J.A.: In Parent-infant interaction, Ciba Foundation Symposium 33, Amsterdam, 1975, Elsevier Publishing Co.

Marshall, R., and Kosmar, C.: Burnout in the neonatal intensive care unit, Pediatrics **65:**1161-1165, 1980.

Martin, P.: Marital breakdown in families of patients with spina bifida cystica, Dev. Med. Child Neurol. **17:**757-764, 1975.

Mason, E.A.: A method of predicting crisis outcome for mothers of premature babies, Public Health Rep. **78:**1031-1035, 1963.

Mata, L.: Personal communication, 1974.

Matheny, A.P., and Vernick, J.: Parents of the mentally retarded child: emotionally overwhelmed or informationally deprived? J. Pediatr. **74:**953-959, 1969.

May, K.A.: A typology of detachment/involvement styles adopted during pregnancy by first-time fathers, J. Nurs. Res. **2**(2):445-453, 1980.

Mayer, A.D., and Rosenblatt, J.S.: Ontogeny of maternal behavior in the laboratory rat: early origins in 18- to 27-day-old young, Dev. Psychobiol. **12:**407-424, 1979.

Mayer, A.D., Freeman, N. C.G., and Rosenblatt, J.S.: Ontogeny of maternal behavior in the laboratory rat: factors underlying changes in responsiveness from 30 to 90 days, Dev. Psychobiol. **12:**425-439, 1979.

McBryde, A.: Compulsory rooming-in in the ward and private newborn serivce at Duke Hospital, J.A.M.A. **145:**625-628, 1951.

McDonald, M.A.: Paternal behavior at first contact with the newborn in a birth environment without intrusions, Birth Fam. J. **5:**123-132, 1978.

McNall, L.K.: Concerns of expectant fathers. In McNall, L.K., and Galeender, J.T., editors: Current practice in obstetrics and gynecology, St. Louis, 1976, The C.V. Mosby Co.

Mehl, L.E., Brendsel, C., and Peterson, G.H.: Children at birth: effects and implications, J. Sex Marital Ther. **3:**274-279, 1977.

Meier, G.W.: Maternal behavior of feral- and laboratory-reared monkeys following the surgical delivery of their infants, Nature **206:** 492-493, 1965.

Meltzoff, A.N., and Moore, M.K.: Imitation of facial and manual gestures by human neonates, Science **198:**75-78, 1977.

Meltzoff, A.N., and Moore, M.K.: Neonate imitation: a test of existence and mechanism. Presented at the Society for Research in Child Development, Denver, 1975.

Mercer, R.T.: Mothers' responses to their infants with defects, Nurs. Res. **23:**133-137, 1974.

Mercer, R.T.: Nursing care for parents at risk, Thorofare, N.J., 1977, Charles B. Slack, Inc.

Mercer, R.T.: One mother's use of negative feedback in coping with her defective infant, Mat. Child Nurs. J. **2:**29-37, 1973.

Merkatz, R.: Prolonged hospitalization of pregnant women: the effects on the family, Birth and the Family Journal **5:**204, 1978.

Miller, F.J.W.: Home nursing of premature babies in Newcastle-on-Tyne, Lancet **2:**703-705, 1948.

Miller, L.G.: Toward a greater understanding of the parents of the mentally retarded child, J. Pediatr. **73:**699-705, 1968.

Mills, N.: Personal communication, 1974.

Minde, K.K., Ford, L., Celhoffer, L., and Boukydis, M.: Interactions of mothers and nurses with premature infants, CMA J. **113:**741-745, 1975.

Minde, K., Marton, P., Manning, D., and Hines, B.: Some determinants of mother-infant interaction in the premature nursery (abstract), J. Am. Acad. Child Psychiatry **19:**1-21, 1980*a*.

Minde, K., Shosenberg, B., Marton, P., Thompson, J., Ripley, J., and Burns, S.: Self-help groups in a premature nursery—a controlled evaluation, J. Pediatr. **96:**933-940, 1980*b*.

Minde, K., Trehub, S., Corter, C., Boukydis, C., Celhoffer, L., and Marton, P.: Mother-child relationships in the premature nursery: an observational study, Pediatrics **61:**373-379, 1978.

Miranda, S., Hack, M., Fanaroff, A.A., and Klaus, M.H.: Neonatal visual pattern fixation: a possible predictor of future mental performance, Pediatr. Res. **8:**463, 1974.

Montagu, A.: Touching: the human significance of the skin, New York, 1971, Columbia University Press.

Moore, T.W., and Ucko, L.E.: Four to six: constructiveness and conflict in meeting doll play problems, J. Child Psychol. Psychiatry **2**:21-47, 1961.

Morris, D.: Parental reactions to perinatal death, Proc. R. Soc. Med. **69**:837, 1976.

Morsbach, G., and Bunting, C.: Maternal recognition of their neonate's cries, Dev. Med. Child Neurol. **21**:178-185, 1979.

Moss, H.A.: Methodological issues in studying mother-infant interaction, Am. J. Orthopsychiatry **35**:482-486, 1965.

Myers, R.E.: Maternal psychological stress and fetal asphyxia: a study in the monkey, Am. J. Obstet. Gynecol. **122**:47-59, 1975.

Nelson, N.M., Enkin, M.W., Saigal, S., Bennett, K.J., Milner, R., and Sackett, D.L.: A randomized clinical trial of the Leboyer approach to childbirth, N. Eng. J. Med. **302**:655-660, 1980.

National Institutes of Health: Cesarean childbirth, Consensus Development Conference Summary, Bethesda, Md., 1980, Vol. 3, no. 6.

Neutra, R.R., Greenland, S., and Friedman, E.A.: Effect of fetal monitoring on cesarean section rates, Obstet. Gynecol. **55**:175-180, 1980.

Newman, L.F.: Parents' perceptions of their low birth weight infants, Paediatrician **9**:182-190, 1980.

Newman, L., and Lind, J.: The child in hospital: early stimulation and therapy through play, Paediatrician **9**:147-150, 1980.

Newton, N.: Parenthood as part of sexual reproduction. In Money, J., and Musaph, H., editors: Handbook of sexology, Amsterdam, 1977, Elsevier/North-Holland Biomedical Press.

Newton, N., and Newton, M.: Mothers' reactions to their newborn babies, J.A.M.A. **181**:206-211, 1962.

Oakley, A.: Women confined, Oxford, 1980, Martin Robertson and Co., Ltd.

O'Connor, S., Vietze, P.M., Sherrod, K.B., Sandler, H.M., and Altemeier, W.A.: Reduced incidence of parenting inadequacy following rooming-in, Pediatrics **66**:176-182, 1980.

Odent, M.: Genèse de l'homme écologique, Paris, 1979, Épi.

O'Driscoll, K.: An obstetrician's view of pain, Br. J. Anaesth. **47**:1053-1059, 1975.

O'Driscoll, K., and Meagher, D.: Active management of labour, London, 1980, The W.B. Saunders Co.

O'Driscoll, K., and Stronge, J.M.: The active management of labour, Clin. Obstet. Gynaecol. **2**:3-17, 1975.

Oliver, J.E., Cox, J., Taylor, A., and Baldwin, J.: Severely ill-treated young children in North-East Wiltshire, Oxford, 1974, Oxford University Unit of Clinical Epidemiology.

Olshansky, S.: Chronic sorrow: a response to having a mentally defective child, Soc. Casework **73**:190-193, 1962.

Orme, R.L.E., and Boxall, J.: The changing pattern of parental involvement in the special-care baby unit in Exeter. In Brimblecombe, F.S.W., et al., editors: Separation and special-care baby units, London, 1978, Heinemann Medical Books.

Parke, R.: Father-infant interaction. In Klaus, M.H., Leger, T., and Trause, M.A., editors: Maternal attachment and mothering disorders: a round table, Sausalito, Calif., 1974, Johnson & Johnson Co.

Parke, R.D.: Perspectives on father-infant interaction. In Osofsky, J.D., editor: The handbook of infant development, New York, 1979, John Wiley & Sons, Inc.

Parke, R.D., Hymel, S., Power, T.G., and Tinsley, B.R.: Fathers and risk: a hospital based model of intervention. In Sawin, D.B., et al., editors: Psychosocial risks in infant-environment transactions, New York, 1980, Bruner/Mazel, Inc.

Parke, R.D., Power, T.G., Tinsley, B.R., and Hymel, S.: The father's role in the family system, Semin. Perinatol. **3**:25-34, 1979.

Parkes, C.M.: Bereavement and mental illness. I. A clinical study of the grief of bereaved psychiatric patients, Br. J. Med. Psychol. **38**:1-12, 1965*a*.

Parkes, C.M.: Bereavement and mental illness. II. A classification of bereavement reactions, Br. J. Med. Psychol. **38**:13-26, 1965*b*.

Parkes, C.M.: The nature of grief, Int. J. Psychiatry **3**:435-438, 1967.

Parkes, C.M.: Bereavement: studies of grief in adult life, New York, 1972, International Universities Press, Inc.

Parmelee, A.H., Kopp, C.B., and Sigman, M.: Selection of developmental assessment techniques for infants at risk, Merrill-Palmer Quarterly **22**:177, 1976.

Parmelee, A.H., Jr., Wenner, W.H., Akiyama, Y., Schultz, M., and Stern, E.: Sleep states in premature infants, Dev. Med. Child Neurol. **9**:70-77, 1967.

Pawlby, S.J.: Imitative interaction. In Schaffer,

H.R., editor: Studies in mother-infant interaction, New York, 1977, Academic Press, Inc.

Pedersen, F.A.: Mother, father and infant as an interactive system. Paper presented at the Annual Convention of the American Psychological Association, Chicago, Sept., 1975.

Peppers, L.G., and Knapp, R.J.: Maternal reactions to involuntary fetal/infant death, Psychiatry **43**:155-159, 1980.

Peppers, L.G., and Knapp, R.J.: Motherhood and mourning, New York, 1980, Praeger Publishers.

Peterson, G.H., and Mehl, L.E.: Some determinants of maternal attachment, Am. J. Psychiatry **135**:1168-1173, 1978.

Phillips, C.R.N.: Neonatal heat loss in heated cribs vs. mothers' arms, J.O.G.N. Nurs. **3**:11-15, 1974.

Phillips, J., and Whitaker, L.A.: The social effects of craniofacial deformity and its correction, Cleft Palate J. **16**:7-15, 1979.

Pittard, W.B.: Breast milk immunology, Am. J. Dis. Child **133**:83-87, 1979.

Poindron, P., and Le Neindre, P.: Hormonal and behavioural basis for establishing maternal behaviour in sheep. In Zichella, L., and Panchari, R., editors: Psychoneuroendocrinology in reproduction, Amsterdam, 1979, Elsevier/North-Holland Biomedical Press.

Poindron, P., and Le Neindre, P.: Endocrine and sensory regulation of maternal behaviour in the ewe. In Rosenblatt, J.S., et al., editors: Advances in the study of behavior, New York, 1980 Academic Press, Inc., Vol. 11.

Poirier, F.E., editor: Primate socialization, New York, 1972, Random House, Inc.

Powell, L.F.: The effect of extra stimulation and maternal involvement on the development of low-birth-weight infants and on maternal behavior, Child Dev. **45**:106-113, 1974.

Prechtl, H., and Beintema, D.: The neurological examination of the full term newborn infant, Clinics in Developmental Medicine, no. 12, London, 1964, Heinemann Medical Books.

Prince, J., Firley, M., and Harvey, D.: Contact between babies in incubators and their caretakers. In Brimblecomb, F.S.W., et al., editors: Separation and special-care baby units, London, 1978, Heinemann Medical Books.

Prugh, D.: Emotional problems of the premature infant's parents, Nurs. Outlook **1**:461-464, 1953.

Raphael, D.: The tender gift: breastfeeding, New York, 1973, Schocken Books.

Rawlings, G., Reynolds, E.O.R., Stewart, A., and Strang, L.B.: Changing prognosis for infants of very low birth weight, Lancet **1**:516-519, 1971.

Renou, P., Chang, A., Anderson, I., and Wood, C.: Controlled trial of fetal intensive care, Am. J. Obstet. Gynecol. **126**:470-476, 1976.

Rheingold, H.R., editor: Maternal behavior in mammals, New York, 1963, John Wiley & Sons, Inc.

Richards, M.P.M.: Possible effects of early separation on later development of children—a review. In Brimblecombe, F.S.W., et al., editors: Separation and special-care baby units, London, 1978, Heinemann Medical Books.

Richards, M.P.M.: Effects on development of early separations for treatment of parents and children. In Shaffer, D., and Dunn, J. editors: The first year of life, New York, 1980, John Wiley & Sons, Inc.

Richards, M.P.M., and Bernal, J.B.: In Schaffer, H.R., editor: The origins of human social relations, New York, 1971, Academic Press, Inc.

Richards, M.P.M., and Roberton, N.R.C.: Admission and discharge policies for special care units. In Brimblecombe, F.S.W., et al., editors: Separation and special-care baby units, London, Heinemann Medical Books.

Richman, L.C.: Parents and teachers: differing views of behavior of cleft palate children, Cleft Palate J. **15**:360-364, 1978.

Richman, L.C., and Harper, D.C.: Observable stigmata and perceived maternal behavior, Cleft Palate J. **15**:215-219, 1978.

Ringler, N.M., Kennell, J.H., Jarvella, R., Navojosky, B.J., and Klaus, M.H.: Mother-to-child speech at 2 years—effects of early postnatal contact, J. Pediatr. **86**:141-144, 1975.

Ringler, N.M., Trause, M.A., and Klaus, M.H.: Mother's speech to her two-year-old, its effect on speech and language comprehension at 5 years, Pediatr. Res. **10**:307, 1976.

Ringler, N.M., Trause, M.A., Klaus, M.H., and Kennell, J.H.: The effects of extra postpartum contact and maternal speech patterns on children's IQs, speech and language comprehension at five, Child Dev. **49**:862-865, 1978.

Rivinus, H., and Katz, S.: Evolution, newborn behavior and maternal attachment, Comments Contemp. Psychiatry **2**:95-104, 1972.

Robertson, J.: A baby in the family: loving and being loved, London, 1982, Penguin Books, Ltd.

Robertson, J., and Robertson, J.: Quality of substitute care as an influence on separation responses, J. Psychosom. Res. **16**:261-265, 1972.

Robertson, J., and Robertson, J.: Young children in brief separation: a fresh look, Psychoanal. Study child **26**:264-315, 1971.

Robson, K.S.: The role of eye-to-eye contact in maternal-infant attachment, J. Child Psychol. Psychiatry **8**:13-25, 1967.

Robson, K., and Kumar, R.: Delayed onset of maternal affection after childbirth, Br. J. Psychiatry **136**:347-353, 1980.

Rödholm, M.: Effects of father-infant postpartum contact on their interaction 3 months after birth, Early Hum. Dev. **5**:79-85, 1981.

Rödholm, M., and Larsson, K.: Father-infant interaction at the first contact after delivery, Early Hum. Dev. **3**:21-27, 1979.

Rödholm, M., and Larsson, K.: The behavior of human male adults at their first contact with a newborn (thesis), Goteborg, Sweden, 1980, University of Goteborg.

Rose, J., Boggs, T., Jr., and Alderstein, A.: The evidence for a syndrome of "mothering disability" consequent to threats to the survival of neonates: a design for hypothesis testing including prevention in a prospective study, Am. J. Dis. Child. **100**:776-777, 1960.

Rosenblatt, J.S.: Nonhormonal basis of maternal behavior in the rat, Science **156**:1512-1514, 1967.

Rosenblatt, J.S.: The development of maternal responsiveness in rats, Am. J. Orthopsychiatry **39**:36-56, 1969.

Rosenblatt, J.S.: In Aronson, L., et al., editors: Development and evolution of behavior: essays in memory of T.C. Schneirla, San Francisco, 1970, W.H. Freeman & Co., Publishers.

Rosenblatt, J.S.: Personal communication,1971.

Rosenblatt, J.S.: In Parent-infant interaction, Ciba Foundation Symposium 33, Amsterdam, 1975, Elsevier Pulishing Co.

Rosenblatt, J.S.: Evolutionary background of human maternal behavior—animal models, Birth Fam. J. **5**:195-199, 1978.

Rosenblatt, J.S., and Lehrman, D.: In Rheingold, H.R., editor: Maternal behavior in mammals, New York, 1963, John Wiley & Sons, Inc.

Rosenblatt, J.S., and Siegel, H.I.: Hysterectomy-induced maternal behavior during pregnancy in the rat, J. Comp. Physiol. Psychol. **89**:685-700, 1975.

Rosenblatt, J.S., and Siegel, H.I.: Factors governing the onset and maintenance of maternal behavior among non primate mammals: the role of hormonal and nonmormonal factors. In Gubernick, D.J., and Klopfer, P.H., editors: Parental care in mammals, New York, Plenum Press, Inc., in press.

Rosenblatt, J.S., Siegel, H.I., and Mayer, A.D.: Progress in the study of maternal behavior in the rat: hormonal, nonhormonal sensory and developmental aspects. In Rosenblatt, J.S., et al., editors: Advances in the study of behavior, New York, 1979, Academic Press, Inc., Vol. 10.

Rosenblum, L.A., and Kaufman, J.C.: In Altmann, S., editor: Social communication among primates, Chicago, 1967, University of Chicago Press.

Rosenfield, A.G.: Visiting in the intensive care nursery, Child Dev. **51**:939-941, 1980.

Roskies, E.: Abnormalities and normalities: the mothering of thalidomide children, New York, 1972, Cornell University Press.

Roth, L., and Rosenblatt, J.S.: Self-licking and mammary development during pregnancy in the rat, J. Endocrinol. **42**:363-378, 1968.

Rubin, R.: Maternal touch, Nurs. Outlook **11**:828-831, 1963.

Rutter, M.: Separation experiences: a new look at an old topic, J. Pediatr. **95**:147-154, 1979.

Ryerson, A.J.: Medical advice on child rearing, 1550-1900, Harvard Ed. Rev. **31**:302, 1961.

Sackett, G.P., and Ruppenthal, G.C.: In Lewis, M., and Rosenblum, L.A., editors: The effect of the infant on its caregiver, New York, 1974, John Wiley & Sons, Inc.

Salariya, E.M., Easton, P.M., and Cater, J.I.: Duration of breast-feeding after early initiation and frequent feeding, Lancet **2**:1141-1143, Nov. 25, 1978.

Salk, L.: The role of the heartbeat in the relations between mother and infant, Sci. Am. **228**:24-29, 1973.

Sameroff, A.J.: In Avery, G.B., editor: Neonatology, Philadelphia, 1975, J.B. Lippincott Co.

Sameroff, A.J., and Chandler, M.J.: Reproductive risk and the continuum of caretaking casualty. In Horowitz, F.D., et al., editors: Review of child development research, Chicago, 1975, University of Chicago Press, Vol. 4.

Sander, L.W., Stechler, G., Burns, P., and Julia, H.: Early mother-infant interaction and 24-hour patterns of activity and sleep, J. Am. Acad. Child Psychiatry **9**:103-123, 1970.

Scarr-Salapatek, S., and Williams, M.L.: The effects of early stimulation on low birth-weight infants, Child Dev. **44:**94-101, 1973.

Schaal, B., Montagner, H., Hertling, E., Bolzoni, D., Moyse, A., and Quichon, R.: Les stimulations olfactives dans les relations entre l'enfant et la mère, Reprod. Nutr. Dev. **20:**843-858, 1980.

Schaffer, H.R., editor: Studies in mother-infant interaction, London, 1977, Academic Press, Ltd.

Schneirla, T.C.: Problems in the biopsychology of social organization, J. Abnorm. Soc. Psychol. **41**(4):385-402, 1946.

Schneirla, T.C., Rosenblatt, J.S., and Tobach, E.: In Rheingold, H.R., editor: Maternal behavior in mammals, New York, 1963, John Wiley & Sons, Inc.

Schoetzer, A.: Effect of viewing distance on looking behavior in neonates, Int. J. Behav. Dev. **2:**121-123, 1979.

Schreiber, J.: Personal communication, 1974.

Schreiner, R., Greshem, E., and Green, M.: Physicians' responsibility to parents after death of an infant, Am. J. Dis. Child. **133:**723-726, 1979.

Seashore, M.H., Leifer, A.D., Barnett, C.R., and Leiderman, P.H.: The effects of denial of early mother-infant interaction on maternal self-confidence, J. Pers. Soc. Psychol. **26:**369-378, 1973.

Segall, M.: Cardiac responsibility to auditory stimulation in premature infants, Nurs. Res. **21:**15-19, 1972.

Selman, E., McEwan, A., and Fisher, E.: Studies on natural sucking in cattle during the first eight hours post partum. I. Behavioral studies (dams), Animal Behav. **18:**276-283, 1970.

Shaffer, D., and Dunn, J., editors: The first year of life, New York, 1979, John Wiley & Sons, Inc.

Shaheen, E., Alexander, D., Truskowsky, M., and Barbero, G.: Failure to thrive—a retrospective profile, Clin. Pediatr. **7:**255-261, 1968.

Shaikh, A.A.: Estrone and estradiol levels in the ovarian venous blood from rats during the estrous cycle and pregnancy, Biol. Reprod. **5:**297-307, 1971.

Shaul, B.: Notes on hand rearing various species of mammals, Int. Zoo Yearbook **4:**300, 1962.

Shearer, M.H., editor: Parent to infant attachment, Cleveland, Nov. 6-9, 1977, Birth Fam. J. **5:**177-260, 1978.

Shereshefsky, P.M., and Yarrow, L.J.: Psychological aspects of a first pregnancy and early postnatal adaptation, New York, 1973, Raven Press.

Sherman, M.: Psychiatry in the neonatal intensive care unit, Clin. Perinatol. **7:** 33-47, 1980.

Shinefield, H.R., Ribble, J.C., Boris, M., and Eichenwald, H.F.: Bacterial interference: its effect on nursery-acquired infection with *Staphylococcus aureus*, Am. J. Dis. Child. **105:**646-654, 1963.

Siegel, E., Bauman, K.E., Schaefer, E.S., Saunders, M.M., and Ingram, D.D.: Hospital and home support during infancy: impact on maternal attachment, child abuse and neglect, and health care utilization, Pediatrics **66:**183-190, 1980.

Siegel, H.I., and Greenwald, M.S.: Effects of mother-litter separation on later maternal responsiveness in the hamster, Physiol. Behav. **21:**147-149, 1978.

Siegel, H.I., Rosenblatt, J.S.: Estrogen-induced maternal behavior in hysterectomized-ovariectomized virgin rats, Physiol. Behav. **14:**465-471, 1975.

Siegel, H.I., and Rosenblatt, J.S.: Duration of estrogen stimulation and progesterone inhibition of maternal behavior in pregnancy-terminated rats, Horm. Behav. **11:**12-19, 1978.

Siegel, H.I., Doerr, H., and Rosenblatt, J.S.: Further studies on estrogen-induced maternal behavior in hysterectomized-ovariectomized nulliparous rats, Physiol. Behav. **21:**99-103, 1978.

Sigman, M., and Parmelee, A.H.: Longitudinal evaluation of the high-risk infant. In Field, T.M. Sostak, A.M., Goldberg, S., and Shuman, H.H., editors: Infants born at risk, New York, 1979, Spectrum Publications, Inc.

Silverman, W.A.: Incubator-baby sideshows, Pediatrics **64:**127, 1979.

Silverman, W.A., and Sinclair, J.C.: Evaluation of precautions before entering a neonatal unit, Pediatrics **40:**900-901, 1967.

Simonds, J.F., and Heimburger, R.E.: Psychiatric evaluation of youth with cleft lip–palate matched with a control group, Cleft Palate J. **15:**193-201, 1978.

Skinner, A., and Castle, R.: Seventy-eight battered children: a retrospective study, London, 1969, National Society for the Prevention of Cruelty to Children.

Solkoff, N., Yaffe, S., Weintraub, D., and Blase, B.: Effects of handling on subsequent development of premature infants, Dev. Psychol. **1:**765-768, 1969.

Solnit, A.J., and Stark, M.H.: Mourning and the birth of a defective child, Psychoanal. Study Child **16:**523-537, 1961.

Sosa, R., Klaus, M.H. Kennell, J.H., and Urrutia, J.J.: The effect of early mother-infant contact on breastfeeding, infection and growth. In Breastfeeding and the mother, Ciba Foundation Symposium 45 (new series), Amsterdam, 1976, Elsevier Publishing Co.

Sosa, R., Kennell, J.H., Klaus, M.H., et al.: The effect of a supportive companion on perinatal problems, length of labor, and mother-infant interaction, N. Engl. J. Med. **303:**597-600, 1980.

Sostek, A., and Read, S.: Reactions to the arrival of an infant sibling. Unpublished manuscript, Washington, D.C., 1979, Georgetown University School of Medicine.

Sousa, P.L.R., Barros, F.C., Gazalle, R.V., Begères, R.M., Pinheiro, G.N., Menezes, S.T., and Arruda, L.A.: Attachment and lactation, Fifteenth International Congress of Pediatrics, Buenos Aires, Oct. 3, 1974.

Spitz, R.A., and Cobliner, W.G.: The first year of life, New York, 1965, International Universities Press, Inc.

Spitz, R.A., and Wolff, K.M.: The smiling response: a contribution to the ontogenesis of social relations, Genet. Psychol. Monogr. **34:**57-125, 1946.

Stechler, G., and Lantz, E.: Some observations on attention and arousal in the human infant, J. Am. Acad. Child Psychiatry **5:**517, 1966.

Stein, S.B.: That new baby, New York, 1974*a*, Walker and Co.

Stein, S.B.: About dying, New York, 1974*b*, Walker and Co.

Stern, D.: In Lewis, M., and Rosenblum, L.A., editors: The effect of the infant on its caregiver, New York, 1974, John Wiley & Sons, Inc.

Stewart, A., and Reynolds, E.O.R.: Improved prognosis for infants of very low birth weight, Pediatrics **54:**724-735, 1974.

Stewart, A.L., Turcan, D.M. Rawlings, G. et al.: Prognosis for infants weighing 1000 g or less at birth, Arch. Dis. Child. **52:**97, 1977.

Sugarman, M.: Paranatal influences on maternal-infant attachment, Am. J. Orthopsychiatry **47:**407-421, 1977.

Sumner, P.E., Wheeler, J.P., and Smith, S.G.: The home-like labor-delivery room, Conn. Med. **40:**319-322, 1976.

Svejda, M.J., Campos, J.J., and Emde, R.N.: Mother-infant bonding: failure to generalize, Child Dev. **51:**775-779, 1980.

Tafari, N., and Ross, S.M.: On the need for organized perinatal care, Ethiop. Med. J. **11:**93-100, 1973.

Tafari, N., and Sterky, G.: Early discharge of low birth-weight infants in a developing country, Environ. Child Health **20:**73-76, 1974.

Taylor, M.K., and Kogan, K.L.: Effects of birth of a sibling on mother-child interactions, Child Psychiatry Hum. Dev. **4:**53-58, 1973.

Taylor, P.M., and Hall, B.L.: Parent-infant bonding: problems and opportunities in a perinatal center, Semin. Perinatol. **3:**73-84, 1979.

Terkel, J., and Rosenblatt, J.S.: Humoral factors underlying maternal behavior at parturition: cross transfusion between freely moving rats, J. Comp. Physiol. Psychol. **80:**365-371, 1972.

Terkel, J., and Rosenblatt, J.S.: Maternal behavior induced by maternal blood plasma injected into virgin rats, J. Comp. Physiol. Psychol. **65:**479-482, 1968.

Thomson, M.E., Hartsock, T.G., and Larson, C.: The importance of immediate postnatal contact: its effect on breastfeeding, Can. Fam. Physician **25:**1374-1378, 1979.

Torres, J.: Personal communication, 1978.

Trause, M.A.: Birth in the hospital: the effect on the sibling, Birth Fam. J. **5:**207-210, 1978.

Trause, M.A., Boslett, M., Voos, D., Kennell, J.H., and Klaus, M.H.: A birth in the hospital: the effect on the sibling, Pediatr. Res. 1977.

Trause, M.A., Kennell, J.H., and Klaus, M.H.: A fresh look at early mother-infant contact (abstract) Pediatr. Res. **12:**376, 1978.

Trenino, F.: Sibling of handicapped children: identifying those at risk. Soc. Casework, pp. 488-493, Oct., 1979.

Trevarthen, C.: Descriptive analyses of infant communicative behaviour. In Schaffer, H.R., editor: Studies in mother-infant interaction, New York, 1977, Academic Press, Inc.

Turnbull, A.C., Patten, P.T., Flint, A.P.F., Keirse, M.J.N.C., Jeremy, J.Y., and Anderson, A.: Significant fall in progesterone and rise in oestradiol levels in human peripheral plasma before onset of labour, Lancet **1:**101-103, 1974.

Urrutia, J.J., Sosa, R., Kennell, J.H., and Klaus,

M.H.: Prevalence of maternal and neonatal infections in a developing country: possible low-cost preventive measures, Ciba Foundation Symposium 77, Amsterdam, 1980, Exerpta Medica.

Van den Daele, L.D.: Modification of infant state by treatment in a rockerbox, J. Psychol. **74**:161-165, 1970.

Van den Daele, L.D.: Infant reactivity to redundant proprioceptive and auditory stimulations: a twin study, J. Psychol. **78**:269-276, 1971.

Vaughan, V.: Personal communication, 1975.

Voysey, M.: Impression management by parents with disabled children, J. Health Soc. Behav. **13**:80-89, 1972.

Walker, A.: Immunology of the gastrointestinal tract, J. Pediatr. **83**:517-530, 1973.

Warkany, J.: Congenital malformations: notes and comments, Chicago, 1971, Year Book Medical Publishers, Inc.

Westbrook, M.T.: The reactions to child-bearing and early maternal experience of women with differing marital relationships, Br. J. Med. Psychol. **51**:191-199, 1978.

Whiten, A.: Assessing the effects of perinatal events on the success of the mother-infant relationship. In Schaffer, H.R., editor: Studies in mother-infant interaction, London, 1977, Academic Press, Ltd.

Whittlestone, W.G.: The physiology of early attachment in mammals: implications for human obstetric care, Med. J. Aust. **1**:50-53, 1978.

Williams, C.P., and Oliver, T.K., Jr.: Nursery routines and staphylococcal colonization of the newborn, Pediatrics **44**:640-646, 1969.

Winnicott, D.W.: The child, the family and the outside world, London, 1957, Tavistock Publications, Ltd.

Winnicott, D.W.: Primary maternal preoccupation. In Collected papers: through paediatrics to psycho-analysis, New York, 1958, Basic Books, Inc., Publishers.

Winnicott, D.W.: The child, the family, and the outside world, New York, 1964, Penguin Books.

Winnicott, D.W.: The contribution of psycho-analysis to midwifery. In The family and individual development, London, 1965, Tavistock Publications, Ltd.

Winnicott, D.W.: The family and individual development, London, 1965, Tavistock Publications, Ltd.

Winnicott, D.W.: Advising parents. In The family and individual development, London, 1965, Tavistock Publications, Ltd.

Winnicott, D.W.: Playing and reality, London, 1971, Tavistock Publications, Ltd.

Winnicott, D.W.: The mirror role of mother and family in child development. In Playing and reality, 1971, Tavistock Publications, Ltd.

Winters, M.: The relationship of time of initial feeding to success of breast-feeding. Unpublished master's thesis, Seattle, 1973, University of Wahsington.

Wolff, J.R., Nielson, P.E., and Schiller, P.: The emotional reaction to a stillbirth, Am. J. Obstet. Gynecol. **108**:73-77, 1970.

Wolff, P.H.: Observations on newborn infants, Psychosom. Med. **21**:110-118, 1959.

Wolff, P.H.: The causes, controls and organization of behavior in the neonate, New York, 1965, International Universities Press, Inc.

Yanover, M.J., Jones, D., and Miller, M.D.: Perinatal care of low-risk mothers and infants: early discharge with home care, N. Engl. J. Med. **294**:702-705, 1976.

Yarrow, L.J.: Maternal deprivation: toward an empirical and conceptual re-evaluation, Psychol. Bull. **58**:459-490, 1961.

Yarrow, L.J.: Separation from parents during early childhood. In Hoffman, L.W., and Hoffman, M.L., editors: Review of child development reasearch, New York, 1964, Russell Sage Foundation, Vol. I.

Yogman, M.W.: Development of the father-infant relationship. In Fitzgerald, H., et al., editors: Theory and research in behavioral pediatrics, New York, 1980, Plenum Press, Inc., Vol. I.

Zahn, M.A.: Incapacity, impotence and invisible impairment: their effects upon interpersonal relations, J. Health Soc. Behav. **14**:115-123, 1973.

Zarrow, M.X., Gandelman, R., and Renenberg, V.: Prolactin: is it an essential hormone for maternal behavior in the mammal? Horm. Behav. **2**:343-354, 1971.

Zuk, G.H.: Religious factor and the role of guilt in parental acceptance of the retarded child, Am. J. Ment. Defic. **64**:139-147, 1959-1960, 1969.

Zuspan, F.P., Cibils, L.A., and Pose, S.V.: Myometrial and cardiovascular responses to alterations in plasma epinephrine and norepinephrine, Am. J. Obstet. Gynecol. **84**:841-851, 1962.

INDEX

□ An italicized page number indicates an illustration; t following a page number indicates a table.

309